T0200727

Vital Accounts

Why did Europeans begin to count births and deaths? How did they collect the numbers and what did they do with them? Through a compelling comparative analysis, *Vital Accounts* charts the work of the physicians, clergymen, and government officials who crafted the sciences of political and medical arithmetic in England and France during the long eighteenth century, before the emergence of statistics and regular government censuses. Andrea A. Rusnock presents a social history of quantification that highlights the development of numerical tables, influential and enduring scientific instruments designed to evaluate smallpox inoculation, to link weather and disease, to compare infant and maternal mortality rates, to identify changes in disease patterns, and to challenge prevailing views about the decline of European population. By focusing on the most important eighteenth-century controversies over health and population, Rusnock shows how vital accounts – the numbers of births and deaths – became the measure of public health and welfare.

Andrea A. Rusnock is Assistant Professor of History at the University of Rhode Island.

Cambridge Studies in the History of Medicine

Edited by

CHARLES ROSENBERG, Professor of History and Sociology of Science, University of Pennsylvania, and COLIN JONES, University of Warwick

Other titles in the series:

Continued on page following the index

Vital Accounts

Quantifying Health and Population in Eighteenth-Century England and France

ANDREA A. RUSNOCK
University of Rhode Island

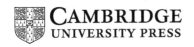

CAMBRIDGE
UNIVERSITY PRESS

CAMBRIDGE
UNIVERSITY PRESS

32 Avenue of the Americas, New York NY 10013-2473, USA

Cambridge University Press is part of the University of Cambridge.

It furthers the University's mission by disseminating knowledge in the pursuit of education, learning and research at the highest international levels of excellence.

www.cambridge.org
Information on this title: www.cambridge.org/9780521803748

© Andrea A. Rusnock 2002

First published 2002

A catalogue record for this publication is available from the British Library

Library of Congress Cataloguing in Publication data
Rusnock, Andrea Alice.
    Vital accounts : quantifying health and population in eighteenth-century England and France / Andrea A. Rusnock.
        p.   cm. – (Cambridge studies in the history of medicine)
        Includes bibliographical references and index.
        ISBN 0-521-80374-8 (hc.)
        1. Medical statistics – England – History.   2. Medical statistics – France –
    History.   3. Mortality – England – History.   4. Mortality – France – History.
    5. Epidemiology – England – History.   6. Epidemiology – France – History.
    7. Public health – England – History.   8. Public health – France – History.
    I. Title.   II. Series.
RA407.5.G7 R87   2002
614.4′241′09033 – dc21

                                                                    2002067063

ISBN 978-0-521-80374-8 Hardback
ISBN 978-0-521-10123-3 Paperback

For Oliver and Rosalind

CONTENTS

ILLUSTRATIONS

ACKNOWLEDGMENTS

This book began as a doctoral dissertation in the Program of History of Science at Princeton University, and I have returned many times to the cardinal questions posed by my astute readers Lorraine Daston, Gerald Geison, and Michael Mahoney. It took a decidely medical turn when I had the pleasure to work at the Wellcome Institute for the History of Medicine in London in 1992–1993. In the richly accoutred building on Euston Road, I benefited from the numerous colloquia and unlimited discussions with Philip Kreager, Susan Lawrence, Andreas Holger Maehle, Molly Sutphen, Andrew Wear, and many other fellows. William Bynum shared his extensive knowledge of the profession of medicine and the history of medicine in all their various guises. The inimitable Roy Porter offered especially valuable and cogent advice at a critical moment during revisions.

This book was supported by a Fellowship for University Teachers from the National Endowment for the Humanities (1996–1997), which allowed for travel to France and time to write. Parts of this book have been presented at the annual meetings of the American Association for the History of Medicine, the American Historical Association, and the History of Science Society and at workshops held at Cambridge University, University of Essex, the Wellcome Institute for the History of Medicine, the Philadelphia College of Physicians, the Clark Library, Princeton University, and Yale University. I thank the participants of these meetings and especially the organizers: Thomas Broman, David Cantor, William Clark, Catherine Crawford, Jan Golinski, Anne Hardy, Eileen Magnello, Simon Schaffer, Mary Terrall, John Harley Warner, and Norton Wise.

Many individuals have helped with specific parts of the book and it is with pleasure that I acknowledge my debts. Colin Jones and Elizabeth Williams generously shared their knowledge of eighteenth-century French medicine and, in particular, the archival resources in Montpellier. Marie-Noelle Bourguet, Laura Mason, and Michael Kwass kept me abreast of the latest scholarship on eighteenth-century French administrative history. Richard Sorrenson introduced me to the archives of the Royal Society (and its elegant cafeteria), and more generally traded notes about eighteenth-century British science. Robert Frank contributed his expertise on English demographic history and pushed me to put my work in a broader political and economic framework. John Carson has remained an incisive critic and encouraging friend since graduate school. Vivien Dietz guided me through the recent work in British history and, more importantly, has offered her warm support and understanding of that essential professional–maternal tension over these many years.

I would also like to thank the archivists and librarians at the Library of the Wellcome Institute for the History of Medicine, the Royal Society, the British Library, the Bibliothèque Nationale, the Académie Royale des Sciences, and the Archives Départementale de l'Hérault. The interlibrary loan staff at Rensselaer Polytechnic Institute and the University of Rhode Island did heroic service. Toby Appel, at the Harvey Cushing/John Hay Whitney Medical Library at Yale University, and Benjamin Weiss, at the Burndy Library of the Dibner Institute for the History of Science and Technology, were very helpful in securing reprints of the tables included in this book. I thank both libraries for their kind permission to reproduce these vital accounts. I am grateful to Editions Rodopi for granting permission to use material from my essays that appeared in *Medicine in the Enlightenment* (edited by Roy Porter) and *The Correspondence of James Jurin*. Princeton University Press kindly allowed me to use material from my essay in *The Values of Precision* (edited by M. Norton Wise).

Theodore Porter, J. Rosser Matthews, and an anonymous reader from Cambridge University Press read the entire manuscript, and their excellent suggestions have made this a richer book. Charles Rosenberg, as series editor, has warmly encouraged me in this project. My colleagues at the University of Rhode Island and Rensselaer Polytechnic Institute, especially P. Thomas Carroll, David Ellison, Joelle Rollo-Koster, Linda Layne, and Marie Schwartz, have provided useful advice. Any errors, of course, remain my own.

Finally, I would like to thank my family: my brother, Paul, for his expansive and entertaining knowledge of eighteenth-century mathematics and philosophy; my mother, Alice, for her unwavering belief in her daughter and for her Scottish commonsense philosophy; and my father, Andrew (an arch quantifier), for his gentle skepticism and unremitting intellectual curiosity. Above all, I am indebted to my husband, Paul Lucier, whose patient support, careful readings (and rereadings!), playful wit, and deep passion for history and science have made the writing of this book both a pleasure and a challenge. It is with the joy of a shared life that I dedicate this book to our children, Oliver and Rosalind.

Wakefield, Rhode Island
April 2002

Vital Accounts

Quantifying Health and Population in Eighteenth-Century England and France

Introduction

This book is about the activity of counting – specifically the counting of births and deaths – during the long eighteenth century. From the 1660s on, the numbers of born or dead, it was argued, would shed light on numerous political and medical issues. Yet despite this emerging desire for numbers, there were almost no government institutions, either at the national or local level, to collect and record these numbers. Rather, it was individuals from rural clergy to metropolitan physicians who did the counting. These political and medical arithmeticians, as they were called, invented ingenious methods of quantifying. They counted not just the number of christenings or burials in a specific geographic area but also, and often more importantly, different groups of individuals identified and classified by particular taxonomic schemes. These activities were as much about *what* to count as about *how* to count: The two were inextricable. Arithmeticians, in this way, brought quantitative analyses to bear on discussions of medical practice and therapy, salubrity and fecundity, and the growth or decline of population. Vital accounts – the numbers of dead and born – became, in short, the quantitative measure of public health and welfare.

Counting, Samuel Johnson told James Boswell in 1783, "brings everything to a certainty, which before floated in the mind indefinitely."[1] Johnson was not the only one to admire the bracing effects of counting. As several scholars have pointed out, quantification was the distinguishing feature of eighteenth-century science, especially in what Thomas Kuhn described as the Baconian sciences, those in which the development and refinement of instruments such as barometers, thermometers, and chemical balances allowed for more exact measurement.[2] The practitioners of political and medical arithmetic shared this

[1] James Boswell, *Life of Samuel Johnson LLD* (1791; reprinted. New York: Modern Library, 1931), p. 1042; quoted in J. Worth Estes, "Quantitative Observations of Fever and Its Treatment before the Advent of Short Clinical Thermometers," *Medical History* 35 (1991): 191.
[2] Thomas Kuhn, "Mathematical versus Experimental Traditions in the Development of Physical Science," in *The Essential Tension* (Chicago: University of Chicago Press, 1977), pp. 31–65; Tore Frängsmyr, J.L. Heilbron, and Robin E. Rider, eds., *The Quantifying Spirit in the 18th Century* (Berkeley:

enthusiasm for quantification and precise measurement, and they focused their efforts on the most basic events of human existence.

When counting births and deaths, eighteenth-century observers used words such as "numbers," "figures," or "accounts," and described their work as political or medical arithmetic. The word quantification was not an eighteenth-century term; it is an analytical concept that refers to the process of representing things by numbers. Quantification can be arrived at by counting, measuring, calculating, estimating, or combining any of these methods. It need not be based on empirical records. (One can construct a quantitative value system by arbitrarily assigning numbers – the judging scale for Olympic figure skating, for example.) The term quantification is useful because it neatly captures an approach that is distinct from mathematics. Mathematics (especially arithmetic) can be employed in quantification, but quantification is not mathematics per se. Mathematics refers to a variety of techniques that relate number and magnitude – it is not referential. Quantification, by contrast, is inherently referential: It is the application of numbers *to* objects, and seventeenth- and eighteenth-century observers recognized this distinction. In 1721, for instance, the English mathematician Edward Hatton described political arithmetic as follows: "This Specie of Arithmetic has nothing new in it, as to the Nature of the Numbers themselves, nor as to the Manner of Operation; but only in the Application or subject about which the Numbers are employ'd. . . . "[3]

Quantification is also distinct from the modern discipline of statistics. In fact, the term "statistics" did not come into widespread use until the 1820s and 1830s.[4]

University of California Press, 1990); J.L. Heilbron, "A Mathematical Mutiny, with Morals," in *World Changes: Thomas Kuhn and the Nature of Science,* ed. Paul Horwich (Cambridge, Mass.: Harvard University Press, 1993), pp. 81–129. Also see M. Norton Wise's helpful introduction to *The Values of Precision,* ed. M. Norton Wise (Princeton, N.J.: Princeton University Press, 1995), pp. 3–13. For quantification and social sciences, see P.F. Lazarsfeld, "Notes on the History of Quantification in Sociology: Trends, Sources and Problems," *Isis* 52 (1961): 277–333.

[3] Edward Hatton, *An Intire System of Arithmetic: Or Arithmetic in All Its Parts* (London, 1721), p. 244.

[4] For histories of statistics, see Theodore M. Porter, *The Rise of Statistical Thinking, 1820–1900* (Princeton, N.J.: Princeton University Press, 1986); Stephen M. Stigler, *The History of Statistics: The Measurement of Uncertainty before 1900* (Cambridge and London: The Belknap Press of Harvard University Press, 1986); Karl Pearson, *The History of Statistics in the 17th and 18th Centuries against the Changing Background of Intellectual, Scientific and Religious Thought,* ed. E.S. Pearson (London: Charles Griffin & Co., 1978); M.J. Cullen, *The Statistical Movement in Early Victorian Britain: The Foundations of Empirical Social Research* (New York: The Harvester Press, 1975). On medical statistics, see Major Greenwood, *Medical Statistics from Graunt to Farr* (Cambridge: Cambridge University Press, 1948); James H. Cassedy, "Medicine and the Rise of Statistics," in *Medicine in Seventeenth-Century England,* ed. Allen G. Debus (Berkeley: University of California Press, 1974), pp. 283–312; James H. Cassedy, *Demography in Early America: Beginnings of the Statistical Mind, 1600–1800* (Cambridge, Mass.: Harvard University Press, 1969); James H. Cassedy, *American Medicine and Statistical Thinking, 1800–1860* (Cambridge, Mass.: Harvard University Press, 1984); J. Rosser Matthews, *Quantification and the Quest for Medical Certainty* (Princeton, N.J.: Princeton University Press, 1995). On quantification and state statistics, see Joshua Cole, *The Power of Large Numbers: Population, Politics, and Gender in Nineteenth-Century France* (Ithaca and London: Cornell University Press, 2000); H. Westergaard, *Contributions to the History of Statistics* (London: P.S. King and Son, 1932); Fernand Faure, "The Development and Progress of Statistics in France," in *The History of Statistics: Memoirs to Commemorate the 75th Anniversary of the American Statistical*

By that time, no one, especially government officials and scientists, questioned the importance of numbers. But seventeenth- and eighteenth-century political and medical arithmeticians had to convince governments, savants, and the literate public of the value of collecting numbers. The eventual overwhelming success of numerical arguments should not obscure the very long and difficult process of establishing what is too easily taken for granted.[5]

In Europe, the first sustained effort at the quantification of things human occurred in Renaissance Italy, and it accelerated during the seventeenth and eighteenth centuries. In trying to account for the increased pace of quantification in early modern Europe, scholars have pointed to large-scale fundamental changes in society. The spur to quantify, for example, has been linked to the growth of capitalism.[6] In the transformation of Europe to a market society where production and consumption became oriented around selling and buying in the marketplace, land, labor, even time, became commodities determined by the calculus of supply and demand and evaluated by the cash nexus. Some sociologists and psychologists have argued that cash supplied the conceptual hinge that allowed for the possibility of turning the qualitative into the quantitative: Assigning something a monetary value remains one of the most fundamental ways of quantifying.[7] The most vivid example of how money promoted the quantification of human society during this period is the slave trade. There, unmistakably, humans were bought, sold, and traded in monetary, quantitative terms.

The demographic revolution – the dramatic growth in population that occurred after 1750 in Britain and France – has also been invoked as a catalyst for quantification.[8] Michel Foucault, for one, argued that increased population encouraged the development of demographic knowledge:

Society (New York: The Macmillan Co., 1918), pp. 219–329; Stuart J. Woolf, "Towards the History of the Origins of Statistics: France, 1789–1815," in Jean-Claude Perrot and Stuart J. Woolf, *State and Society in France, 1789–1815* (New York: Harwood Academic Publishers, 1984).
5 Simon Schaffer argued that mathematization and quantification were not inevitable and "demand a social history." Simon Schaffer, "A Social History of Plausibility: Country, City and Calculation in Augustan Britain," in *Rethinking Social History: English Society, 1570–1920, and Its Interpretation,* ed. Adrian Wilson (Manchester and New York: Manchester University Press, 1993), pp. 128–157.
6 Patricia Cline Cohen, *A Calculating People – The Spread of Numeracy in Early America* (Chicago: University of Chicago Press, 1982), esp. pp. 41–47.
7 See Georg Simmel, *The Philosophy of Money,* trans. Tom Bootmore and David Frisby (1907; London: Routledge & Kegan Paul, 1978). Simmel wrote: "Within the historical-psychological sphere, money by its very nature becomes the most perfect representative of a cognitive tendency in modern science as a whole: the reduction of qualitative determinations to quantitative ones" (p. 277). It is interesting to note that Russian psychologists in the 1920s found that rural villagers could solve certain logical and mathematical problems if and only if the problems were described as monetary transactions. See A.R. Luria, "Towards the Problem of the Historical Nature of Psychological Processes," *International Journal of Psychology* 6 (1971): 259–272.
8 James C. Riley analyzed various discussions of population during the period of the demographic revolution in his *Population Thought in the Age of the Demographic Revolution* (Durham, N.C.: Carolina Academic Press, 1985). I examine many of the same works as Riley. While he focused primarily on the ideas of these writers, I have concentrated on their *methods.*

The great eighteenth-century demographic upswing in Western Europe, the necessity for co-ordinating and integrating it into the apparatus of production and the urgency of controlling it with finer and more adequate power mechanisms cause 'population,' with its numerical variables of space and chronology, longevity and health, to emerge not only as a problem but as an object of surveillance, analysis, intervention, modification, etc.[9]

Under the rubric "biopower," Foucault sketched two levels of techniques used by the state to exercise power over human beings.[10] At the individual level (anatomo-politics), a person's body is subject to disciplinary practices.[11] The second level (biopolitics) concerns the aggregate, where a population is controlled through the sciences of demography and statistics.[12] Biopolitics assumed its power only in the nineteenth century with the growth of hospitals, schools, prisons, and state bureaucracies, institutions that recorded and monitored information about their populations. Its origins, Foucault noted in passing, were to be found in the eighteenth century, and not in any particular state institution but, rather, as a diffuse cultural problem associated with the social and economic repercussions of population growth.

For eighteenth-century English and French writers, the demographic problem was not one of overabundance but, rather, insufficient numbers of persons. The Malthusian fear of overpopulation so present just under the surface of Foucault's writings – where population becomes something to watch and discipline – was a demon of the future. The eighteenth-century challenge was how to encourage growth, not restrict it. More important from an analytical perspective is the historical point: Population – the entity itself – had first to be created before it could be controlled. Thus, in contrast to those scholars who have suggested that European society needed to change (as a result of capitalism or population growth) before quantification could become possible at all,[13] this book takes the approach that the large economic, demographic, social, and political transformations and the increasing measurement of the world occurred simultaneously.[14] The modern concept of population and its measurement were mutually constitutive.

---

[9] Michel Foucault, "The Politics of Health in the Eighteenth Century," in *Power/Knowledge – Selected Interviews and Other Writings, 1972–1977,* ed. Colin Gordon, trans. Colin Gordon, Leo Marshall, John Mepham, and Kate Soper (New York: Pantheon Books 1980), p. 171.

[10] For a critical discussion of Foucault's idea of biopower, see Michael Donnelly, "On Foucault's Uses of the Notion 'Biopower,'" in *Michel Foucault, Philosopher,* trans. Timothy J. Armstrong (New York: Routledge, 1992), pp. 199–203.

[11] This has best been shown in Foucault's analysis of the prison in *Discipline and Punish: The Birth of the Prison,* trans. Alan Sheridan (New York: Vintage Books, 1979).

[12] He only briefly outlined this second level of biopower in his essay on eighteenth-century health and later in *The History of Sexuality*; Foucault, "The Politics of Health"; Foucault, *The History of Sexuality,* Vol. 1: *An Introduction,* trans. Robert Hurley (1976; New York: Vintage Books, 1980), pp. 139–145.

[13] Lorraine Daston, *Classical Probability in the Enlightenment* (Princeton, N.J.: Princeton University Press, 1988), pp. 51–52.

[14] Recent studies in the history and sociology of science have emphasized the coconstructed character of the modern measured world. Bruno Latour characterized this process as metrology. Bruno Latour, *Science in Action* (Cambridge, Mass.: Harvard University Press, 1987). Also see Theodore Porter, *Trust in Numbers: The Pursuit of Objectivity in Science and Public Life* (Princeton,N.J.: Princeton

Part of that constitutive process can be traced directly to the central role that population played in political economy, particularly in the theory of mercantilism. For mercantilists and other political philosophers, such as Jean Bodin, a nation-state's wealth and strength depended in part on the size of population. A few of the early mercantilist writers supplied numbers of the total population of a given state; however, they did so without any evidence whatsoever of how they arrived at their figures.[15] Only in the mid–seventeenth century did commentators begin to provide numerical estimates of population based on empirical records. This development had a snowball effect. Population figures facilitated comparison between states, which in turn provoked questions about the accuracy and source of the numbers. Comparison also led to the creation of new measures of population. Total population, for instance, measured the greatness of France, while across the Channel, population density or favorable hospital mortality rates demonstrated the strength and health of England.[16]

METHOD OF TABLES

The work of political and medical arithmeticians depended on the creation of methods to collect, sort, and record numerical information and then to display that information. The proliferation of newspapers, pamphlets, and periodicals – essential components of the emerging public sphere – increased the flow of information, contributed to the spread of numeracy, and proved critical to the exchange, debate, and refinement of quantitative methods.[17] In addition, the circulation of private letters and the growing use of correspondence – the Republic of Letters – encouraged the free exchange of information among quantifiers, who frequently collected and distributed numbers about local populations.[18] In practice, medical and political arithmeticians became individual

University Press, 1995); and Ian Hacking, *The Taming of Chance* (Cambridge: Cambridge University Press, 1990).

[15] For a general introduction to population doctrines, see Charles Emil Stangeland, *Pre-Malthusian Doctrines of Population: A Study in the History of Economic Thought* (New York: Columbia University Press, 1904).

[16] In the mid–eighteenth century, the population of England was roughly 6 million and of France, 26 million. See E.A. Wrigley and R.S. Schofield, *The Population History of England, 1541–1871* (Cambridge, Mass.: Harvard University Press, 1981); Jacques Dupâquier, ed., *Histoire de la population française,* Vol. 2: *De la Renaissance à 1789* (Paris: Presses Universitaires de France, 1988).

[17] Riley underscored the importance of counting populations to the extension of numeracy; see Riley, *Population Thought,* p. xvii; for discussions of numeracy, see Cohen, *A Calculating People*; and Keith Thomas, "Numeracy in Early Modern England," *Transactions of the Royal Historical Society,* 5th ser. 37 (1977): 103–132.

[18] For recent discussions of the Republic of Letters, see Lorraine Daston, "The Ideal and Reality of the Republic of Letters in the Enlightenment," *Science in Context* 2 (1991): 367–386; Anne Goldgar, *Impolite Learning: Conduct and Community in the Republic of Letters, 1680–1750* (New Haven and London: Yale University Press, 1995); and Dena Goodman, *The Republic of Letters: A Cultural History of the French Enlightenment* (Ithaca and London: Cornell University Press, 1994).

centers of calculation; they digested bits of information gathered by many hands into a single product, a table or set of tables.[19]

The table itself was the most important technology for collecting and displaying quantitative information, and its development constitutes one of the central themes of this book.[20] Tables were used extensively and effectively in arguments over the health and wealth of the population. They were heralded as a new method for organizing and displaying knowledge about the natural and social worlds. For Francis Bacon, their most famous advocate, tables were not only persuasive new instruments but also the best means for recording and ordering observations of a world overflowing with facts. Significantly, Bacon's tables did not contain numbers. Nonetheless, his insistence on the role of tables as instruments of discovery strongly influenced John Graunt and William Petty, the first political and medical arithmeticians, who made extensive use of *numerical* tables in their writings.

Building on Graunt's and Petty's work, eighteenth-century arithmeticians stressed the advantages of tables of numbers or accounts. Although numbers embedded in text certainly conveyed information, comparison between figures was not immediate nor easy if numbers were separated by words. Tables displayed numbers in a way that partially eliminated these difficulties. But all tables were not alike. Some were easier to comprehend than others; clearly, a balance had to be struck between the desire to convey as much information as possible and the complexity of the form. Various conventions or styles proved differently convincing and valued, and tables, like other instruments, could be manipulated.

[19] Centers of calculation is Bruno Latour's phrase; Latour, *Science in Action,* chap. 6.
[20] Tables are literary technologies, a term that refers to the ways in which experimental results were communicated to those who had not witnessed an experiment or partaken in the collection of information; the use of the word technology underlines the written account as a "knowledge-producing tool." See Steven Shapin and Simon Schaffer, *Leviathan and the Air-Pump: Hobbes, Boyle, and the Experimental Life* (Princeton, N.J.: Princeton University Press, 1985), p. 25. Michel Foucault placed great emphasis on the table as a place where knowledge was ordered and displayed during the Classical episteme; Foucault, *The Order of Things: An Archaeology of the Human Sciences,* trans. anon. (1966; New York: Vintage Books, 1973), esp. pp. 71–76. William Clark has developed the Foucauldian idea of the table as a disciplinary tool in his "On the Table Manners of Academic Examination," in *Wissenschaft als kulturelle Praxis, 1750–1900,* ed. Hans Erich Bödecker, Peter Hanns Reill, and Jürgen Schlumbohm (Göttingen: Vandenhoeck & Ruprecht, 1999), pp. 33–67. Mary Poovey argued that separating numbers from narrative contributed to the idea that numbers form a distinct and special type of evidence; Poovey, *A History of the Modern Fact* (Chicago: University of Chicago Press, 1998), pp. xi–xv, and chap. 2, pp. 29–91; finally Edward Tufte has examined the changing conventions of tables and graphs; Edward Tufte, *The Visual Display of Quantitative Information* (Cheshire, Conn.: Graphics Press, 1983). On the role of visual representation in science more generally, see the fine set of essays in Brian S. Baigrie, ed., *Picturing Knowledge: Historical and Philosophical Problems Concerning the Use of Art in Science* (Toronto: University of Toronto Press, 1996), and Martin Rudwick, "The Emergence of a Visual Language of Geology, 1760–1840," *History of Science* 14 (1976): 149–195. Also see Bruno Latour, "Visualization and Cognition: Thinking with Eyes and Hands," *Knowledge and Society: Studies in the Sociology of Culture Past and Present* 6 (1986): 1–40.

METHOD OF COMPARISON

Quantification and the method of tables facilitated the process of comparison, and comparison was fundamental to medical and political arithmetic.[21] Rational judgments, arithmeticians agreed, could be based on numerical measures: Was Paris larger than London? Was smallpox inoculation less risky than natural smallpox? Were mountainous regions healthier than marshy lands? Comparison, of course, was not limited to medical and political issues; it was key to John Locke's and Étienne Bonnot de Condillac's theories of knowledge, and Bacon, too, had viewed comparison as essential to natural philosophy.

Certain liabilities, however, attended the marriage of quantification and comparison. Of central importance was the problem of classification: what to count. The starting point in any quantitative inquiry was to determine which categories to enumerate. As many recent studies have shown, classificatory schemes are highly culturally specific and frequently political.[22] Classifying deaths was of particular importance to arithmeticians, whether by disease, casualty, age, sex, location, or some combination of these. Moreover, few of these categories were stable; disease, for example, was constantly redefined, and popular and elite classifications increasingly diverged over the course of the eighteenth century. Even when categories were seemingly equivalent, or were construed as equivalent by particular authors − a significant achievement itself − their comparability was frequently challenged by others.[23]

To highlight the cultural and political contingencies of quantification, this book compares political and medical arithmetic in England and France during the long eighteenth century, roughly 1660 to 1800.[24] As several recent studies have emphasized, Britain and France created and expanded the apparatus of the modern nation-state, including standing armies, new forms of taxation, and their concomitant bureaucracies. These developments, especially taxation

[21] Sergio Moravia argued that comparison (*comparaison*) as a method was central to the Enlightenment and critical to the development of the human sciences; Moravia, "The Enlightenment and the Sciences of Man," *History of Science* 18 (1980): 247−268.

[22] Mary Douglas, *How Institutions Think* (Syracuse, N.Y.: Syracuse University Press, 1986), chap. 8; Foucault, *The Order of Things*; Hacking, *The Taming of Chance*; Porter, *Trust in Numbers,* chap. 2; and Geoffrey C. Bowker and Susan Leigh Star, *Sorting Things Out: Classification and Its Consequences* (Cambridge and London: The MIT Press, 1999).

[23] In her study of Napoleonic statistics, Marie-Noëlle Bourguet demonstrated that individual communities in France created their own categories (despite explicit instructions from the central government), which made comparison between communities difficult, if not impossible; Bourguet, *Déchiffrer la France: La statistique départementale à l'époque napoléonienne* (Paris: Édition des archives contemporaines, 1988). Witold Kula also demonstrated how socially embedded quantitative measures could be in early modern Europe. See Witold Kula, *Measures and Men,* trans. Richard Szreter (Princeton, N.J.: Princeton University Press, 1986).

[24] Important work was also done in Sweden and Prussia, especially by Pehr Wargentin and Johann Peter Süssmilch; see Karin Johannisson, "Society in Numbers: The Debate over Quantification in Eighteenth Century Political Economy," in *The Quantifying Spirit in the Eighteenth Century,* pp. 343−362; Hacking, *The Taming of Chance,* chap. 3.

and methods of accounting, encouraged quantification.[25] Yet the substantive political and social differences between the two countries cannot be overstated. France was an absolute monarchy, Britain a constitutional one. France was a *société d'ordres,* where privileges were legally defined; England was a burgeoning commercial society based on common law that emphasized the individual over the corporative. In France, the Catholic Church held considerable power, and the boundaries between ecclesiastical and royal authority were ill-defined and overlapping. In England, the Anglican Church was under state control. Religious intolerance was more pronounced in France, especially after the revocation of the Edict of Nantes in 1685, which ended a royal policy of toleration toward Protestantism. In England, Dissenters found their paths to participation in local and national government blocked by the Corporation Act of 1661 and the Test Act of 1673.

Culturally, the upper classes in both countries shared standards of living, education, and manners. Many embraced the Enlightenment attack on the irrational and superstitious, and supported the promotion of happiness by looking for ways to decrease poverty, disease, and crime. Indeed, some of the most characteristic and lasting contributions to Enlightenment thought grew out of exchanges between French and English savants. Their leading scientific institutions, established within four years of each other, the Royal Society of London in 1662 and the Paris Académie Royale des Sciences in 1666, played highly influential roles in shaping the pursuit of natural philosophy. On the other hand, the two could not have been more different. The London society served as a dues-paying gentlemen's club with a Royal Charter; the Paris academy functioned as an extension of the French state, complete with hierarchical membership and pensioned positions.[26] Although each scientific body published a journal, a quick glance at their contents reveals their divergent interests and approaches. The *Philosophical Transactions* contained a hodgepodge

---

[25] Ken Alder, *Engineering the Revolution: Arms and Enlightenment in France, 1763–1815* (Princeton, N.J.: Princeton University Press, 1997); Keith Baker, *Inventing the French Revolution* (Cambridge: Cambridge University Press, 1990); John Brewer, *The Sinews of Power* (New York: Alfred A. Knopf, 1988), chap. 8; Éric Brian, *La mesure de l'état: Administrateurs et géomètres au XVIIIe siècle* (Paris: Albin Michel, 1994), Part 2; Alain Desrosières, *La politique des grand nombres: Histoire de la raison statistique* (Paris: Éditions la Découverte, 1993), chap. 1; Julian Hoppit, "Political Arithmetic in Eighteenth-Century England," *Economic History Review* 49 (1996): 516–540; Philip Kreager, "Quand une population est-elle une nation? Quand une nation est-elle un état? La démographie et l'émergence d'un dilemme moderne, 1770–1870," *Population* 6 (1992): 1639–1656; Michael Kwass, *Privilege and the Politics of Taxation in Eighteenth-Century France: Liberté, Égalité, Fiscalité* (Cambridge: Cambridge University Press, 2000); and Jacques Revel, "Knowledge of the Territory," *Science in Context* 4 (1991): 133–161.

[26] In Charles Gillispie's concise formulation, the Académie Royale des Sciences was an official organization, the Royal Society a voluntary one; see Charles C. Gillispie, *Science and Polity in France at the End of the Old Regime* (Princeton, N.J.: Princeton University Press, 1980), pp. 78–80. Margaret C. Jacob also provided an incisive comparison between English and French natural philosophy; Margaret C. Jacob, *Scientific Culture and the Making of the Industrial West* (New York and Oxford: Oxford University Press, 1997).

of short accounts of two-headed monstrous births and other natural wonders, followed by learned mathematical treatises penned in Latin. The *Histoire et Mémoires* presented a well-organized collection of polished scientific articles arranged by subject. "Soldiers who are under a regular Discipline and besides well paid," Voltaire remarked of the members of both societies, "must necessarily, at last, perform more glorious Atchievements than others who are mere Volunteers."[27]

If the natural philosophers could be divided between the regulars and the volunteers, so too could the physicians. In France, local corporations controlled medical practice to a far greater extent than in England, where medical entrepreneurship flourished.[28] In both countries, medicine provided a route to social advancement in terms of status and income, but religion constrained individual careers. In France, after 1685, Protestants were by regulation excluded not only from university and medical corporations but also from practice. A few Protestant physicians nonetheless created successful practices in France; this became increasingly possible later in the eighteenth century with the growth of religious tolerance.[29] In England, one had to be an Anglican to attend the two medical schools at Oxford and Cambridge, but many Dissenters obtained their MDs at Edinburgh or Leiden and then practiced freely in London and throughout England (although they could not become Fellows of the Royal College of Physicians). Physicians in both countries played prominent roles in the Republic of Letters and the Enlightenment; many of the contributors to the *Encyclopédie,* for example, were physicians. And during the second half of the eighteenth century, the establishment of several new medical and scientific societies, both in the capitals and in provincial cities, encouraged enlightened activities and promoted humanitarian ideals.[30]

These national contours help to explain the particular trajectories of political and medical arithmetic and the course of quantification in each country. Political arithmetic took shape during the Restoration in England where its chief spokesman, William Petty, viewed it as a method to shore up monarchical authority in the wake of England's civil war. In France, the chief advocate of

---

[27] Voltaire, Letter XXIV, "On the Royal Society and Other Academies," in *Letters Concerning the English Nation,* ed. with notes and introduction by Nicholas Cronk (1733; Oxford: Oxford University Press, 1994), p. 117.

[28] On French medicine, see Laurence Brockliss and Colin Jones, *The Medical World of Early Modern France* (Oxford: Clarendon Press, 1997); on English medicine, see Harold Cook, *The Decline of the Old Medical Regime in Stuart London* (Ithaca, N.Y.: Cornell University Press, 1986); Susan C. Lawrence, *Charitable Knowledge: Hospital Pupils and Practitioners in Eighteenth-Century London* (Cambridge: Cambridge University Press, 1996); and Dorothy Porter and Roy Porter, *Patients and Practitioners: Doctors and Doctoring in Eighteenth-Century England* (Stanford, Calif.: Stanford University Press, 1989).

[29] Brockliss and Jones, *The Medical World of Early Modern France,* pp. 483–485.

[30] Shelby T. McCloy, *The Humanitarian Movement in Eighteenth-Century France* (Lexington: University of Kentucky Press, 1957); Francis M. Lobo, "John Haygarth, Smallpox and Religious Dissent in Eighteenth-Century England," in *The Medical Enlightenment of the Eighteenth Century,* ed. Andrew Cunningham and Roger French (Cambridge: Cambridge University Press, 1990), pp. 217–253.

quantification in the late seventeenth century, Sébastien Le Prestre de Vauban, one of Louis XIV's close advisors, regarded regular censuses as valuable resources for the monarchy. After 1750 in England, political arithmetic became primarily a republican activity practiced by Dissenters who, because of their faith, remained outside of government.[31] In France, enlightened intendants – that is, royal bureaucrats – took up political arithmetic in an effort to reform the French monarchy. Thus, in both countries the politics of political arithmetic changed over the course of the eighteenth century, while the location of the practitioners remained distinct.

Central to this political shift were the medical arithmeticians. The work done by physicians and others to improve public and individual health – central goals of the Enlightenment – recast the ideology and practice of political arithmetic. Living conditions in France and England were horrendous, by modern standards, throughout the eighteenth century. The majority of inhabitants in both countries were poor, illiterate, malnourished, and often starving (an estimated one-fifth of the French population died in the 1709–1710 famine). But there were some glimmers of hope. Bubonic plague, a recurrent feature of European life from the mid-fourteenth century, had disappeared, according to late-eighteenth-century commentators. Smallpox emerged as the most dreaded disease, but here, too, there was room for optimism: Inoculation provided physicians with a technique to reduce mortality.[32] Medical arithmeticians furnished the means for evaluating and encouraging these improvements.

METHOD OF CONTROVERSY

The three most important controversies concerning health and population in eighteenth-century England and France were smallpox inoculation, environmental medicine, and depopulation. An analysis of the types of arguments used in these controversies illustrates and illuminates several styles or patterns of thought. More important, studying these controversies reveals the changes in those styles or patterns, as well as the mechanism (the controversy itself) for change.[33] For the sociology of scientific knowledge, controversies serve as

[31] Peter Buck, "People Who Counted: Political Arithmetic in the Eighteenth Century," *Isis* 73 (1982): 29. Also see Peter Buck, "Seventeenth-Century Political Arithmetic: Civil Strife and Vital Statistics," *Isis* 68 (1977): 67–84. Buck attributes the shifting politics of political arithmetic to a renewed expression of classical republican ideology that emerged out of the unlikely alliance between the political aims of Dissenters and landed gentry.
[32] Peter Gay emphasized the link between medicine and optimism during the Enlightenment; Peter Gay, *The Enlightenment*, Vol. 2: *The Science of Freedom* (New York: Norton, 1969), pp. 8–23.
[33] The French historian Jean-Claude Perrot has recently suggested that "la querelle" – or controversy – played a significant role in the development of ideas during the eighteenth century, in the "history of the conditions of thought." Michel Foucault had earlier written that such an approach (an examination

important sites for research precisely because in these moments, scientists articulate their tacit assumptions, unfamiliar practices, and unchallenged knowledge claims.[34] Political and medical arithmeticians felt impelled and were compelled by outside observers to explain and justify their methods and conclusions.

The order of the controversies is roughly chronological. The debates surrounding smallpox inoculation, which peaked in England in the 1720s and in France in the 1750s, are analyzed in Part I (Chapters 2, 3 and 4). Throughout the eighteenth century, smallpox was a deadly and disfiguring disease. It struck the rich and poor alike, and its sudden and lethal attack on many members of European royalty led in some cases to political crises. The hope that inoculation, introduced into Europe at the beginning of the eighteenth century, could prevent smallpox propelled the practice to the center of public debate. Some advocates of inoculation constructed numerical accounts showing the risks of dying from inoculation to be far smaller than the risks of dying from natural smallpox. This is arguably the first use of numbers to evaluate a medical procedure.

Chapter 2 examines the construction of these numerical risks through a close study of the work of James Jurin, physician and secretary to the Royal Society. As secretary, Jurin solicited and collected accounts of inoculation in correspondence from individuals throughout England during the 1720s; from these accounts he calculated the risks of dying from inoculated smallpox. The chapter details the difficulties Jurin encountered and the kind of work he had to do to make the accounts comparable and thus quantifiable. Many of the techniques Jurin developed were used by later medical and political arithmeticians.

Chapter 3 discusses numerical arguments in French debates over inoculation. Unlike in England, where physicians took the lead in promoting inoculation, most French physicians opposed the practice until midcentury. *Philosophes* from Voltaire to Charles-Marie de La Condamine campaigned to have the procedure accepted. Numerical arguments played a relatively minor role in the debates, except for the well-publicized exchange at the Paris Académie des Sciences between Jean d'Alembert and Daniel Bernoulli. Although both supported inoculation, they disagreed about how to calculate the risks involved. The degree of mathematical specialization evidenced in this exchange discouraged the use and acceptance of quantification by the French medical community during the eighteenth century.

---

of controversies) would result in "only a history of opinions," not in an understanding of the "general system of thought" – the episteme. See Jean-Claude Perrot, "Les économistes, les philosophes et la population," in *Histoire de la population française*, Vol. 2: *De la Renaissance à 1789*, p. 545; and Michel Foucault, *The Order of Things*, p. 75. My use of the terms styles or patterns of thought is closer to Perrot's "conditions of thought" than to Foucault's more restrictive "episteme."

[34] For a recent discussion of controversy studies, see Jan Golinski, *Making Natural Knowledge: Constructivism and the History of Science* (Cambridge: Cambridge University Press, 1998), chap. 1, pp. 13–46.

Chapter 4 looks at numerical arguments in English debates of the 1770s over whether to inoculate the urban poor. Taking figures from the London bills of mortality, physicians constructed a variety of tables to ascertain if smallpox mortality had increased or remained the same over the course of the eighteenth century. Opponents of inoculating the poor argued that their tables demonstrated that smallpox mortality had increased precisely because of the indiscriminate practice of inoculation; that is, inoculated individuals had spread the contagion (unless they had been isolated for two to three weeks). By contrast, advocates used their tables to argue that smallpox mortality (as measured by the London bills) had remained more or less constant over the course of the eighteenth century, and they concluded that inoculating the poor would do more good than harm. In this case, tables failed to secure consensus and instead underlined the malleability of this type of argument.

Controversy about environmental medicine – how the environment affected health – is the focus of Part II (Chapters 5 and 6).[35] Debates were stimulated by the growing recognition of changes in disease patterns (most markedly the disappearance of widespread, epidemic plague from Western Europe after 1721) and the seeming success of inoculation, both of which brought a sense of optimism to the understanding and prevention of disease.[36]

One way to make sense of the effects of the environment was to examine the links between weather and health. Chapter 5 treats attempts to craft a science of medical meteorology, including the proposed techniques to collect, record, and display observations. Like Jurin's inoculation project, medical meteorology projects encountered difficulties in securing accurate and complete information from volunteers. The relatively new and unstandardized meteorological instruments such as barometers and thermometers hindered comparison, and the tabular format proved insufficient to the task of recording two very different phenomena: weather and disease.

Efforts to use mortality figures to address issues of health and geography are the subject of Chapter 6. Contemporaries frequently remarked on the expansion of London and Paris, and many felt that it came at the expense of the population in the countryside. They associated many problems with greater numbers of people within a small compass: higher incidence of disease, breakdown of traditional mores (complaints about luxury and immorality), and anonymity. Debate centered on variations in and causes of salubrity. Physicians began to collect and use mortality and morbidity data (displayed in various tables) in

---

[35] For an overview of environmental medicine in the eighteenth century, see James C. Riley, *The Eighteenth-Century Campaign to Avoid Disease* (New York: Macmillan, 1987).

[36] For a recent discussion about the changing epidemiology of eighteenth-century England, see Alex Mercer, *Disease, Mortality and Population in Transition: Epidemiological-Demographic Change in England since the Eighteenth Century as Part of a Global Phenomenon* (Leicester, London & New York: Leicester University Press, 1990).

order to assess the salubrity of different geographies, seasons, and groups of individuals. Much of this project was descriptive, but not all. Several policy recommendations were suggested by this approach, which one contemporary labeled medical arithmetic.

Finally, Part III (Chapter 7) looks at the depopulation controversy that flourished in the last decades of the eighteenth century. Most observers believed that the English, French, and indeed the entire European population had declined in numbers since antiquity, and especially over the course of the eighteenth century. The causes and consequences of this depopulation generated vigorous debate. In the inoculation controversy, arithmeticians had established that 10 percent of the population died from smallpox. This number – once agreed upon and thereby stabilized as a scientific fact[37] – was invoked by subsequent commentators as one of the principal causes of population decline. Another commonly held belief was that cities were more deadly than the countryside; this was cited in conjunction with the visible growth of cities as evidence of depopulation.[38] By one theory, overall mortality rates were higher because more people were living (and dying) in unhealthy cities than in the salubrious countryside. During the last decades of the eighteenth century, arithmeticians began to evaluate numerically these depopulationists' claims. They expanded methods of collecting vital accounts and developed techniques to calculate population. Their work generally indicated population growth, rather than decline, but criticisms about the accuracy of their calculations abounded. The methods and the meaning of quantification were once again contested.

Epistemologically, there is something special about quantification. Numbers allow for comparison, even if the grounds of comparison are not always level. The importance of comparison cannot be overstressed: Once quantified, things can be put on a numerical scale, from lesser to greater. They can be displayed in tables, which themselves promote certain kinds of comparison. Numbers have an inherent order to them that words often do not. Quantification can thus be a powerful tool, but its profound consequences were neither

---

[37] There is a stimulating debate about the emergence of the fact as an epistemological category. See Lorraine Daston, "Baconian Facts, Academic Civility, and the Prehistory of Objectivity," *Annals of Science* 8 (1991): 337–364; Poovey, *A History of the Modern Fact;* Steven Shapin and Simon Schaffer, *Leviathan and the Air-Pump: Hobbes, Boyle, and the Experimental Life* (Princeton, N.J.: Princeton University Press, 1985); Steven Shapin, *A Social History of Truth: Civility and Science in Seventeenth Century England* (Chicago: University of Chicago Press, 1994); and Barbara J. Shapiro, *A Culture of Fact: England 1550–1720* (Ithaca and London: Cornell University Press, 2000).

[38] For a discussion of the beliefs surrounding health and environment in early modern England, see Andrew Wear, "Making Sense of Health and the Environment in Early Modern England," in *Medicine in Society: Historical Essays,* ed. Andrew Wear (Cambridge: Cambridge University Press, 1992), pp. 119–147; Mary J. Dobson, *Contours of Death and Disease in Early Modern England* (Cambridge: Cambridge University Press, 1997), chaps. 1 and 2, pp. 9–77.

easily anticipated nor fully understood. Nor were the virtues of quantification (inherent scale, easy comparison, association with certainty) universally or readily accepted. A close examination of the debates over smallpox inoculation, environmental medicine, and depopulation makes clear that quantification and numerical tables were controversial techniques for producing new knowledge.

1

A New Science: Political Arithmetic

> [Algebra] came out of Arabia by the Moores into Spaine and from thence hither, and W[illiam] P[etty] hath applyed it to other than purely mathematicall matters, viz.: to policy by the name of Politicall Arithmetick, by reducing many termes of matter to termes of number, weight, and measure, in order to be handled mathematically.
>
> William Petty[1]

The origin of quantitative studies of population is most often traced to a single book: John Graunt's *Natural and Political Observations Made upon the Bills of Mortality* published in 1662. In this modest volume, Graunt, a London tradesman, argued that "Trade and Government may be made more certain and Regular" through the application of arithmetic, and that knowledge of "how many People there be of each Sex, State, Age, Religion, Trade, Rank, or Degree, &c." provided a fair method "to balance Parties and Factions both in Church and State."[2] Writing in the immediate aftermath of the English Civil War, Graunt was keenly aware of the suffering caused by religious intolerance and economic turmoil. He also felt the widespread desire for order and stability after Charles II's ascension to the throne. Through quantification, Graunt sought to construct a new form of knowledge that could provide a trustworthy resource for reducing conflict, maintaining political equilibrium, and cultivating commercial prosperity.[3]

Graunt's friend and patron William Petty fervently embraced the new project and coined a name for Graunt's method: political arithmetic. Petty shared Graunt's confidence in the certainty and regularity of mathematics. "God send

---

[1] *The Petty Papers: Some Unpublished Writings of Sir William Petty*, ed. Marquis of Lansdowne, 2 vols. (London: Constable & Co., 1927), vol. 2, p. 15.

[2] John Graunt, *Natural and Political Observations Made upon the Bills of Mortality*, 5th ed. much Enlarged (London, 1676); reprinted in *The Economic Writings of Sir William Petty*, ed. Charles Henry Hull (Cambridge: Cambridge University Press, 1899), pp. 396–397. Future references are to this edition except when otherwise indicated.

[3] Peter Buck, "Seventeenth-Century Political Arithmetic: Civil Strife and Vital Statistics," *Isis* 68 (1977): 67–84.

mee the use of things, and notions, whose foundations are sense and the super-structure mathematicall reasoning," Petty pleaded, "for wont of which props so many Governments doe reel and stagger, and crush the honest subjects that live under them."[4] Mathematics would secure good and proper government.

Together, Graunt and Petty laid the foundations for the sciences of polit-ical and medical arithmetic. Their ideas found an immediate and receptive audience among members of the Royal Society. Established in 1662, this small group of natural philosophers enthusiastically pursued empirical and mathemat-ical approaches to natural phenomena. For the Fellows, mathematics proved a useful tool in commerce and natural philosophy, and it seemed only common sense to extend it to natural and political questions.[5] This institutional sup-port was critical to the introduction and development of quantitative studies of population.

CRAFTING A NEW METHOD: NUMERICAL TABLES

An important aspect of Graunt's and Petty's work was their use of tables as a method or instrument of investigation and discovery. Tables, of course, have been around a long time. They first gained widespread distribution with the advent of the printing press, which ensured that they could be reproduced more accurately and quickly than those copied by hand.[6] By the seventeenth century, several types of published numerical tables existed: 1) astronomical and astrological tables, often found in almanacs; 2) mathematical tables, for example, multiplication tables or tables of weight and currency exchanges; and 3) tables in accounting books. While scholars have discussed Graunt's and Petty's writings extensively, especially as prefiguring the disciplines of statistics and economics, they have paid little attention to the tables.[7] Numerical tables, both Graunt and

---

[4] *Petty Papers*, vol. 1, p. 111.
[5] Mary Poovey emphasized Petty's role as a "go-between" of the natural philosophical community and those interested in trade and wealth; Poovey, *A History of the Modern Fact: Problems of Knowledge in the Sciences of Wealth and Society* (Chicago and London: The University of Chicago Press, 1998), chap. 3, pp. 92–143.
[6] See Elizabeth Eisenstein, *The Printing Press as an Agent of Change; Communications and Cultural Trans-formations in Early-Modern Europe* (Cambridge: Cambridge University Press, 1979), vol. 2, pp. 461, 466–468. For a recent critique of Eisenstein, see Adrian Johns, *The Nature of the Book: Print and Knowledge in the Making* (Chicago: University of Chicago Press, 1998).
[7] Graunt has been called the "true Father of Statistics" by Karl Pearson; see Pearson, *The History of Statistics*, p. 10. For other discussions of Graunt's work, see D.V. Glass, "John Graunt and his 'Natural and Political Observations,' " *Notes and Records of the Royal Society* 19 (1964): 63–100; Anders Hald, *A History of Probability and Statistics and their Applications before 1750* (New York: John Wiley & Sons, 1990), pp. 81–105; Robert Kargon, "John Graunt, Francis Bacon, and the Royal Society: The Reception of Statistics," *Journal of the History of Medicine* 18 (1963): 337–348; Philip Kreager, "New Light on Graunt," *Population Studies* 42 (1988): 129–140; J. Sutherland, "John Graunt: A Tercentenary Tribute," *Journal of the Royal Statistical Society, Series A* 126 (1963): 536–556. Karl Marx hailed Petty, rather than Adam Smith, as the "father of English Political Economy" in recognition of Petty's ideas on the value of labor; see Karl Marx, *A Contribution to the Critique of Political Economy*, trans. from

Petty argued, would yield reliable and useful observations about the natural and political world. This new method combined tabular forms of presentation with quantification.

Tables had been championed by Francis Bacon as the method for improving knowledge about the natural world. Tables would aid the memory, provide a way to summarize information, and make that information more accessible. The compilation of natural histories in tables would help observers inquire into the relations among observations.[8] Tables were thus a vital first step in the process of induction. "So after long and anxious thought," Bacon realized that "the first thing necessary was to set forth Tables of Discovery or, as it were, formulae of a legitimate mode of research, in certain fields, to serve as an example and to be a sort of visible embodiment of the work to be done."[9]

Graunt cited Bacon admiringly and explicitly compared his natural and political observations to Bacon's natural histories: for both, tables were crucial.[10] Graunt "reduced several great confused *Volumes* into a few perspicuous *Tables,*" and underscored the power of tables to bring clarity and conciseness to specific topics.[11] Tables had the additional virtue of allowing anyone who so desired to re-create and evaluate the manner in which the initial conclusions had been drawn. "I have taken the pains, and been at the charge," Graunt admitted, "of setting out those *Tables*, whereby all men may both correct my *Positions*, and raise others of their own."[12] Here, then, is the essence of this new method and instrument: A thorough presentation of the data provided the means for independent assessment and discovery.[13]

Graunt's tables, in contrast to Bacon's, were entirely quantitative. Bacon had not included quantitative information in his tables and, in general, did not

second German edition by N.I. Stone (New York: International Library Publishing Co., 1904), pp. 58–60. Classical economists, including Adam Smith, dismissed Petty's work. "I have no great faith in Political Arithmetic," Smith wrote in *An Inquiry into the Nature and Causes of the Wealth of Nations,* (1776; reprint ed. Edwin Cannan, New York: The Modern Library, 1937), p. 501. For other evaluations of Petty's contributions to economics, see William L. Bevan, *Sir William Petty: A Study in English Economic Literature* (Baltimore: American Economic Association, 1894); Maurice Pasquier, *Sir William Petty: Ses Idées Économiques* (New York: Burt Franklin, 1971 [1903]); and William Letwin, *The Origins of Scientific Economics – English Economic Thought, 1660–1776* (London: Methuen, 1963). In a more recent study, Juri Mykkänen has used Foucault's ideas of governmentality to analyze Petty's work. Mykkänen, "'To methodize and regulate them': William Petty's Governmental Science of Statistics," *History of the Human Sciences* 7 (1994): 65–88.

8 For discussions of Bacon's method, see Paolo Rossi, *Francis Bacon: From Magic to Science,* trans. Sacha Rabinovitch (Chicago: University of Chicago Press, 1968), esp. p. 205; and Lisa Jardine, *Francis Bacon: Discovery and the Art of Discourse* (Cambridge: Cambridge University Press, 1974).

9 Francis Bacon, *Cogitata et Visa* (1607); quoted in Rossi, *Francis Bacon,* p. 205.

10 For a discussion of Bacon's influence on Graunt, see Kreager, "New Light on Graunt"; and Kargon, "John Graunt, Francis Bacon, and the Royal Society."

11 Graunt, *Natural and Political Observations,* p. 320.

12 Graunt, *Natural and Political Observations,* p. 334.

13 On the functions of Boyle's writing strategies, see Steven Shapin and Simon Schaffer, *Leviathan and the Air-Pump: Hobbes, Boyle, and the Experimental Life* (Princeton, N.J.: Princeton University Press, 1985).

envision a primary role for mathematics because he regarded numbers and quantity as accidental, not essential, qualities (following Aristotelian metaphysics).[14] Graunt thought otherwise. The inspiration for his quantitative accounts came from his long experience as a London tradesman; in his own words, the tables depended "upon the Mathematicks of my Shop-Arithmetick."[15] Graunt's work thus drew on and was shaped explicitly by shop arithmetic, that is, contemporary bookkeeping and accounting techniques.[16]

This marriage of Baconian natural history and accounting is clearly revealed in Petty's "Materialls for a New History of Life and Death." Modeled on the style of Bacon's *History of Life and Death,* Petty's queries asked for numerical answers. The first two read:

1. Of 100 birthes, how many live to bee 10, 20, 30 &c. – to 100?
2. Of 100 persons now alive, how many are aged between 1 and 10, between 10 and 20 &c. – to between 90 and 100?[17]

Petty's near obsession with quantification was more philosophical in origin than Graunt's, whose attachment to arithmetic was rooted in day-to-day practice. Petty regarded the virtues of quantification as self-evident and took his mission to quantify seriously. At a meeting of the Royal Society, he scolded another member for using imprecise language, such as "considerably bigger," and "cautioned, that no word might be used but what marks either number, weight, or measure."[18] Quantification allowed for precise and exact treatment of whatever problems were at hand, although Petty realized the limitations of his form of arithmetic, particularly its claims to certainty: "I know these are not so perfect Demonstrations as are required in pure Mathematicks; but they are such as our superiors may work with, as well as Wheelwrights and Clockmakers do work without the Quadrature of a Circle."[19] Like skilled craftsmen, political arithmeticians could produce useful knowledge without the benefit of geometrical certainty.

If numerical tables provided the method, the London bills of mortality provided the raw materials for Graunt's and Petty's work. The bills of mortality were initially published in the mid–fifteenth century to warn Londoners of an

---

[14] Jardine, *Francis Bacon,* pp. 78–79.
[15] Graunt, *Natural and Political Observations,* Epistle Dedicatory, p. 323.
[16] Philip Kreager has carefully analyzed Graunt's reliance on contemporary accounting techniques. See Kreager, "New Light on Graunt."
[17] Petty, "Materialls for a New History of Life and Death," *Petty Papers,* vol. 1, p. 187.
[18] Thomas Birch, *The History of the Royal Society of London* (London, 1756–1757), vol. 4, p. 193, (March 14, 1682/3). Petty's project can be regarded as part of the movement to make language clear and precise as, for example, in the universal language schemes. See Mary Slaughter, *Universal Languages and Scientific Taxonomy in the Seventeenth Century* (Cambridge: Cambridge University Press, 1982).
[19] Petty, *Treatise of Ireland* (written in 1687, not published until 1899), in *The Economic Writings of Sir William Petty,* p. 611.

impending plague epidemic.[20] "The *Bill of Mortality* is of very great use and necessity," wrote John Bell, clerk to the Company of Parish Clerks, during the great plague epidemic of 1665, "in that it giveth a general notice of the *Plague*, and a particular Accompt of the places which are therewith infected, to the end such places may be shunned and avoided."[21] In 1611, James I incorporated the Company of Parish Clerks and gave them sole responsibility for drawing up the weekly bills.[22] Instructed to tally the number of deaths from plague, as well as the total number of parishioners who had died each week, parish clerks sent these numbers to the Clerk of the Company, who thereupon totaled the figures and published a weekly bill of mortality. Parish clerks received information about deaths within their parishes from the Searchers, who typically were older women paid by the parish to examine corpses and ascertain causes of death. Graunt provided a detailed description of the process:

When any one dies, then, either by tolling, or ringing of a Bell, or by bespeaking of a Grave of the Sexton, the same is known to the Searchers, corresponding with the said Sexton.

The Searchers hereupon (who are antient Matrons, sworn to their Office) repair to the place where the dead Corps lies, and by view of the same, and by other enquiries, they examine by what Disease, or Casualty the corps died. Hereupon they make their Report to the Parish-Clerk, and he, every Tuesday night, carries in an Accompt of all the Burials, and Christnings, happening that Week, to the Clerk of the Hall. On Wednesday the general Accompt is made up and printed, and on Thursday published and dispersed to the several families who will pay four shillings per Annum for them.[23]

The earliest known bill of mortality, from sometime in the mid–fifteenth century, listed parishes with the plague deaths noted in roman numerals. Beginning in 1603, the bills of mortality appeared regularly and assumed a form retained with only minor changes throughout the seventeenth and eighteenth centuries. A comparison of a mid–fifteenth-century bill and a 1624 bill reveals the advantages of arabic numerals (at least to the modern eye) and a table format for quickly comprehending the information presented. (See Figures 1.1 and 1.2.) Figure 1.1 presents a weekly bill of mortality from the mid–fifteenth century, which recorded that 34 persons died of plague and that 32 died of other diseases ("oder sekenes"), for a total of 66 deaths in London. Figure 1.2

---

[20] One writer, however, has claimed that the "almost sole purpose" for the publication of the bills in Elizabeth's reign "was that of frightening persons away from the metropolis. The Queen and her Government had a great dread of the inordinate growth of the city...." See Cornelius Walford, "Early Bills of Mortality," *Transactions of the Royal Historical Society* 7 (1878): 217.
[21] John Bell, *London Remembrancer, or a True Account of Christnings and Mortality in All the Years of the Pestilence* (London, 1665), n.p.
[22] Charles H. Hull long ago provided what is still the most complete discussion of these bills. See his "Introduction" to *The Economic Writings of Sir William Petty*, pp. lxxx–xci. Also see Walford, "Early Bills of Mortality," and William Ogle, "An Inquiry into the Trustworthiness of the Old Bills of Mortality," *Journal of the Royal Statistical Society* 55 (1892): 437–460.
[23] Graunt, *Natural and Political Observations*, p. 346.

Syns the xvjth day of November unto the xxiij day of the same month ys deed. In the citie and fredom yong and old thes mayny folowyng of the plage and oder dyseases.

In primys benetts grace churche j of ye plage
S buttolls without bysshops gate j corse
S nycholas flesshammuls^M j of ye plage
S peturs in cornell j of the plage
   Mary Wolnorth j corse
All halowes barkyng. ij corses
Kateryne colmane j of the plage
Mary aldermanebery j corse
Michaels in cornelle iij one of ye plage
Alle halowes ye moore ij   j of the plagee
S gylez iiij corses iij of the plage
S dunstons in ye west iiij of ye plage
Stevens in colmane strete j corse
Alle halowys lumbert strete j corse
Martens owute whiche^M j corse
Mergett moyses j of the plage
Kateryne crechurche ij of the plage
Martens in ye vyntre ij corses
Buttolls without algate iiij corses
S olavus in hert strete ij corses
S Andros in holborne ij of ye plage
S peters at powls wharff ij of ye plage
S ffeythes j corse of ye plage
S alphes j corse of the plage
S Mathews in fryday strete j of the plag
Aldermary ij corses
Sepulcres iiij corses j of the plage
S thomas appostells ij of the plage
S leonerds faster lane j of ye plage
Michaels in ye ryalle ij corses
S alborowes j corse of the plage
Swytthyns ij corses of ye plage
Mary somersetts j corse

S bryds v corses j of the plage
S benetts powls wharff j of the plage
Alle halows in ye walle j of ye plage
Mary Hylle j corse

sum of ye plage xxxiiij persons
sum of oder sekenes xxxij persons
        the holle sum iij^{xx} and vj.
and ther is this weke clere.

iij^{xx} and iij parysh as by thes
   bills dothe appere

1.1 Fifteenth-century London bill of mortality. *Source:* William Ogle, "An Inquiry into the Trustworthiness of the Old Bills of Mortality," *Journal of the Royal Statistical Society* 55 (1892): 437–460.

1624. 1625.

A general, or great Bill for this Year, of the whole number of Burials, which have been buried of all Diseases, and also of the *Plague* in every Parish within the City of *London*, and the Liberties thereof; as also in the nine out-Parishes adjoyning to the said City; with the Pest-house belonging to the same. From *Thursday* the 16. day of *December*, 1624. to *Thursday* the 15 day of *December*, 1625. According to the Report, made to the king's most Excellent Majesty, by the Company of Parish-Clerks of *London*.

LONDON,	Bur.	Plag.	LONDON.	Bur.	Plag.
Albanes in Woodstreet	188	78	Gabriel Fen church	71	54
Alhallows Barking	397	263	George Botolphs-lane	30	19
Alhallows Breadstreet	34	14	Gregories by Pauls	196	196
Alhallows the Great	442	302	Hellens in Bishopsgatest.	136	71
Alhallows Hony-lane	16	8	James by Garlickhithe	180	109
Alhallows the less	259	205	John Baptist	122	79
Alhal. in Lumberdstreet	86	44	John Evangelist	7	0
Alhallows Stainings	183	138	John Zacharies	143	97
Alhallows the Wall	301	155	James Duks place	310	254
Alphage Cripple-gate	240	190	Katherine Coleman	163	175
Andrew-Hubbard	146	101	Katherine Cree-church	886	373
Andrews Undershaft	219	149	Lawrence in the Jewrie	91	55
Andrews by Wardrobe	373	191	Lawrence Pountney	106	117
Annes at Aldersgate	196	118	Leonards Eastcheap	55	26
Annes Black-Friers	336	215	Leonards Fosterlane	192	209
Antholins Parish	62	31	Magnus Parish by Bridge	137	85
Austins Parish	72	40	Margarets Lothbury	114	64
Barthol. at the Exchange	52	24	Margarets Moses	37	25
Bennets Fink	108	57	Margarets new Fishstreet	123	82
Bennets Grace-Church	48	14	Margarets Pattons	77	50
Bennets at Pauls Wharf	226	131	Mary Ab-church	98	58
Bennets Shereheg	24	8	Mary Aldermanbury	126	79
Botolps Billings-gate	99	66	Mary Aldermary	92	54
Christ's Church Parish	611	371	Mary le Bow	35	19
Christopher's Parish	48	28	Mary Bothaw	22	14
Clements by Eastcheap	87	72	Mary Colechurch	26	11
Dyonis Black-Church	99	59	Mary at the Hill	152	84
Dunstans in the East	335	235	Mary Mounthaw	76	58
Edmunds Lumberdstreet	78	49	Mary Sommerset	270	192
Ethelborow in Bishopsg.	205	101	Mary Stainings	70	44
St. Faiths	89	45	Mary Woolchurch	58	25
St. Fosters in Foster-lane	149	102	Mary Woolnoth	82	50
					Martins

1.2 London bill of mortality (1624–1625). *Source:* John Graunt, *Natural and Political Observations Made upon the Bills of Mortality* (London, 1662).

L O N D O N.	Bur.	Pla.	L O N D O N.	Bur.	Pla.
Martins Ironmonger-lane	25	18	Nicholas Acons———	33	13
Martins at Ludgate————	254	164	Nicholas Cole-Abby —	87	67
Martins Organs ————	88	47	Nicholas Olaves ——·—	70	43
Martins Outwich ———	60	30	Olaves in Hartftreet——·	266	195
Martins in the Vintry —	339	208	Olaves in the Jewry——	43	25
Matthew Fridayftreet —	24	11	Olaves in Silverftreet —	174	103
Maudlins in Milkftreet —	401	23	Pancras by Soperlane—	17	8
Maudlins Oldfifh-ftreet--	225	142	Peter in Cheap———	68	44
Michael Baffifhaw ———	199	139	Peters in Corn-hill ——	318	78
Michael Corn-Hill ———	159	79	Peters at Pauls Wharf.—	97	68
Michael Crooked-lane —	144	91	Peters poor in Broadftreet-	52	27
Michael Queenhithe ——	215	157	Stevens in Colemanftreet.	506	350
Michael in the Quern —	53	30	Stevens in Walbrook——	25	13
Michael in the Ryal———	111	61	Swithins at Londonftone-	99	60
Michael in Woodftreet—	189	68	Thomas Apoftles ————	141	107
Mildreds Breadftreet —	60	44	Trinity Parifh —·— ———	148	87
Mildreds Poultrey——	94	45			

Buried within the 97. Parifhes within the Walls of, all Difeafes.—14340.
Whereof, of the Plague. ———·— —·— ——— ——— 9197.

	Bur.	Pla.		Bur.	Pla.
Andrews in Holborn —	2190	1636	Georges Southwark—	1608	912
Bartholmew the Great—	516	360	Giles Cripplegate————	3988	2338
Bartholmew the lefs —	111	65	Olaves in Southwark--	3689	2609
Brides Parifh ————	1481	1031	Saviours in Southwark--	2746	1671
Botolph Algate ————	2573	1653	Sepulchres Parifn ——	3425	2420
Bridewel Precinct————	213	152	Thomas in Southwark—	335	277
Bottolph Bifhopgate —	2334	714	Trinity in the Minories-	131	87
Botolph Alderfgate —	578	307	At the Pefthoufe———	194	189
Dunftanes the Weft—	860	642			

Buried in the 16 Parifhes without the Walls, ftanding part within
the Liberties, and part without: in Middlefex, and Surrey, and 26972
at the Pefthoufe. ———— ——
Whereof, of the Plague ——— ·—·——— —— ——— ——— 17153

Buried in the nine out-Parifhes.

	Bur.	Pla.		Bur.	Pla.
Clements Templebar—	1284	755	Martins in the Fields—	1470	973
Giles in the Fields —	1333	947	Mary White-chappel —	3305	2172
James at Clarkenwell—	1191	903	Magdalens Bermondfey-	1127	889
Katherins by the Tower-	998	744	Savoy Parifh ———	250	176
Leonards in Shorditch--	1995	1407			

Buried in the nine out Parifhes, in Middlefex, and Surrey———12953
Whereof, of the Plague ——— ·——— ——— —— ——— 9067

1.2 *(cont.)*

presents an annual summary compiled from weekly bills of mortality for the
year 1624, a year that plague struck London. Plague accounted for more than
half the deaths that year (35,417 out of 54,265), and the proportion was even
higher in the parishes within the walls (9,197 of 14,340 burials) and the nine
out-parishes (9,067 of 12,953 burials).

The Diſeaſes, and Caſualties this year being 1632.

Abortive, and Stilborn	445	Jaundies	43
Affrighted	1	Jawfaln	8
Aged	628	Impoſtume	74
Ague	43	Kil'd by ſeveral accidents	46
Apoplex, and Meagrom	17	King's Evil	38
Bit with a mad dog	1	Lethargie	2
Bleeding	3	Livergrown	87
Bloody flux, ſcowring, and flux	348	Lunatique	5
Bruſed, Iſſues, ſores, and ulcers	28	Made away themſelves	15
Burnt, and Scalded	5	Meaſles	80
Burſt, and Rupture	9	Murthered	7
Cancer, and Wolf	10	Over-laid, and ſtarved at nurſe	7
Canker	1	Pallie	25
Childbed	171	Piles	1
Chriſomes, and Infants	2268	Plague	8
Cold, and Cough	55	Planet	13
Colick, Stone, and Strangury	56	Pleuriſie, and Spleen	36
Conſumption	1797	Purples, and ſpotted Feaver	38
Convulſion	241	Quinſie	7
Cut of the Stone	5	Riſing of the Lights	98
Dead in the ſtreet, and ſtarved	6	Sciatica	1
Dropſie, and Swelling	267	Scurvey, and Itch	9
Drowned	34	Suddenly	62
Executed, and preſt to death	18	Surfet	86
Falling Sickneſs	7	Swine Pox	6
Fever	1108	Teeth	470
Fiſtula	13	Thruſh, and Sore mouth	40
Flocks, and ſmall Pox	531	Tympany	13
French Pox	12	Tiſſick	34
Gangrene	5	Vomiting	1
Gout	4	Worms	27
Grief	11		

Chriſtened ⎰ Males—4994, Females—4590, In all—9584 ⎱   Buried ⎰ Males—4932, Females—4603, In all—9535 ⎱ Whereof, of the Plague 8

Increaſed in the Burials in the 122 Pariſhes, and at the Peſthouſe this year 331
Decreaſed of the Plague in the 122 Pariſhes, and at the Peſthouſe this year 266

1.3 Table of casualties from the 1632 London bill of mortality. *Source:* John Graunt, *Natural and Political Observations Made upon the Bills of Mortality* (London, 1662).

In these two early examples, the bills of mortality listed each parish separately, reflecting a concern for geographical specificity. Beginning in 1629, the bills included other causes of death besides plague and divided the total number of burials and christenings by sex. Figure 1.3, a portion of the bill of mortality for the year 1632, illustrates these new additions. In contrast to the bill of 1624, that of 1632 was relatively low in overall mortality. Only 8 persons died of plague, compared to the 35,417 in 1624. During the eighteenth century, the only major change to the London bills of mortality was the inclusion of the age of death, beginning in 1728. The bills continued to be printed until 1837, when the General Register Office took over the task of vital registration.

In his *Observations,* Graunt remarked on how little use was made of the bills of mortality, other "than to look at the foot, how the Burials increased, or decreased."[24] He admitted that the bills had their faults, in particular the Searchers' abilities to determine cause of death, and he sought to make "Corrections upon the, perhaps, ignorant and careless Searchers Reports."[25] Not only carelessness marred the reliability of the numbers reported in the bills. Comparing the low number of deaths attributed to syphilis and the large number of individuals complaining of the disease, Graunt reasoned that many who died from syphilis were listed as dying from other diseases. "The Old-Women Searchers," he charged, "after the mist of a Cup of Ale, and the bribe of a two-grout fee . . . cannot tell whether this emaciation or leanness were from a phthisis, or from an Hectick Fever, Atrophy &c. or from an Infection of the Spermatick parts." After interviewing several parish clerks, Graunt concluded "that onely hated persons, and such, whose very Noses were eaten off were reported by the Searchers to have died of this too frequent Malady."[26]

Graunt tempered his criticism of the Searchers' willful and wanton over-sights with a strong dose of pragmatism: "I say, it is enough if we know from the Searchers but the most predominant Symptoms; . . . if one died suddenly, the matter is not great, whether it be reported in the Bills, Suddenly, Apoplexie, or Planet-strucken &c."[27] In this practical vein, Graunt analyzed the bills of mortality into two sets of issues: the natural, that is, those "concerning the Air, Countries, Seasons, Fruitfulness, Health, Diseases, Longevity, and the proportions between the Sex, and Ages of Mankind"; and the political, those "concerning Trade and Government."[28]

NATURAL OBSERVATIONS

Little is known about John Graunt beyond the barest facts of his life. Born in 1620 in the Parish of St. Michael Cornhill in London where his father Henry Graunt was a draper, John was "educated while a Boy in English learning" and apprenticed to a haberdasher. He became a tradesman of some standing and served the city government in various capacities, rising to the level of a common councilman.[29] In 1662 he published his only book, *Natural and Political*

---

[24] Graunt, *Natural and Political Observations,* p. 333.
[25] Graunt, *Natural and Political Observations,* p. 347.
[26] Graunt, *Natural and Political Observations,* pp. 356–357.
[27] Graunt, *Natural and Political Observations,* p. 348.
[28] Graunt, *Natural and Political Observations,* p. 322.
[29] See Anthony Wood, *Athenae Oxonienses: An Exact History of All the Writers and Bishops Who Have Had Their Education in the Most Antient and Famous University of Oxford* (London: Knaplock, Midwinter

Observations Made upon the Bills of Mortality, which enjoyed immediate popularity; four editions were issued within five years of its first printing.[30] This book also led to his election as Fellow of the Royal Society upon the direct recommendation of Charles II. The early historian and publicist of the Royal Society Thomas Sprat commented on this unusual event: "[I]t was so farr from being a prejudice, that he was a Shop-keeper of London; that His Majesty gave this particular charge to His Society, that if they found any more such Tradesmen, they should be sure to admit them all, without any more ado."[31] In 1671–1672, Graunt was appointed warden of the Draper's Company. After that, he was rumored to have converted to Catholicism, and he died in poverty in 1674.

Graunt employed his shopkeeper's arithmetic in drawing up his Table of Casualties, in which he condensed twenty years of the London bills of mortality into a single table. (See Figure 1.4.) This significant innovation enabled Graunt to compare annual mortality figures for a variety of diseases. "I had reduced into Tables" the weekly London bills, Graunt wrote, "so as to have a view of the whole together, in order to *the more ready comparing* of one Year, Season, Parish, or other Division of the City, with another, in respect of all the Burials and Christenings, and of all the Diseases, and Casualties, happening in each of them respectively."[32] Graunt's Table of Casualties facilitated comparison, as he himself noted: "I did then begin not only to examine the Conceits, Opinions, and Conjectures, which upon view of a few scattered Bills I had taken up, but did also admit new ones, as I found reason, and occasion from my Tables."[33]

Graunt signaled the novelty of his approach by including explicit instructions for how to read his tables. Entitled "Advertisements for the better understanding of the several tables," the instructions carefully described the columns in

and Tonson, 1721 edition), vol. 1, p. 311; quoted in Karl Pearson, *The History of Statistics in the 17th and 18th Centuries against the Changing Background of Intellectual, Scientific and Religious Thought,* ed. E.S. Pearson (London: Charles Griffin & Co., 1978), p. 11. There are some further references to Graunt in Samuel Pepys's diary and in John Aubrey's writings. See Pearson (pp. 22–29) for a catalog. Also see scattered references in *The Diary of Robert Hooke, M.A., M.O., F.R.S., 1672–1680,* ed. Henry W. Robinson and Walter Adams (London: Taylor & Francis, 1935). D.V. Glass provided a thorough biography of Graunt in "John Graunt and His *Natural and Political Observations,*" *Notes and Records of the Royal Society of London* 19 (1964): 63–100.

[30] There were five editions published during his lifetime: 1st ed., London, 1662; 2d ed., London, 1662; 3d ed., London 1665; 4th ed., Oxford, 1665; and 5th ed., London, 1676. The 1st and 2d editions are identical; the 3d and 4th editions contain an appendix in which Graunt added observations on bills of mortality from Dublin and Amsterdam. He also presented timely estimates of plague mortalities from many different cities, including Cairo, Leyden, Prague, and Constantinople. In the 5th edition, a further appendix was added in which Graunt compared the bills of mortality from London and Paris, and noted the proportion of Protestants to Catholics. He also included the total number of deaths from London's 1665 plague epidemic.

[31] Thomas Sprat, *History of the Royal Society* (1667; reprint edited with critical appratus by Jackson I. Cope and Harold Whitmore Jones, St. Louis: Washington University Studies, 1959), p. 67.

[32] Emphasis added. Graunt, *Natural and Political Observations,* pp. 333–334.

[33] Graunt, *Natural and Political Observations,* pp. 333–334.

The Years of our Lord	1647	1648	1649	1650	1651	1652	1653	1654	1655	1656	1657	1658
Abortive and Stil-born	335	329	327	351	389	381	384	433	483	419	463	467
Aged	916	835	889	696	780	834	864	974	743	892	869	1176
Ague and Fever	1260	884	751	970	1038	1212	282	1371	689	875	999	1800
Apoplex and Suddenly	68	74	64	74	106	111	118	86	92	102	113	138
Bleach			1	3	7	2				1		
Blasted	4	1			6	6			4		5	5
Bleeding	3	2	5		1	3	4	3	2	7	3	5
Bloody Flux, Scouring and Flux	155	176	802	289	833	762	200	386	168	368	362	233
Burnt and Scalded	3	6	10	5	11	8	5	7	10	5	7	4
Calenture	1			1		2	1	1			3	
Cancer, Gangrene and Fistula	26	29	31	19	31	53	36	37	73	31	24	35
Wolf				8								
Canker, Sore-mouth and Thrush	66	28	54	42	68	51	53	72	44	81	19	27
Child-bed	161	106	114	117	206	213	158	192	177	201	236	225
Chrisoms and Infants	1369	1254	1065	990	1237	1280	1050	1343	1089	1393	1162	1144
Colick and Wind	103	71	85	82	76	102	80	101	85	120	113	179
Cold and Cough							41	36	21	58	30	31
Consumption and Cough	2423	2200	2388	1988	2350	2410	2286	2868	2606	3184	2757	3610
Convulsion	684	491	530	493	569	653	606	828	702	1027	807	841
Cramp			1									
Cut of the Stone		2	1		3		1	1	2	4	1	3
Dropsie and Tympany	185	434	421	508	444	556	617	704	660	706	631	931
Drowned	47	40	30	27	49	50	53	30	43	49	63	60
Excessive drinking			2									
Executed	8	17	29	43	24	12	19	21	19	22	20	18
Fainted in a Bath					1							
Falling-Sickness	3	2	2	3		3	4	1	4	3	1	
Flox[1] and small Pox	139	400	1190	184	525	1279	139	812	1294	823	835	409
Found dead in the Streets	6	6	9	8	7	9	14	4	3	4	9	11
French-Pox	18	29	15	18	21	20	20	20	29	23	25	53
Frighted	4	4			3		2		1	1		
Gout	9	5	12	9	7	7	5	6	8	7	8	13
Grief	12	13	16	7	17	14	11	17	10	13	10	12
Hanged, and made-away themselves	11	10	13	14	9	14	15	9	14	16	24	18
Head-Ach		1	11	2					5	3	4	5
Jaundice	57	35	39	49	41	43	57	71	61	41	46	77
Jaw-faln	1	1			3				2	2	3	1
Impostume	75	61	65	59	80	105	79	90	92	122	80	134
Itch			1									
Killed by several Accidents	27	57	39	94	47	45	57	58	52	43	52	47
King's Evil	27	26	22	19	22	20	26	26	27	24	23	28
Lethargy	3	4		4	4	4	3	10	9		6	2
Leprosie			1									1
Liver-grown, Spleen and Rickets	53	46	56	59	65	72	67	65	52	50	38	51
Lunatick	12	18	6		11	7	9	12	6	7	13	5
Meagrom	12	13				6	6	14	3	6	7	6
Measles	5	92		3	33	33	62	8	52	11	153	80
Mother	2						1	1	2	3		3
Murdered	3	2	7	5	4	3	3	3	3	6	5	7
Overlaid and Starved at Nurse	25	22	36	28	28	29	30	36	58	53	44	50
Palsie	27	21	19	20	23	16	29	18	22	23	20	22
Plague	3597	611	67	15	23	16	6	16	9	6	4	14
Plague in the Guts					1		110	32	87	315	446	
Pleurisie	30	26	13	20	23	19	17	23	10	9	17	16
Poisoned		3			7							
Purples and Spotted Fever	145	47	43	65	54	60	75	89	56	52	56	126
Quinsie and Sore-throat	14	11	12	17	24	20	18	9	15	13	7	10
Rickets	150	224	216	190	260	329	229	372	347	458	317	476
Mother, rising of the Lights	150	92	115	120	134	138	135	178	166	212	203	228
Rupture	16	7	7	6	7	16	7	15	11	20	19	18
Scal'd head	2				1				2			
Scurvy	32	20	21	21	29	43	41	44	103	71	82	82
Smothered and stifled			2									
Sores, ulcers, broken and bruised	15	17	17	16	26	32	25	32	23	34	40	47
Shot (Limbs							13	13		6	2	5
Spleen	12	17										
Shingles												
Starved		4	8	7	1	2	1	1	3	1	3	6
Stitch				1								
Stone and Strangury	45	42	29	28	50	41	44	38	49	57	72	69
Sciatica												
Stopping of the Stomach	29	29	30	33	55	67	66	107	94	145	129	277
Surfet	217	137	136	123	104	177	178	212	128	161	137	218
Swine-Pox	4	4	3				1		4	2	1	1
Teeth and Worms	767	597	540	598	709	905	691	1131	803	1198	878	1036
Tissick	62	47										
Thrush											57	66
Vomiting		6	3	7	4	6	3	14	7	27	16	19
Worms	147	107	105	65	85	86	53					
Wen	1		1							1		2
Suddenly												

[1] Probably a name for confluent small

1.4 John Graunt's table of casualties (1629–1660). *Source:* John Graunt, *Natural and Political Observations Made upon the Bills of Mortality* (London, 1662).

UALTIES.

1659	1660	1629	1630	1631	1632	1633	1634	1635	1636	1629–1632	1633–1636	1647–1650	1651–1654	1655–1658	1629 / 1659	In 20 Years
421	544	499	439	410	445	500	475	507	523	1793	2005	1342	1587	1832	1247	8559
909	1095	579	712	661	671	704	623	794	714	2475	2814	3336	3452	3680	2377	15759
2303	2148	956	1091	1115	1108	953	1279	1622	2360	4418	6235	3865	4903	4363	4010	23784
91	67	22	36		17	24	35	26		75	85	280	421	445	177	1306
												4	9	1	1	15
3	8	13	8	10	13	6	4		4	54	14	5	12	14	16	99
7	2	5	2	5	4	4	3			16	7	11	12	19	17	65
346	251	449	438	352	348	278	512	346	330	1587	1466	1422	2181	1161	1597	7818
6	6	3	10	7	5	1	3	12	3	25	19	24	31	26	19	125
								1	3		4	2	4	3		13
63	52	20	14	23	28	27	30	24	30	85	112	105	157	150	114	609
											8					8
73	68	6	4	4	1			5	74	15	79	190	244	161	133	689
226	194	150	157	112	171	132	143	163	230	590	668	498	769	839	490	3364
858	1123	2596	2378	2035	2268	2130	2315	2113	1895	9277	8453	4678	4910	4788	4519	32106
116	167	48	57					37	50	105	87	341	359	497	247	1389
33	24	10	58	51	55	45	54	50	57	174	207	00	77	140	43	598
2982	3414	1827	1910	1713	1797	1754	1955	2080	2477	5157	8266	8999	9914	12157	7197	44487
742	1031	52	87	18	241	221	386	418	709	498	1734	2198	2656	3377	1324	9073
				1	0	0	0	0	0	01	00	01	0	0	1	2
6	4				5	1	5	2	2	5	10	6	4	13	47	38
646	872	235	252	279	280	266	250	329	389	1048	1734	1538	2321	2982	1302	9623
57	48	43	33	29	34	37	32	32	45	139	147	144	182	215	130	827
												2		2	2	2
7	18	19	13	12	18	13	13	13	13	62	52	97	76	79	55	384
																1
4	5	3	10	7	7	2	5	6	8	27	21	10	8	8	9	74
1523	354	72	40	58	531	72	1354	293	127	701	1846	1913	2755	3361	2785	10576
2	6	18	33	20	6	13	8	24	24	83	69	29	34	27	29	243
51	31	17	12	12	12	7	17	12	22	53	48	80	81	130	83	392
	9	1			1				3	2	3	9	5	2	2	21
14	2	2	5	3	4	4	5	7	8	14	24	35	25	36	28	134
13	4	18	20	22	11	14	17	5	20	71	56	48	59	45	47	279
11	36	8	8	6	15		3	8	7	37	18	48	47	72	32	222
35	26							4	2	0	6	14	14	17	46	051
102	76	47	59	35	43	35	45	54	63	184	197	180	212	225	188	998
		10	16	13	8	10	10	4	11	47	35	02	5	6	10	95
105	96	58	76	73	74	50	62	73	130	282	315	260	35	428	228	1639
						10				00	10	01				11
55	47	54	55	47	46	49	41	51	60	202	201	217	207	194	148	1021
28	54	16	25	18	38	35	20	20	69	97	150	94	94	102	66	537
6	4	1		2	2	3		2	2	5	7	13	21	21	9	67
		2						2	2	2	2	1		1		06
8	15	94	12	99	87	82	77	98	99	392	356	213	269	191	158	1421
14	14	6	11	6	5	4	2	2	5	28	13	47	39	31	26	158
5	4			24					22	24	22	30	34	22	05	132
6	74	42	2	3	80	21	33	27	12	127	83	133	155	259	51	757
1	8	1							3	01	3	2	4	8	02	18
70	20				3	7		6	8	10	1	17	13	27	77	86
46	43	4	10	13	7	7	8	14	14	34	46	111	123	215	86	529
17	21	17	23	17	25	14	21	25	17	82	77	87	90	87	53	423
36	14		1317	274	8		1		10400	1599	10401	4290	61	33	103	16384
253	402									00	00	61	142	844	253	991
12	10	26	24	26	36	21		45	24	112	90	89	72	52	51	415
						2			2	00	4	10	00	00	00	14
368	146	32	58	58	38	24	125	245	397	186	791	300	278	290	243	1845
21	14	01	8	6	7	24	04	5	22	22	55	54	71	45	34	247
441	521					14	49	50	00	00	113	780	1190	1598	657	3681
210	249	44	72	99	98	60	84	72	104	309	220	777	585	809	369	2700
12	28	2	6	4	9	4	3	10	13	21	30	36	45	68	21	201
												2	1	2		05
95	12	5	7	9		9			25	33	34	94	132	300	115	593
			24							24		2			2	26
61	48	23		20	48	19	19	22	29	91	89	65	115	144	141	504
7	20											29	26	13	07	27
7	7														07	68
1						1									1	2
7	14									14		19	5	13	29	51
												1				1
22	30	35	39	58	50	58	49	33	45	114	185	144	173	247	51	937
					1	3		1	6	1	4				2	13
186	214								6		6	121	295	247	216	669
202	192	63	157	149	86	104	114	132	371	445	721	613	671	644	401	3094
2		5	8	4	6	3		10		23	13	11	5	5	10	57
839	1008	440	506	335	470	432	454	539	1207	1751	2632	2502	3436	3915	1819	14236
		8	12	14	34	23	15	27		68	65	109			8	242
		15	23	17	40	28	31	34		95	93			123	15	211
8	10	1	4	1	1	2	5	6	3	7	16	17	27	69	12	136
1		19	31	28	27	19	28	27		105	74	424	224		124	830
				1		4				1	4	2	4	4	2	15
1	1	63	59	37	62	58	62	78	34	221	233				63	454
															34190	229250

pox. See Creighton, i., 462—463.

I.4 (cont.)

each table, as well as what the numbers in each column represented.[34] Graunt thought the instructions necessary, in large part because the arrangement of his table was not immediately obvious.[35] The table displayed the number of burials attributed to various diseases and casualties (listed alphabetically, just as they were in the London bills) for twenty years, but the columns were not arranged chronologically. The first fourteen columns covered the years 1647 to 1660; Graunt referred to them as containing "two of the last Septenaries of years, which being the latest are set down first." Here Graunt assumed that the most recent figures would be of most interest. The next eight columns listed figures for the years 1629 (the first year that diseases other than plague were included in the bills) through 1636. Graunt then omitted the years between 1636 and 1647 "as containing nothing Extraordinary, and as not consistent with the Incapacity of a Sheet." Thus, two considerations apparently determined what would be excluded from Graunt's table: 1) the ordinariness of the observations; and 2) the size of the paper. As with all scientific instruments, the table was constrained by theory (here, considerations of what was ordinary vs. extraordinary) and by material (the paper).

The next five columns contained sums of various four-year periods ("Quarternions"). He gave no rationale for these quarternions except in order "that Comparison might be made between each 4 years taken together, as well as each single year apart." The next column displayed the sum of mortalities for the three years 1629, 1649, and 1659 so "that the distant years, as well as consequent, might be compared with the whole 20, each of the 5 Quarternions." Again he gave no explanation for why he chose these three specific years, nor why he did not choose a fourth in order to make this column more comparable with the other five quarternions. There are other inconsistencies between this table and other tables Graunt included in his work, and Graunt's apparent lack of precision can be attributed to the general seventeenth-century accounting practices characterized by informal and approximate calculations.[36]

Graunt's Table of Casualties demonstrated the large variation in yearly plague mortality (1,317 burials in 1630, 1 in 1634, 10,400 in 1636, 3,597 in 1647, and 6 in 1653), while the mortality attributed to other diseases appeared more constant, for instance, jaundice, for which the number of burials ranged from 35 to 102.

---

[34] In the first edition of Graunt's *Natural and Political Observations* that I consulted at the Library of the Wellcome Institute for the History of Medicine, the "Advertisement" was appended at the end of the tables. In the 1973 reprint of this edition of Graunt's book, the "Advertisement" is missing. It is included in Hull's edition of Graunt's and Petty's work, pp. 429–431.

[35] John Bell, clerk to the Company of Parish Clerks, took up Graunt's innovation in his *London's Rembrancer, or a True Account of Christnings and Mortality in All the Years of the Pestilence*, a study of the plague epidemic of 1665. Bell, like Graunt, included "Instructions for the better understanding of the following Tables." See Bell, *London's Rembrancer*, "To the Reader," n.p.

[36] Kreager, "New Light on Graunt," pp. 133–134.

Observations such as these led Graunt to classify diseases reported in the bills into four groups: those affecting children; chronic; acute or epidemic; and external injuries or "outward griefs."

Graunt identified the high mortality rate among children – one of the most prominent demographic features of the early modern period – by grouping together all casualties generally afflicting only them, specifically "Thrush, Convulsion, Rickets, Teeth, and Worms; and as Abortives, Chrysomes, Infants, Liver-grown, and Over-laid." He concluded "That about one-third of the whole died of those Diseases, which we guess did all light upon children under four or five Years old."[37] In other words, infants and children accounted for one-third of all deaths in London. A certain fatalism attended this observation; Graunt said little about how to improve the situation. Arithmeticians in the eighteenth century, however, began to suggest ways to reduce mortality among infants and children.[38]

Chronic diseases "whereunto the City is most subject," and some accidents, Graunt noted, "bear a constant proportion unto the whole number of burials." Included in this category were consumption, dropsy, jaundice, and gout, and more surprising, "some accidents, as Grief, Drowning, Men's making away themselves, and being Kill'd by several Accidents, &c. do the like. . . ."[39] Mortality associated with acute or epidemic diseases, such as plague, smallpox, and measles, by contrast, varied dramatically from year to year and depended on the climate and alterations in the air. Prevailing medical theory emphasized the idea that bad airs, or miasma, were responsible for epidemic disease, which happened "suddenly and vehemently."[40] Graunt measured these variations by constructing ratios of the deaths due to acute and chronic diseases to the total number of deaths. Out of a total of 229,250 deaths, roughly 50,000 were caused by acute and epidemic diseases, while only 70 were due to chronic diseases. "For as the proportion of Acute and Epidemical Diseases shews the aptness of the Air to suddain and vehement Impressions," he wrote, "so the Chronical Diseases shew the ordinary temper of the Place, so that upon the proportion of Chronical Diseases seems to hang the judgment of the fitness of the Country for long Life."[41] Here, then, was Graunt's measure for salubrity; acute and epidemic diseases indicated the "healthfulness of the air," chronic diseases the

---

[37] Graunt, *Observations Natural and Political*, p. 349.

[38] See Chapter 6. Some historians have argued that it was not until the mid–nineteenth century that physicians and others concerned with public health questioned and sought to change this appallingly high figure of infant mortality. Mortality statistics played a critical role in focusing physicians' concern on this issue.

[39] Graunt, *Natural and Political Observations*, p. 352. In this passage, Graunt realized the regular frequency of suicides – "Men's making away with themselves" – an observation that for the most part was ignored until the nineteenth century, when Durkheim and Quetelet made it famous.

[40] Graunt, *Natural and Political Observations*, p. 350.

[41] Graunt, *Natural and Political Observations*, p. 350.

Table of notorious Diseases.

Apoplex	1306
Cut of the Stone	38
Falling Sickness	74
Dead in the Streets	243
Gout	134
Head-ach	51
Jaundice	998
Lethargy	67
Leprosie	6
Lunatick	158
Overlaid and Starved	529
Palsie	423
Rupture	201
Stone and Strangury	863
Sciatica	5
Suddenly	454 ‖

1.5 John Graunt's table of notorious diseases. *Source:* John Graunt, *Natural and Political Observations Made upon the Bills of Mortality* (London, 1662).

"wholesomeness of the Food." He later suggested that longevity was the best measure of salubrity.[42]

In his chapter on "The Sickliness, Healthfulness, and Fruitfulness of Seasons," Graunt identified years with high mortality as important so "that the World may see by what spaces and intervals we may hereafter expect such times again."[43] The table format itself suggested this possibility of extrapolation; past patterns of mortality might yield reliable information about future epidemics. Underlying this approach was the assumption that epidemics were cyclical, certainly an understandable assumption, given London's experience with plague. Graunt also used his Table of Casualties to confront the widespread fear of certain dreaded diseases: "Whereas many persons live in great fear and apprehension of some of the more formidable and notorious Diseases following; I shall only set down how many died of each: that the respective numbers, being compared with the total 229250, those persons may the better understand the hazard they are in."[44] Thus, Graunt hoped that his tables would persuade individuals that many of the "formidable and notorious Diseases" they most feared were in fact relatively uncommon – that is, their fears were exaggerated. (See Figure 1.5.)

Graunt's table also enabled him to evaluate the consistencies and inconsistencies in the Searchers' reporting and recording deaths. One striking example appears in his discussion of the diseases livergrown and rickets. He discovered

---

[42] Graunt, *Natural and Political Observations*, pp. 351–352.
[43] Graunt, *Natural and Political Observations*, p. 368.
[44] Graunt, *Natural and Political Observations*, p. 350.

that a decrease in the number of deaths attributed to livergrown corresponded to an increase in the number attributed to rickets. By establishing that the proportion of livergrown and rickets deaths, taken together, to total mortality remained roughly the same over this twenty-year period, Graunt reasoned that they were, in fact, the same disease. The import of this observation was profound. Graunt had assumed the stability over time of the disease phenomenon (livergrown-rickets), as compared to the instability of the name given to that disease phenomenon. A comparison of the numbers in his table, he reasoned, demonstrated this fact: The phenomenon was regular and quantifiable; its classification should be, too.[45]

Whereas Graunt provided detailed discussion of variations in disease and mortality patterns, Petty addressed medical concerns only in passing. One example comes from Petty's *Observations upon the Dublin Bills of Mortality,* published in 1683. In this pamphlet, Petty adopted Graunt's method of compiling mortality figures over a period of years and recording them into a set of tables. He took the number of burials and christenings from fifteen years of the Dublin bills of mortality and "digested [it] into the one *Table* or Sheet annexed."[46] Petty, however, found the Dublin bills wanting and suggested several ways to improve them. Thus, he went one step further than Graunt by proposing what kinds of information the government should collect about its subjects.

Petty prepared model forms for weekly and quarterly bills of mortality that would supply more useful information. (See Figures 1.6 and 1.7.) He asked for the following quantitative information from each parish: births (total, male, and female), burials (total, under age 16, over age 16), and burials due to specific diseases (plague, smallpox, measles, and spotted fever). From this list, it is clear that Petty considered the incidence of epidemic diseases (plague, smallpox, measles, spotted fever) of primary importance to considerations of salubrity. Petty's "ideal" quarterly bill of mortality differed from its weekly counterpart in that it further divided deaths into three categories: contagious, acute, and chronic. He created these categories "in order to know how the different Scituation, Soil and way of living in each Parish, doth dispose Men to each of the said three species."[47] Thus, enumerations of deaths by contagious, acute, and chronic diseases for each parish provided a geographical depiction of salubrity. Besides the three categories of diseases, the quarterly bill included the number of marriages, deaths under 2, under 16, over 60, and over 70 years of age. The number of deaths under two years of age was a way of measuring infant mortality for Petty (something Graunt had pointed out); the ages between 16 and 60

[45] Graunt, *Natural and Political Observations,* pp. 357–358. Kreager emphasized the ideas of balance found in contemporary bookkeeping procedures in Graunt's evaluation of the bills of mortality; Kreager, "New Light on Graunt," pp. 136–137; also see Lloyd G. Stevenson, "'New Diseases' in the Seventeenth Century," *Bulletin of the History of Medicine* 39 (1965): 1–21.
[46] Petty, *Observations upon the Dublin Bills of Mortality* (London, 1683); reprinted in *The Economic Writings of Sir William Petty,* p. 481.
[47] Petty, *Observations on the Dublin Bills,* p. 491.

A Weekly Bill of Mortality for the City of *Dublin,*

Ending the   day of   1681.

PARISHES NAMES.	Births.	Males.	Females.	Burials.	Under 16 years old.	Above 16 years old.	Plague.	Small Pox.	Measels.	Spotted Fever.
1 St. *Katherins* and St. *James,*										
2 St. *Nicholas* without,										
3 St. *Michans,*										
4 St. *Andrews* with *Donabrook,*										
5 St. *Bridgets,*										
6 St. *Johns,*										
7 St. *Warbrough,*										
8 St. *Audaens,*										
9 St. *Michael,*										
10 St. *Keavens.*										
11 St. *Nicholas* within,										
12 St. *Patrick*'s Liberties,										
13 Christ-Church and *Trinity*-Colledge										
Totals,										

1.6 William Petty's proposed weekly bill of mortality for Dublin. *Source:* William Petty, *Observations upon the Dublin Bills of Mortality* (London, 1683).

A Quarterly Bill of Mortality,

Beginning   and ending   for the City of *Dublin.*

PARISHES Names	Births. 1.	Marriages. 2.	Buried of			Plague. Small Pox, Spotted Fever, Measels.	Stone. Gout, Dropsie, Consumption,	Plague. Quinsey, Pleurisie, Fever.	Sudden Death.	Aged above 70 years old.	Infants under 2 years old.	All other Casualties.
			Above 60 years old.	Under 16 years old.								
1 St. *Katherins* and St. *James,*												
2 St. *Nicholas* without,												
3 St. *Michans,*												
4 St. *Andrews* with *Donabrook,*												
5 St. *Bridgets,*												
6 St. *Johns,*												
7 St. *Warbrough,*												
8 St. *Audaens,*												
9 St. *Michael,*												
10 St. *Keavens,*												
11 St. *Nicholas* within,												
12 St. *Patrick*'s Liberties												
13 Christ-Church and *Trinity*-Colledge												
Totals,												

1.7 William Petty's proposed quarterly bill of mortality for Dublin. *Source:* William Petty, *Observations upon the Dublin Bills of Mortality* (London, 1683).

Petty considered to be the most productive, and the distinction between deaths above 60 and above 70 allowed him to calculate longevity, which he held to be a measure of salubrity.

Numerical tables, then, were critical to Graunt's and Petty's inquiries into the health of the people. Using their tables, they could identify variations in mortality by seasons, years, and period of life; analyze the relative impact of acute and chronic diseases on mortality; and evaluate the salubrity of different places. Tables, thus, facilitated comparison among places, years, and, diseases and, further, they allowed readers to evaluate for themselves the conclusions drawn from the tables.

POLITICAL OBSERVATIONS

"I have been several times in company with men of great experience in this City," Graunt remarked, "and have heard them talk seldom under Millions of People to be in London."[48] Believing this figure to be much too high, Graunt began to calculate the number of inhabitants of London. This subject formed the core of his political observations on the London bills of mortality, and both he and Petty developed several ways to determine population.

Graunt's method for measuring the population was based on a series of assumptions, several of which became common features of later political arithmetical calculations; therefore, it is important to go through Graunt's calculation step-by-step. First, he reasoned that the number of childbearing women was roughly twice the number of christenings in a year (a number Graunt could take from the bills of mortality), based on the common experience that a fertile woman had, on average, one child every two years. Second, he computed the number of families by doubling the number of childbearing women. (Graunt estimated the total number of adult women [ages 16 to 70] to be roughly twice the number of childbearing women [ages 16 to 40].) Third, he judged that a family consisted of eight persons (husband, wife, three children, and three servants/lodgers). And last, he multiplied the number of families by the number of persons per family, thus arriving at 384,000 as the total number of inhabitants of London – considerably less than the "millions" of which his contemporaries boasted.[49]

Graunt was also interested in the number of fighting men in London, and he developed a different method for calculating this figure. He took the ratio of 14 males to 13 females from the number of christenings listed in the London bills and asserted that this ratio was constant throughout the population at all ages. Graunt admitted that more men "die violent deaths," and were "slain in Wars, killed by Mischance, drowned at Sea," or "go to the Colonies, and travel

---

[48] Graunt, *Natural and Political Observations,* p. 383.
[49] Graunt supplemented this estimate with other calculations based on the number of families and houses; Graunt, *Natural and Political Observations,* pp. 385–386.

into Forein parts."[50] Still, this did "not prejudice the due proportion between them and Females," and no woman would ever go without a husband. Another example of Graunt's fluid bookkeeping, it was also a novel numerical indictment of the "irreligious" and "irrational" proposals "to multiply the people by polygamy."[51] During the English Revolution, many radical ideas had surfaced about the nature of society and the structure it should take, including discussions of polygamy.[52] The Puritan response to this issue had been to emphasize monogamy, and Graunt constructed a numerical argument to support this position. "That Christian Religion, prohibiting Polygamy, is more agreeable to the Law of Nature, that is, the Law of God, than Mahumetism, and others, that allow it; for one man his having many Women, or Wives, by Law, signifies nothing, unless there were many Women to one Man in Nature also."[53] The natural result was that of the 384,000 inhabitants of London, 199,112 were men, and 184,186 were women (a 14 to 13 ratio).

Of this number of men, Graunt's next step was to determine how many were eligible for military service (that is, between the ages of 16 and 56). To do this, he created a new type of table, what later became known as a life table, to indicate how many individuals out of a population of 100 were alive at any given age.[54](See Figure 1.8.) Because he did not know the age of death (this was not included in the bills until 1728), he had to estimate the number of individuals of a given population that died at each age. He described his procedure for generating this table:

Whereas we found, that of 100 quick Conceptions about 36 of them die before they be six years old, and that perhaps but one surviveth 76; we having seven Decads between six and 76, we sought six mean proportional numbers between 64, the remainder, living at six years, and the one, which survives 76, and find, that the numbers following are practically near enough to the truth; for men do not die in exact Proportions, nor in Fractions, from whence arises this Table following.[55]

[50] Graunt, *Natural and Political Observations*, p. 375.

[51] Graunt, *Natural and Political Observations*, p. 320.

[52] Christopher Hill, *The World Turned Upside Down* (New York: Penguin Books, 1975), chap. 15, esp. pp. 313–314.

[53] Graunt, *Natural and Political Observations*, p. 374. The language that Graunt employed (i.e., "Law of Nature" and "Law of God") fitted into the more general development of the concept of laws of nature during the seventeenth century; see Joseph Needham, "Human Laws and Laws of Nature in China and the West," *Journal of the History of Ideas* 12 (1951): 3–30; Francis Oakley, "Christian Theology and the Newtonian Science: The Rise of the Concept of the Laws of Nature," *Church History* 30 (1961): 433–457; and Edgar Zilsel, "The Genesis of the Concept of Physical Law," *Philosophical Review* 51 (1942): 242–279.

[54] For histories of life tables, see L. Behar, "Des Tables de mortalité aux XVIIe et XVIIIe siècles; Histoire – signification," *Annales de Démographie Historique,* 1976, pp. 173–200; Lorraine Daston, *Classical Probability in the Enlightenment* (Princeton, N.J.: Princeton University Press, 1988), esp. 132–138; Jacques and Michel Dupâquier, *Histoire de la démographie* (Paris: Librairie Académique Perrin, 1985), esp. chap. 6; Ian Hacking, *The Emergence of Probability* (Cambridge: Cambridge University Press, 1975), esp. chap. 13; Pearson, *The History of Statistics,* esp. chaps. 3, 5, 6.

[55] Graunt, *Natural and Political Observations*, p. 386. "Quick Conceptions" referred to pregnancies where the mother had felt the fetus move. This was the most accepted sign of pregnancy at the time.

Viz. of 100 there dies, The fourth —————6
within the first six years 36 | The next ——————4
The next ten years, or | The next ——————3
Decad ——.——— 24 | The next ——.———2
The second *Decad* — 15 | The next ——.———1
The third *Decad* ——09 |

　10. From whence it follows, that of the said 100 conceived there remains alive at six years end 64.

At Sixteen years end 40 | At Fifty six ——.——— 6
At Twenty six ——— 25 | At Sixty six ——— 3
At Tirty six ———— 16 | At Seventy six ——— 1
At Fourty six ——.— 10 | At Eighty ——————0

1.8 John Graunt's life table. *Source:* John Graunt, *Natural and Political Observations Made upon the Bills of Mortality* (London, 1662).

From this table, Graunt could read how many individuals were alive at any given age and then calculate the number of men between ages 16 and 56 by using the 14 to 13 ratio. It followed that "67694, viz. near 70000" fighting men resided in London, "the truth whereof," Graunt confidently noted, "I leave to examination."[56]

Graunt's life table, like his table of casualties, was a significant innovation that later became an essential tool for life insurance and demography.[57] Over the course of the late seventeenth and eighteenth centuries, mathematicians, such as Edmond Halley and Antoine Déparcieux, refined the life tables.[58] The distinguishing feature of these improved tables was that they were based on empirical sources that recorded the age of death – information Graunt could not get from the London bills of mortality.

If the modest shopkeeper Graunt was the one who furnished the new numerical techniques to measure population, it was the flamboyant virtuoso William Petty who burnished them with a catchy name: political arithmetic. Through his voluminous writings, Petty publicized political arithmetic but added little to Graunt's careful calculations. For Petty, economic theory outweighed a close analysis of the numbers; nonetheless, his enthusiasm for quantification found a happy object in Graunt's *Observations*.

Self-confident and seldom one to pass up opportunity, Petty became famous in his lifetime.[59] Son of a cloth worker and tailor, Petty was born in Romsey,

---

[56] Graunt, *Natural and Political Observations*, p. 387.
[57] Major Greenwood called Graunt's life table "his greatest achievement." Greenwood, *Medical Statistics from Graunt to Farr* (Cambridge: Cambridge University Press, 1948), p. 30. On life tables and life insurance, see Geoffrey Clark, *Betting on Lives: The Culture of Life Insurance in England, 1695–1775* (Manchester and New York: Manchester University Press, 1999).
[58] See Chapter 7, "Counting the People: Censuses and Vital Registration."
[59] There are two biographies of Petty: Lord Edmond Fitzmaurice, *The Life of Sir William Petty, 1623–1687* (London: John Murray, 1895), and E. Strauss, *Sir William Petty – Portrait of a Genius* (London: The Bodley Head, 1954).

Hampshire, in 1623. According to the seventeenth-century biographer John Aubrey, Petty's "greatest delight was to be looking on the artificers, e.g. smiths, the watchmakers, carpenters, joiners, etc.: and at twelve years old [Petty] could have worked at any of these trades."[60] At age 13 he became a cabin boy on a merchant ship, but upon breaking his leg at sea was put ashore on the French coast near Caen, where he enrolled in a Jesuit school and soon mastered Latin, Greek, and French. Petty returned to England to serve with the navy until the outbreak of the Civil War, whereupon he traveled to the Netherlands to study medicine at Utrecht, Leiden, and Amsterdam. In 1645 he journeyed to Paris where he read Vesalius with Thomas Hobbes, who introduced him to the Parisian scientific society centered around Marin Mersenne.

By 1646 Petty had returned to England, and two years later published a small tract on education entitled *The Advice of W.P. to Mr. S. Hartlib for the Advancement of Some Particular Parts of Learning* (1648), which signaled his close connection with the virtuosi associated with Samuel Hartlib. The following year, Petty resumed his studies in medicine at Oxford, and in 1650 he received his doctorate of medicine and soon thereafter was appointed professor of anatomy at Brasenose College. His reputation as a physician spread quickly, helped along by his sensational revival of the murderess Anne Green. Green had been hanged for infanticide, but when Petty was about to dissect her, he discovered that she was still alive. Petty revived and treated her until she fully recovered.[61]

In 1652, Petty left the university to become physician-general to Oliver Cromwell's army in Ireland, where he became involved with and soon directed the Downs Survey, the first systematic survey of Ireland. Demonstrating a flair for management, Petty organized the army to carry out a thorough land reconnaissance in just one year. In the process, he acquired an immense amount of property, especially in County Kerry. Much of the rest of his life was devoted to managing these lands and securing them against many legal claims made during the Restoration. In April 1661, Petty was knighted by Charles II. In 1667 he married Elizabeth Fenton, with whom he had many children, but only two sons and a daughter survived infancy.

Petty was a charter member of the Royal Society of London and an active participant until his death in 1687. He was also one of the founders and the first president of the Dublin Philosophical Society.[62] An incredibly prolific writer, he boasted of "53 chests" full of manuscripts.[63] Although only a small portion

---

[60] John Aubrey, *Brief Lives*, ed. Richard Barber (London: The Boydell Press, 1982), p. 242.

[61] For Petty's own self-aggrandizing account, see *Petty Papers*, vol. 2, pp. 157–167.

[62] See *Petty Papers*, vol. 2, pp. 87–92, for Petty's "Rules for the Dublin Society" and "Advertisements to the Dublin Society." Also see K. Theodore Hoppen, *The Common Scientist in the Seventeenth Century: A Study of the Dublin Philosophical Society, 1683–1708* (Charlottesville: The University Press of Virginia, 1970).

[63] "I have rummaged and methodized my papers which amount to 53 chests, and are so many monuments of my Labours and Misfortunes." *The Petty–Southwell Correspondence*, ed. Marquis of Lansdowne

of these were published during his lifetime, a steady stream of posthumous publications edited by relatives and historians began shortly after his death, when his son published *Political Arithmetick* in 1690.

Petty put great emphasis on a large and growing population and the necessity of *measuring* it. He developed these views most clearly in his two essays, *Political Arithmetick* (1677/1690) and *Another Essay on Political Arithmetick* (1682), although he referred to the subject in almost all of his writing.[64] Petty's political and nationalist agenda amounted to a numerical demonstration of the superiority of England over France. In *Political Arithmetick,* chapters entitled "That France cannot, by reason of Natural and Perpetual Impediments, be more powerful at Sea, than the English, or Hollanders" and "That the King of England's Subjects, have Stock, competent, and convenient to drive the Trade of the whole Commercial World" drove this point home.[65] Petty's jingoism hindered the publication of *Political Arithmetick,* as his son explained: "Had not the Doctrines of this Essay offended France, they had long since seen the light."[66]

Petty listed four reasons why "thick-peopled" areas (such as Holland) were better than "thin-peopled" areas (such as France). First, he noted that government administration was more manageable in densely populated areas (presumably because communication was easier). Second, mutual defense against invasion, robbers, and thieves was facilitated. Third, laws were more efficiently enforced because "Witnesses and Parties may be easily summoned."[67] And finally, he asserted that "those who live in Solitary places, must be their own Soldiers, Divines, Physicians, and Lawyers; and must have their Houses stored with necessary Provisions (like a ship going upon a long Voyage,) to the great waste, and needless expense of such Provisions."[68] Petty elaborated his views on the advantages of "thick-peopled" countries in *Another Essay in Political Arithmetick* (1682), in which he added the following benefits: gain in foreign commerce, making internal commerce and travel more expeditious, preventing beggars and thieves,[69] and advancement of learning.[70] His populationist doctrines operated both at the production and consumption levels, and

(London: Constable & Co., 1928), p. 138. For a list of Petty's publications, see Sir Geoffrey Langdon Keynes, *A Bibliography of Sir William Petty F.R.S. and of the Observations on the Bills of Mortality by John Graunt F.R.S.* (Oxford: Clarendon Press, 1971).

[64] Petty began *Political Arithmetick* in 1671 and probably completed it in 1676–7. Many manuscript copies were circulated, several of which survive. For details, see *The Economic Writings of Sir William Petty,* pp. 235–238.

[65] Petty, *Political Arithmetick*; reprinted in *The Economic Writings of Sir William Petty,* pp. 247–248.

[66] Petty, *Political Arithmetick,* Dedication by Petty's son, p. 240.

[67] Petty, *Political Arithmetick,* p. 255.   [68] Petty, *Political Arithmetick,* pp. 255–256.

[69] Petty wrote: "As for Thievery, it is affixt to all thin-peopled Countries, such as Ireland is, where there cannot be many Eyes to prevent such Crimes; and where what is stolen, is easily hidden and eaten; and where 'tis easy to burn the House, or violate the Persons of those who prosecute these Crimes, and where thin-peopled Countries are govern'd by the Laws that were made and first fitted to thick-peopled Countries. . . ." Petty, *Political Anatomy of Ireland* (London, 1691); reprinted in *The Economic Writings of Sir William Petty,* p. 202.

[70] Petty, *Another Essay in Political Arithmetick* (1682); reprinted in *The Economic Writings of Sir William Petty,* pp. 470–471.

he relied upon psychological arguments to make his point. "So when England shall be thicker peopled," Petty argued, "the very same people shall then spend more, than when they lived more sordidly and inurbanely, and further asunder, and more out of the sight, observation, and emulation of each other; every Man desiring to put better Apparel when he appears in Company, than when he had no occasion to be seen."[71] For Petty, "encrease of Trade depends chiefly and naturally upon encrease of people and luxury in their consumption."[72]

While such populationist sentiments were widely shared among his contemporaries, Petty distinguished himself by his desire to *measure* the population. "[A]n Exact Account of the People is Necessary in this Matter," he asserted, and because such an account was not available, he had to develop one.[73] "Till a better Rule can be obtained," he admitted, "we conceive that the Proportion of the People may be sufficiently Measured by the Proportion of the Burials in such Years as were neither remarkable for extraordinary Healthfullness or Sickliness."[74] A year later, Petty had changed his mind. "Births are the best way," he decided, because burials were "subject to more contingencies and variety of causes."[75] He mentioned the number of marriages as well, "expecting in such Observations to read the improvement of the Nation."[76] Marriages bred children, if not contentment.

Several years later, in his *Two Essays in Political Arithmetick* (1687) and *Five Essays in Political Arithmetick* (1687), Petty returned to the topic of population and presented three ways to estimate population: "1. By the Houses, and Families, and Heads in each. 2. By the number of Burials in healthfull times, and by the proportion of those that live, to those that die. 3. By the number of those who die of the plague in Pestilential years, in proportion to those that scape."[77] The first method involved using information from the Hearth Office; the second and third relied upon the bills of mortality. In the first method, Petty multiplied the number of dwellings by the number of individuals per family (which he estimated at 6 – less than Graunt's estimate of 8). In the second method, he took the average number of burials for two healthy years and then multiplied this by the number 30, in effect relying upon the crude empirical rule that approximately 1 of every 30 persons dies every year. "[T]ill I see another round number, grounded upon many observations, nearer than 30," Petty admitted, "I hope to have done pretty well in multiplying our burials by 30, to find the number of the People."[78] The third method was the most speculative, and was not pursued in later works.

[71] Petty, *Political Arithmetick,* p. 290.   [72] Petty, unpublished manuscript, *Petty Papers,* vol. 1, p. 247.
[73] Petty, *Another Essay in Political Arithmetick,* p. 456.
[74] Petty, *Another Essay in Political Arithmetick,* p. 458.
[75] Petty, *Observations upon the Dublin Bills,* p. 482.   [76] Petty, *Observations upon the Dublin Bills,* p. 491.
[77] Petty, *Five Essays in Political Arithmetick* (1687); reprinted in *The Economic Writings of Sir William Petty,* p. 533.
[78] Petty, *Five Essays in Political Arithmetick,* pp. 535–536.

Besides his interest in total population, Petty wanted to classify different groups within the population. In an unpublished piece entitled "Magnalia Regni" (1687), he designed several tables to be used by parish clerks to register the number of persons who were "male, female, under 10, over 70, impotent, freeholders, barristers, catholics, dissenters, laborers, surgeons" and so on.[79] In general, Petty called for "A Stock of Materialls for Politicall Arithmetick; with the art of Reducing and Stating all propositions and questions in terms of number, weight, and measure, and at last into numbers, soe as to make them Demonstrable."[80] Only with categorized and quantified information could governments make rational decisions and policies.

Petty, like Graunt, situated his work within the context of supporting and consolidating government power. Throughout much of the seventeenth and eighteenth centuries, population was considered an essential component of the wealth of nations. A growing population would increase trade and production and allow for more efficient manufacture through the division of labor. It would increase the base for taxation and the supply of militarily fit men, and it would lead to progress through the decrease of rural isolation and the increase of general commerce.[81] Governments later adopted policies to encourage marriage and children, and political writers of different stripes argued about the ways to increase population. Petty and Graunt emphasized both the importance of population and accurate accounts of it.

"It may be now asked, to what purpose tends all this laborious buzzling, and groping?"[82] The answer, Graunt thought, was straightforward and significant.[83] He and many others wanted to know the numbers of people – men and women, married and single, christened and buried, teeming and fighting – what years were fruitful and mortal, and which areas were salubrious and prosperous. More important from an historical perspective, Graunt and Petty had provided the methods to gain this knowledge. These methods depended upon the construction of numerical tables that would provide "a clear knowledge of all [the] particulars and many more." But, Graunt cautioned, "whether the knowledge thereof be necessary to many, or fit for others," he left to future consideration.[84] As we will see in the following chapters, many found this knowledge useful, reliable, and suitable for the public.

---

[79] *Petty Papers,* vol. 1, p. 180.   [80] *Petty Papers,* vol. 1, p. 276.
[81] Leslie Tuttle, " 'Sacred and Politic Unions': Natalism, Families, and the State in Old Regime France, 1666–1789," Ph.D. thesis, Princeton University, 2000.
[82] Graunt, *Natural and Political Observations,* p. 394.
[83] Actually, Graunt's answer was somewhat surly: "To this I might answer in general, by saying, that those who cannot apprehend the reason of these Enquiries, are unfit to trouble themselves to ask them." Graunt, *Natural and Political Observations,* p. 395.
[84] Graunt, *Natural and Political Observations,* p. 395.

PART ONE

Smallpox Inoculation and Medical Arithmetic

2

A Measure of Safety: English Debates over Inoculation in the 1720s

> A Practice which brings the Mortality of the *Small Pox* from one in ten to one in a hundred, if it obtain'd universally would save to the City of *London* at least 1500 People Yearly; and the same Odds wou'd be a sufficient prudential Motive to any private Person to proceed upon.
>
> [John Arbuthnot] 1722[1]

Just as the fear of plague led to the collection and publication of the London bills of mortality, which Graunt had so creatively used in his *Natural and Political Observations,* smallpox stimulated the development of medical arithmetic during the eighteenth century. Although smallpox had a significantly lower fatality rate than plague, its impact on public life was almost as great. Numerous members of the royalty succumbed to smallpox, including Queen Mary of England in 1694 and Louis XV of France in 1774. Smallpox caused disfigurement, blindness, and widespread suffering, which haunted the popular imagination. But it was not just the experience or fear of smallpox that led individuals to analyze its mortality rates. As with plague, the hope of preventive measures to offset the incidence of smallpox played an important role. Quarantine and fleeing potentially risky environments for safer climes were standard public health measures used to prevent or at least to limit plague epidemics. However, there existed a more potent preventive measure for smallpox: inoculation.

Inoculation provided an individual with a measure of safety – of immunity – against future smallpox epidemics. It had long been a folk practice in Turkey, Africa, China, and even parts of Wales before it came to the attention of Europe's elite in the early eighteenth century. The actual procedure consisted of making a scratch or small incision, typically on two limbs (some combination of arms and legs), and placing a thread covered with the pus from a virulent pock on that incision. (Later in the century, pocky matter was taken from an individual with inoculated smallpox in the belief that this produced a less dangerous case of the

---

[1] [John Arbuthnot], *Mr. Maitland's Account of Inoculating the Smallpox Vindicated, from Dr. Wagstaffe's Misrepresentations of That Practice, with Some Remarks on Mr. Massey's Sermon* (London, 1722), p. 21.

disease.) The scratch was covered with bandages for a day or so to ensure that the graft would take. The incisions would become inflamed approximately four days after they were made. The inoculee would then develop a fever on the seventh or eighth day, and a few pocks on the tenth or eleventh day. The individual normally recovered by the fifteenth or sixteenth day. Reactions varied, and in the worst cases, a few individuals contracted such a severe case of smallpox that they died.[2]

The best-known publicist for the procedure in the early eighteenth century was Lady Mary Wortley Montagu, who first became aware of inoculation while living in Constantinople where her husband was posted as an ambassador for England. An aristocrat with extensive connections, Montagu had her three-year-old daughter inoculated in April 1721, and she helped persuade Caroline, the Princess of Wales, to inoculate two of her daughters, Princess Amelia (age 11) and Princess Caroline (age 9), in April 1722.[3] The royal inoculations were critical to the acceptance of inoculation by the English public, but they did not convince everyone of its benefits, especially in the wake of two well-publicized deaths related to inoculation in the spring of 1722.[4]

Besides Montagu's advocacy and the actions of the royal family, two London-based physicians, John Arbuthnot (1665–1735) and James Jurin (1684–1750), argued the case for inoculation by using a novel method of quantification. Presenting comparative mortality figures for natural and inoculated smallpox, they showed that the hazard of dying from inoculated smallpox was much less than that of dying from natural smallpox. Theirs was arguably the first use of numerical evidence to evaluate a medical practice, and it was to play a decisive role not only in the debates over inoculation but also in subsequent evaluations of medical knowledge and practice.

Arbuthnot's and Jurin's quantitative arguments in favor of inoculation found a receptive audience among the fellows of the Royal Society of London. While physicians' corporations remained silent (such as the Royal College of Physicians) or hostile (the Paris Faculté de Médecine) to inoculation, the Royal Society provided a relatively open arena for discussion and evaluation of this

---

[2] For accounts of inoculation in England, see Deborah Brunton, "'Pox Britannica': Smallpox Inoculation in Britain, 1721–1830," Ph.D. thesis, University of Pennsylvania, 1990; Charles Creighton, *A History of Epidemics in Britain,* 2 vols. (Cambridge, 1894); Maisie May, "Inoculating the Urban Poor in the Late Eighteenth Century," *British Journal for the History of Science* 30 (1997): 291–305; Genevieve Miller, *The Adoption of Inoculation for Smallpox in England and France* (Philadelphia: University of Pennsylvania Press, 1957); and Peter Razzell, *The Conquest of Smallpox: The Impact of Inoculation on Smallpox Mortality in Eighteenth Century Britain* (Sussex: Caliban Books, 1977).

[3] On the royal inoculations, see Miller, *The Adoption of Inoculation,* pp. 96–98. For contrasting views on Montagu's influence, see Isobel Grundy, "Medical Advance and Female Fame: Inoculation and Its After-Effects," *Lumen* 13 (94): 13–42; and Genevieve Miller, "Putting Lady Mary in Her Place: A Discussion of Historical Causation," *Bulletin of the History of Medicine* 55 (1981): 2–16.

[4] Miller, *The Adoption of Inoculation,* pp. 96–98.

new medical practice.[5] Fellows of the Society became informed about inoculation in 1713 and 1714 from reports by Italian physicians practicing in Constantinople. These accounts were read before the members and later published in the *Philosophical Transactions*; they became authoritative accounts of the procedure.[6]

Lady Montagu's campaign on behalf of inoculation brought a new sense of urgency to the evaluation of the procedure, and several Fellows became active participants in the public trial of inoculation made on six Newgate prisoners in August 1721. The trial was made at the instigation of the royal family, prior to the inoculation of the royal princesses. Six prisoners were selected, three men and three women, with the understanding that if they survived they would be released. All six recovered, and they left Newgate on 6 September 1721.[7]

Despite the results of this trial and the royal inoculations in 1722, a heated controversy ensued.[8] An extensive pamphlet war took place during the early 1720s involving the religious, medical, and nationalist objections to the practice. Religious leaders argued that inoculation interfered with divine providence, while medical opponents focused on its ethics. Inoculation could not properly be classified as a therapy: What physician would give an illness to prevent an illness? This action certainly transgressed the Hippocratic maxim to do no harm. Because of its non-European origins, some such as the physician William Wagstaffe, author of the influential pamphlet *A Letter to Dr. Freind Shewing the Danger and Uncertainty of Inoculating the Small Pox* (1722), disparaged inoculation because it was practiced "by a few *ignorant women*, amongst an illiterate and unthinking People."[9] And finally, English nationalists raised Hippocratic objections to a practice developed in a foreign land (Turkey) for a foreign people: It could not possibly suit the needs of the Christian, meat-eating, English.[10]

It was into this storm that Arbuthnot and Jurin launched their new approach. Both were mathematically inclined London physicians who were at home among other men who fashioned similarly successful careers by combining

[5] Miller highlighted the role played by the Royal Society in the encouragement of inoculation. Miller, *The Adoption of Inoculation*, pp. 123–133. On the hostility of the Paris Faculté de Médecine, see Miller, pp. 185–187.
[6] Emanuele Timoni, "An Account, or History, of the Procuring the Small Pox by Incision, or Inoculation; As It Has for Some Time Been Practised at Constantinople. Being the Extract of a Letter from Emanuel Timonius, Oxon. & Patav. M.D. F.R.S. Dated at Constantinople, December 1713. Communicated to the Royal Society by John Woodward, M.D. Profes. Med. Gresh. and F.R.S.," *Philosophical Transactions* 29 (1714): 72–82; Jacob Pylarini, "Nova et tuta variolas excitandi per transplantionem methodus; nuper inventa et in usum tracta: qua rite peracta immunia in posterum praeservantur ab hujusmodi contagio corpora," *Philosophical Transactions* 29 (1716): 393–399. Miller provided a list of eighteenth-century editions of these works; Miller, *The Adoption of Inoculation,* Appendix B.
[7] On the Newgate experiment, see Miller, *The Adoption of Inoculation,* pp. 80–91.
[8] The pamphlet literature on inoculation is extensive and for the most part repetitive. See Miller's book for a bibliography of English and French pamphlets. Miller, *The Adoption of Inoculation.*
[9] William Wagstaffe, *A Letter to Dr. Freind Shewing the Danger and Uncertainty of Inoculating the Small Pox* (London, 1722), p. 5.
[10] Wagstaffe, *Letter to Dr. Freind,* p. 7.

interests in the new natural philosophy with lucrative medical practices. London proved an exciting and creative milieu where informal exchanges in coffee-houses among merchants, physicians, writers, and instrument makers comple-mented more formal activities among gentlemen at the Royal Society. Natural philosophy was prestigious and fashionable, and participating in various scien-tific efforts frequently enhanced an individual's status among the London elite. Further, natural philosophy enjoyed wide support among the general public who attended lectures and demonstrations.[11] For Arbuthnot and Jurin, medicine and natural philosophy were the means to prosperous public and private lives.

ARBUTHNOT'S VINDICATION

Born in Kinkardineshire, Scotland, Arbuthnot studied medicine at St. Andrews in Aberdeen and received his degree in 1696. Moving to London the following year, he first gave private lessons in mathematics and eventually established a lucrative medical practice attending London's elite, including the royal family. (He became physician to Queen Anne in 1705.) Numbering among his friends Alexander Pope and Jonathan Swift, Arbuthnot penned satires with John Gay, and together they created the portly character John Bull to represent England. Besides his remarkable literary skills, Arbuthnot wrote several important medi-cal and natural philosophical works. He became Fellow of the Royal Society in 1704 and Fellow of the Royal College of Physicians in 1710. An active member of both societies, he served on the Council of the Royal Society for several years.[12]

Early in his career, Arbuthnot published on mathematical topics. In 1692 he did a partial translation of Christiaan Huygens's treatise *De ratiociniis in ludo Aleae* [*Of the Laws of Chance*], and nine years later he published *An Essay on the Usefulness of Mathematical Learning* (1701). In these writings, Arbuthnot under-lined the importance of mathematics to the search for certain knowledge.[13] He asserted:

There are very few things which we know, which are not capable of being reduced to a mathematical reasoning, and when they cannot, it is a sign the knowledge of them is very small and confused; and, when a mathematical reason can be had, it is as great a folly to

---

[11] Many recent works focusing on medicine and natural philosophy have captured the dynamism of London during the eighteenth century. See especially Larry Stewart, *The Rise of Public Science: Rhetoric, Technology, and Natural Philosophy in Newtonian Britain, 1660–1750* (Cambridge: Cambridge University Press, 1992); and Susan Lawrence, *Charitable Knowledge: Hospital Pupils and Practitioners in Eighteenth-Century London* (Cambridge: Cambridge University Press, 1996).

[12] For a biography, see Lester M. Beattie, *John Arbuthnot – Mathematician and Satirist* (Cambridge, Mass.: Harvard University Press, 1935).

[13] See John Arbuthnot, *An Essay on the Usefulness of Mathematical Learning in a Letter from a Gentleman in the City to His Friend in Oxford*, 2d ed. (1st ed. 1701; Oxford, 1721).

make use of any other, as to grope for a thing in the dark when you have a candle standing by you.[14]

Arbuthnot shared John Graunt's and William Petty's view that mathematics would bring clarity and greater understanding.

Reflecting this conviction, Arbuthnot brought mathematics to bear on topics not typically treated quantitatively. In an influential essay, "An Argument for Divine Providence," he used baptism figures from a series of 82 years of the London bills of mortality to establish the ratio of male to female christenings, just as Graunt had done. Arbuthnot arrived at a proportion of 13 to 12, in contrast to Graunt's of 14 to 13. Arbuthnot argued that this excess cannot be due to chance, but instead attributed it to divine providence. Drawing an analogy between a two-sided die and the two sexes, Arbuthnot reasoned that without divine intervention there would be an equality between males and females, just as a toss of the two-sided die yielded equal numbers of each side over a long number of trials. Divine providence was needed, Arbuthnot asserted, because boys and men were subject to more accidents and diseases than were girls and women.[15] (Graunt had not relied on divine providence to explain the source of the inequality, nor had he made use of the die analogy.) Accepting this ratio as a natural fact, Arbuthnot reached the same conclusion as Graunt:

From hence it follows that polygamy is contrary to the Law of Nature and Justice, and to the Propagation of the Human Race; for where Males and Females are in equal number, if one Man takes Twenty Wives, nineteen Men must live in Celibacy, which is repugnant to the Design of Nature; nor is it probable that Twenty Women will be so well impregnated by one Man as by Twenty.[16]

Here was the divine economy of procreation spelled out in numerical simplicity.

Arbuthnot's contribution to the inoculation debates was made anonymously and employed satire as well as mathematics to undermine opponents of inoculation.[17] Entitled *Mr. Maitland's Account of Inoculating the Smallpox Vindicated, from Dr. Wagstaffe's Misrepresentations of That Practice, with Some Remarks on Mr. Massey's Sermon,* Arbuthnot's pamphlet went through two editions in 1722, indicating that it enjoyed some popularity. The first two-thirds of the pamphlet

[14] John Arbuthnot, *Of the Laws of Chance* (London, 1692); quoted in William Black, *Observations Medical and Political: On the Small-pox and Inoculation; and on the Decrease of Mankind at Every Age with a Comparative View of the Diseases Most Fatal to London during Ninety Years* (London, 1781), pp. 35–36.

[15] For discussions of Arbuthnot's argument, see Ian Hacking, *The Emergence of Probability* (Cambridge: Cambridge University Press, 1975), chap. 18; and Anders Hald, *A History of Probability and Statistics and Their Applications before 1750* (New York: John Wiley & Sons, 1990), pp. 275–285.

[16] Arbuthnot, "An Argument for Divine Providence Taken from the Regularity Observ'd in the Birth of Both Sexes," *Philosophical Transactions* 27(1710 to 1712): 186–190. Quotation is on p. 189.

[17] Arbuthnot's authorship was revealed in a letter from the surgeon Claude Amyand to the French physician Jean Delacoste. See Miller, *The Adoption of Inoculation,* p. 106. Delacoste reprinted this letter in his pamphlet *Lettre sur l'Inoculation de la Petite Vérole comme elle se pratique en Turquie et en Angleterre* (Paris, 1723), p. 25.

Dy'd of all *Diſeaſes*.   Dy'd of the *SmallPox*.

1707.	21600	-	-	-	1707.	1078
	21291	-	-	-		1687
	21800	-	-	-		1024
	24620	-	-	-		3138
	19833	-	-	-		0915
	21198	-	-	-		1943
	21057	-	-	-		1614
	26569	-	-	-		2810
	22232	-	-	-		1057
	24436	-	-	-		2427
	23446	-	-	-		2211
1718.	26523	-	-	-	1718.	1884
	274605					**21788**

2.1 John Arbuthnot's table of smallpox deaths from the London bills (1707–1718). *Source:* [John Arbuthnot], *Mr. Maitland's Account of Inoculating the Smallpox Vindicated* (London, 1722). Yale University, Harvey Cushing/John Hay Whitney Medical Library.

refuted Wagstaffe's objections; the last 20 pages responded to Edmund Massey's *A Sermon against the Dangerous and Sinful Practice of Inoculation. Preached at St. Andrew's Holborn, on Sunday, July 8th, 1722.* In his discussion of Wagstaffe's tract, Arbuthnot developed quantitative arguments that pointed to two conclusions: (1) that inoculation was less risky than a natural case of smallpox, and (2) that the population as a whole would benefit from the reduced mortality if inoculation were adopted universally.

To establish the risks of natural smallpox, Arbuthnot followed the same method Graunt had used in his *Natural and Political Observations*. Arbuthnot combed through the London bills of mortality and created a table with columns for total burials and burials attributed to smallpox for the years 1707 to 1718, inclusive. (See Figure 2.1.) From this table, Arbuthnot calculated the average proportion of smallpox deaths to total deaths in London and arrived at the figure of 1 of 12 deaths. The next steps in Arbuthnot's argument were less clear. First, he adjusted this ratio by incorporating Graunt's observation about the high rate of infant mortality. Arbuthnot reasoned that roughly 8 of 9 infants died before having been exposed to smallpox, so that the actual mortality of smallpox was greater than the ratio originally calculated. He estimated that roughly 1 of 10 deaths over the age of one were due to smallpox, and he argued that because everyone in London would be exposed to smallpox at some point in their lives, 1 of 10 people who contracted smallpox would die. Arbuthnot compared this figure with an estimate of mortality due to inoculation, which he gave (without evidence) as 1 of 100. Thus, in Arbuthnot's words, "A Practice which brings the

Mortality of the *Small Pox* from one in ten to one in a hundred, if it obtain'd universally would save to the City of *London* at least 1500 People Yearly; and the same Odds wou'd be a sufficient prudential Motive to any private Person to proceed upon."[18]

This last argument, characteristic of the political arithmetic promoted by Graunt and Petty, emphasized the interests of the state by indicating how inoculation would increase population. Unlike the early arithmeticians, however, Arbuthnot was also interested in shaping individual behavior. Over the course of the eighteenth century, statist arguments became restricted to discussions about the desirability of inoculating the poor, and Arbuthnot's contemporaries for the most part refrained from including similar calculations, and instead focused on the risks and benefits to the individual. The pamphlet was Arbuthnot's only contribution to the inoculation debates, and it was published anonymously, perhaps to protect his medical practice. It was Arbuthnot's younger colleague, Jurin, who developed and diffused the numerical evaluation of inoculation.

JURIN'S ACCOUNTS

A descendent of Huguenots, Jurin was born in London, attended Christ's Hospital and earned a scholarship to Trinity College, Cambridge.[19] At Trinity he studied Newtonian natural philosophy with Roger Cotes and William Whiston during the years 1703 through 1708 and became a skilled mathematician. Upon the recommendation of Richard Bentley, Chancellor to Trinity, he took up the position of schoolmaster at the grammar school of Newcastle-upon-Tyne. While in Newcastle, he offered a series of public lectures and courses on mathematics and natural philosophy. In 1715 he returned to Cambridge and received an MD the following year, whereupon he removed to London.

Jurin wasted little time in advancing his position both as a physician and a natural philosopher. He attended his first meeting of the Royal Society on 25 October 1716 and became a fellow in 1717; in 1719, he was elected a fellow of the Royal College of Physicians. During his first years in the Royal Society, he contributed several papers and performed numerous experimental demonstrations at weekly meetings. Elected secretary to the Society in November 1721, Jurin became one of its most active secretaries: He cultivated and expanded the Society's correspondence and published volumes 31 through 34 of the *Philosophical Transactions*. Jurin served as secretary during the last years of Newton's presidency, and he rose to prominence as one of the leading spokesmen for the Newtonian program in natural philosophy and as a staunch advocate for the application of mathematics to medical topics.

---

[18] [Arbuthnot], *Mr. Maitland's Account . . . Vindicated*, p. 21.
[19] For a biography of Jurin, see *The Correspondence of James Jurin (1684–1750), Physician and Secretary to the Royal Society,* ed. Andrea Rusnock (Amsterdam and Atlanta: Rodopi Press, 1996), pp. 3–61.

It is something of a paradox that Jurin's ardent Newtonianism would end his career as secretary. When Newton died in March 1727, two men stepped forward to replace him: Martin Folkes, a mathematician and polymath, whom Newton had appointed vice-president of the Royal Society; and Sir Hans Sloane, physician to George II, former secretary to the Society, collector, and natural historian. Politics entered into the election over the issue of how the Royal Society should address the Hanoverian king and prince. (It seems that Newton's distrust of the Hanoverian rulers – because of Leibniz's association with Hanover – carried over to his followers.)[20] John Byrom, teacher of a method of shorthand and Fellow of the Society, was particularly outspoken about Hanoverian rule. A German surgeon attending the Society's meeting made a great display of writing Byrom's name down after Byrom had made some potentially critical remarks. Folkes and Jurin supported Byrom on the grounds "that every member of this Society had a right to speak his mind upon occasion," but rumors began to circulate through the London coffeehouses. "It has been said there were Jacobites in the Society," commented one Fellow.[21]

Political divisions were amplified by philosophical differences. The philomaths rallied around Folkes, who sought to maintain the Newtonian research program, with its emphasis on mechanics, astronomy, iatromechanics, and the new mathematics. Sloane, on the other hand, promoted natural history and put less stock in mathematical pursuits. One observer noted, "It has been the whole talk of the town; and there had been as much canvassing and intrigue made use of, as if the fate of the Kingdome depended on it."[22] It seems that Jurin followed his Newtonian allegiances, rather than his obligations to his medical patron Sloane, who had helped him to establish his practice. Folkes and Jurin were very good friends – Folkes had proposed Jurin for fellowship – and Jurin supported Folkes's bid for the presidency.

On election day, 30 November 1727, Sloane won by a considerable majority, and consequently Jurin lost his position as secretary and was replaced by the physician William Rutty. Jurin was not content to go quietly, however; his dedication to Folkes in his final volume of the *Philosophical Transactions* was a ringing endorsement of Newtonian natural philosophy, and a not very subtle rebuke of Sloane and his program of natural history. After noting that the great man himself had appointed Folkes vice-president for his "singular Attainments in those noble and manly Sciences, to which the Glory of *Sir Isaac Newton,* and the Reputation of the *Royal Society* is solely and entirely owing," Jurin went on to spell out the differences between Newton and Sloane. Newton

[20] John Heilbron provided an account of this episode. See J.L. Heilbron, *Physics at the Royal Society during Newton's Presidency* (Los Angeles: William Andrews Clark Memorial Library, 1983), p. 37.

[21] John Byrom, *The Private Journal and Literary Remains of John Byrom,* ed. Richard Parkinson (Manchester: Chetham Society, 1854), vol. 1, pp. 253–254.

[22] Letter from Richard Richardson to Samuel Brewer dated 14 December 1727; quoted in G.R. de Beer, *Sir Hans Sloane and the British Museum* (Oxford: Oxford University Press, 1953), p. 92.

was "sensible, that something more than knowing the Name, the Shape and obvious Qualities of an Insect, a Pebble, a Plant, or a Shell, was requisite to form a Philosopher, even of the lowest rank, much more to qualifie one to sit at the Head of so great and learned a Body." A low blow indeed to Sloane, but Jurin went further: "We all of us remember that Saying so frequently in his [Newton's] Mouth, That *Natural History might indeed furnish Materials for Natural Philosophy; but, however, Natural History was not Natural Philosophy.*"[23] After this episode, Jurin continued to advocate Newtonian ideas, most famously in the *Analyst* controversy, where under the pseudonym Philalethes Cantabrigiensis, he defended Newtonian fluxions from George Berkeley's criticisms.

In a series of pamphlets published between 1723 and 1727, Jurin argued the case for inoculation using a novel method of quantification. Presenting comparative mortality figures for natural and inoculated smallpox, he showed that the hazard of dying from inoculated smallpox was much less than dying from natural smallpox.[24] Unlike Arbuthnot, Jurin based his figures for inoculated smallpox on empirical sources, and because of this, Jurin's writings on inoculation enjoyed great popularity. His ratios were widely cited in England and on the Continent, and his method was adopted by subsequent arithmeticians.

Jurin showed an interest in inoculation as early as 1722, when he published "An Account of a Remarkable Instance of the Infection of the Small Pox" in the *Philosophical Transactions,* but it was correspondence with the Yorkshire physician Thomas Nettleton that immediately triggered Jurin's foray into the controversy.[25] Nettleton had begun to practice inoculation in Halifax after having learned of it solely from the *Philosophical Transactions.* As one of the first to inoculate individuals outside of London, Nettleton was driven to adopt such a radical procedure because of the suffering he encountered while trying to treat individuals with the disease. Because of his sense of isolation, he wrote about his efforts to a fellow Yorkshire physician, William Whitaker, who as a member

---

[23] *Philosophical Transactions* 34 (1727), Dedication.

[24] See James Jurin: "A Letter to the Learned Caleb Cotesworth, MD, FRS, of the College of Physicians, and Physician to St. Thomas's Hospital, Containing a Comparison between the Mortality of the Natural Small Pox, and That Given by Inoculation," *Philosophical Transactions* 32, no. 374 (1722–1723): 213–224, and published separately as a pamphlet with additions, *A Letter to the Learned Caleb Cotesworth . . . Which is Subjoined an Account of the Success of Inoculation in New-England; As Likewise an Extract from Several Letters concerning a Like Method of Communicating the Small Pox, That Has Been Used Time Out of Mind in South Wales* (London, 1723); *An Account of the Success of Inoculating the Small Pox in Great Britain with a Comparison between the Miscarriages in that Practice, and the Mortality of the Natural Small Pox* (London, 1724); *An Account of the Success of Inoculating the Small Pox for the Year 1724* (London, 1725); *An Account of the Success of Inoculating the Small Pox for the Year 1725* (London, 1726); *An Account of the Success of Inoculating the Small Pox for the Year 1726* (London 1727). John Gasper Scheuchzer took over Jurin's project in 1727 and published *An Account of the Success of Inoculating the Small-Pox in Great Britain, for the years 1727 and 1728* (London, 1729).

[25] Miller underscored Nettleton's role in suggesting a statistical analysis. See Miller, *The Adoption of Inoculation,* pp. 111–116.

of the Royal Society passed the letter on to Jurin. This initiated a fruitful eight-year correspondence between Jurin and Nettleton, which provided Nettleton with a sense of community and support and supplied Jurin with information about the practice of inoculation in northern England.[26]

In one of his early letters, Nettleton suggested that the only way inoculation could be established in Britain against the prejudices it faced was "by making a Comparison so far as our Experience will extend" of the dangers of inoculated and natural smallpox.[27] Jurin agreed and penned an 11-page pamphlet addressing precisely Nettleton's suggestion.[28] Jurin narrowed the comparison posed by Nettleton to the risks of dying from inoculated versus natural smallpox; he excluded morbidity associated with natural smallpox and inoculation. Just as Arbuthnot had done, Jurin turned to the London bills of mortality to find evidence for the chances of dying from natural smallpox. He examined two 12-year periods and constructed the following tables, which he placed at the heart of his first pamphlet on inoculation. (See Figures 2.2 and 2.3.) The first table indicated mortality figures for the years 1667–1686, and the second for the period 1701–1722. He omitted the intervening years (1687–1700) because deaths due to smallpox and measles were counted together.

Jurin's tables differed from Arbuthnot's in the addition of the two columns at the right. While Arbuthnot had simply recorded the number of burials, Jurin included calculations based on those numbers for each year. By doing this, Jurin invited the reader to survey the variations in smallpox mortality in two ways: 1) the number of deaths due to smallpox per 1,000 deaths (much closer to today's common use of percentages); and 2) the proportion of deaths due to smallpox compared to all deaths with the number one in the numerator. This latter form of expressing a ratio predominated throughout the course of the eighteenth century. From these tables, Jurin initially concluded that 1 of 14 died of natural smallpox, but he went on to adjust these odds in light of mortality patterns characteristic of London.

Like Graunt and Arbuthnot before him, Jurin recognized that the high infant mortality rate might skew the odds. He concluded:

For since one fourteenth part of Mankind die of the Small Pox, and the other thirteen parts die of other Diseases; if these thirteen have all had the Small Pox, and recover'd from it, before they fell ill of those other Diseases of which they died, then just thirteen will have recover'd from the Small Pox, for one that dies of that Distemper: but, as it is notorious, that great numbers, especially of young Children, die of other Diseases, without ever having the Small Pox, it is plain, that fewer than thirteen must recover from this Distemper, for one that dies of it.[29]

[26] Their correspondence is preserved in the Royal Society Inoculation Papers and the Library of the Wellcome Institute for the History of Medicine. It is published in *The Correspondence of James Jurin*.
[27] Nettleton to Jurin, 16 December 1722, RS Early Letters N.1.94; published in *Correspondence of James Jurin*, p. 118.
[28] James Jurin, "A Letter to the Learned Caleb Cotesworth."
[29] Jurin, "A Letter to the Learned Caleb Cotesworth," p. 219.

TABLE I.

Years	Total No. of Burials	Died of the Small Pox. In all.	In 1000	In Proportion.
1667	15842	1196	75	$\frac{1}{13}$
1668	17278	1987	115	$\frac{1}{9}$
1669	19432	951	49	$\frac{1}{20}$
1670	20198	1465	73	$\frac{1}{14}$
1671	15729	696	44	$\frac{1}{23}$
1672	18230	1116	61	$\frac{1}{16}$
1673	17504	853	49	$\frac{1}{21}$
1674	21201	2507	118	$\frac{1}{8}$
1675	17244	997	58	$\frac{1}{17}$
1676	18732	359	19	$\frac{1}{52}$
1677	19067	1678	88	$\frac{1}{11}$
1678	20678	1798	87	$\frac{1}{12}$
1679	21730	1967	91	$\frac{1}{11}$
1680	21053	689	33	$\frac{1}{31}$
1681	23971	2982	125	$\frac{1}{8}$
1682	20691	1408	68	$\frac{1}{15}$
1683	20587	2096	102	$\frac{1}{10}$
1684	23202	156	7	$\frac{1}{149}$
1685	23222	2496	107	$\frac{1}{9}$
1686	22609	1062	47	$\frac{1}{21}$
20 Years	398200	28459	$71\frac{1}{7}$	$\frac{1}{14}$
Each Year at a *Medium*	19910	1423	$71\frac{1}{7}$	$\frac{1}{14}$

2.2 James Jurin's table of smallpox mortality from the London bills (1667–1686). *Source:* James Jurin, "A Letter to the Learned Dr. Caleb Cotesworth, . . ." *Philosophical Transactions* 32, no. 374 (1722–1723): 17. Burndy Library, Dibner Institute for the History of Science and Technology.

Again like Graunt and Arbuthnot, Jurin subtracted the number of deaths due to certain diseases associated with infants, for example, "Overlaid, Chrysoms and Infants, Convulsions, Horseshoehead, Headmoldshot, Teeth," which together amounted to 386 deaths per 1,000 over the 22-year period. Thus, deaths due to smallpox must now be reckoned as a fraction of the remaining 614 deaths per 1,000. Jurin made the further assumption that everyone after two years of age contracted smallpox at some point in his or her life.[30] The adjusted figures revealed that 1 of 7 or 8 persons who had contracted smallpox died, a significantly greater mortality rate than Arbuthnot's 1 of 10.

To calculate the risks of dying from inoculated smallpox, Jurin drew on the experience of several London inoculators during the years 1721 and 1722,

[30] Jurin, "A Letter to the Learned Caleb Cotesworth," p. 220.

T A B L E II.

Years	Total No of Burials	Died of the Small Pox.		
		In all.	In 1000	In Proportion.
1701	20471	1095	53	$\frac{1}{19}$
1702	19481	311	16	$\frac{1}{61}$
1703	20720	898	43	$\frac{1}{21}$
1704	22684	1501	66	$\frac{1}{15}$
1705	22097	1095	50	$\frac{1}{20}$
1706	19847	721	36	$\frac{1}{28}$
1707	21600	1078	50	$\frac{1}{20}$
1708	21291	1687	79	$\frac{1}{13}$
1709	21800	1024	47	$\frac{1}{21}$
1710	24620	3138	127	$\frac{1}{8}$
1711	19833	915	46	$\frac{1}{22}$
1712	21198	1943	92	$\frac{1}{11}$
1713	21057	1614	77	$\frac{1}{13}$
1714	26569	2810	106	$\frac{1}{9}$
1715	22232	1057	48	$\frac{1}{21}$
1716	24436	2427	99	$\frac{1}{10}$
1717	23446	2211	94	$\frac{1}{11}$
1718	26523	1884	71	$\frac{1}{14}$
1719	28347	3229	114	$\frac{1}{9}$
1720	25454	1440	57	$\frac{1}{18}$
1721	26142	2375	91	$\frac{1}{11}$
1722	25750	2167	84	$\frac{1}{12}$
22 Years	505598	36620	72	$\frac{1}{14}$
Each Year at a *Medium*.	22982	1665	72	$1\frac{1}{4}$
42 Years	903798	65079	72	$\frac{1}{14}$
Each Year in 42 at a *Medium*.	21519	1550	72	$\frac{1}{14}$

2.3 James Jurin's table of smallpox mortality from the London bills (1701–1722). *Source:* James Jurin, "A Letter to the Learned Dr. Caleb Cotesworth, ..." *Philosophical Transactions* 32, no. 374 (1722–1723): 18. Burndy Library, Dibner Institute for the History of Science and Technology.

made familiar to him through presentations at meetings of the Royal Society. He also incorporated reports from Boston, Massachusetts, where inoculation had been practiced during a severe smallpox epidemic in 1721.[31] Jurin based his calculations on these known and specific instances and arrived at the ratio

[31] 13 June 1723, RS Journal Books XII, p. 371; 31 October 1723, RS Journal Books XII, pp. 392–393. In his article, Jurin referred to a letter dated 10 March 1721 from Cotton Mather, who reported that 5 or 6 of 300 inoculated individuals died. Mather attributed some of these deaths to the fact that many persons were inoculated in Boston regardless of their condition, including many pregnant women and ill individuals. See Jurin, "A Letter to the Learned Caleb Cotesworth," p. 215.

that 1 of 91 individuals died from inoculation, close to Arbuthnot's estimate (1 of 100), but grounded on experience.[32]

BUILDING A CORRESPONDENCE NETWORK

Jurin's account, initially published in the *Philosophical Transactions,* was warmly received, and he issued it separately with additions in 1723.[33] Encouraged, he decided to solicit accounts of inoculation through correspondence and placed an advertisement in two volumes of the *Philosophical Transactions* and in his pamphlet, *A Letter to the Learned Caleb Cotesworth;* it was also reissued in each annual pamphlet entitled *An Account of the Success of Inoculating the Smallpox for the Year....*[34] (See Figure 2.4.) Numerous individuals throughout the British Isles replied, and they supplied Jurin with a wealth of information about the practice, risks, and success of inoculation.[35]

Many difficulties beset Jurin's numerical investigations in medicine. To construct mortality ratios, he had to collect and collate case histories from an extensive correspondence with a group of geographically widespread practitioners. Building such a network took considerable effort, and maintaining the goodwill of voluntary correspondents required diplomatic skill. The creation of standard narratives from the numerous individual case histories involved the extraction of consistent, quantifiable information, which then had to be tallied and tabulated in established categories. Jurin's ratios of the number of inoculated and natural smallpox cases were thus the result of an arduous and, at times, controversial process of soliciting, selecting, and sorting varied case histories. The process of creating and extending metrology is a deliberate and resource-intensive activity.[36]

Complete, faithful, and accurate case histories were central to Jurin's project, especially in the first year or so when inoculation was an unfamiliar procedure to most people in Britain. In his 1724 *Account of the Success of Inoculating the Small Pox,* Jurin gave a composite account of the procedure and the typical course of illness in an inoculated patient. "I shall here give some Account of what is to be done, and what is usually observ'd in Inoculation," Jurin instructed, "as I have extracted it from a careful Examination and Comparison of

---

[32] Jurin, "A Letter to the Learned Caleb Cotesworth," pp. 214–215.

[33] James Jurin, *A Letter to the Learned Caleb Cotesworth.*

[34] See *Philosophical Transactions* 32 (1723), no. 378, unnumbered last page; 33 (1724), no. 383, unnumbered last page.

[35] Much of the following is drawn from Andrea A. Rusnock, "The Weight of Evidence and the Burden of Authority: Case Histories, Medical Statistics and Smallpox Inoculation," in *Medicine in the Enlightenment,* ed. Roy Porter, Wellcome Clio Medica Series, (Amsterdam and Atlanta: Rodopi Press, 1995), pp. 289–315.

[36] Theodore Porter, *Trust in Numbers: The Pursuit of Objectivity in Science and Public Life* (Princeton, N. J.: Princeton University Press, 1995); Bruno Latour, *Science in Action* (Cambridge, Mass.: Harvard University Press, 1987).

ADVERTISEMENT.

THE Practice of inoculating the SMALL POX being now extended into many Parts of the Kingdom, and it being highly requisite that the Publick should be faithfully inform'd of the Success of that Method, whether Good or Bad ; It is defir'd, that all PHYSICIANS, SURGEONS, APOTHECARIES, and others therein concern'd, will be pleas'd to tranfmit to Dr. *Jurin*, Secretary to the ROYAL SOCIETY, a particular Account, fpecifying the Name and Age of every Perfon by them inoculated, the Place where it was done, the Manner of the Operation, whether it took Effect or no, what Sort of Diftemper it produced, on what Day from Inoculation the Eruption appear'd ; and, laftly, whether the Patient died or recover'd. They are defired to comprehend in their Accounts all Perfons inoculated by them, from the Beginning of this Practice among us to the End of the prefent Year, and to fend them fome Time in *January* or *February* next.

IN cafe this be comply'd with, the ADVERTISER promifes to give the Publick an exact Account of the whole Number of Perfons inoculated in *Great Britain*, diftinguifhing them into Claffes according to their feveral Ages ; as likewife of thofe that it has had no Effect upon, and of thofe that have died of it.

AND he farther promifes to preferve the Original Accounts, that fhall be fent him, and to give a Sight of them to any Gentleman who fhall defire it, that in cafe any of thofe, who have been inoculated, fhall afterwards have the SMALL POX in the natural Way, it may be known, whether fuch Perfon had before received the SMALL POX by Inoculation, or not.

N. B. THE Names of the Perfons inoculated fhall not be printed without Leave of the Parties concern'd.

Dec. 11th. 1723.

JAMES JURIN.

2.4 James Jurin's advertisement soliciting accounts of inoculation (1723). *Source: Philosophical Transactions* 32, no. 374 (1722–1723); unnumbered last page. Burndy Library, Dibner Institute for the History of Science and Technology.

the several Relations transmitted to me."[37] This section was excluded in his subsequent pamphlets, presumably because inoculation had become fairly well known.

Respondents to Jurin's advertisement ranged socially and geographically. Medical men – apothecaries, surgeons, and physicians – were by far the majority of contributors, but there were also letters from the gentry (Sir Thomas Lyttleton and Lady Catherine Percivall provided detailed accounts of their children's inoculations), from local ministers who vouched for the legitimacy of

[37] Jurin, *Account* (1724), p. 12.

certain reports, and from a weaver turned medical practitioner who became embroiled in a particularly disputed case, to be discussed below in this chapter.

Certainly, part of Jurin's success in collecting inoculation accounts must be attributed to his position as secretary to the Royal Society. The Society provided crucial institutional support for such mundane, but necessary, matters as covering postage costs, as well as for such less tangible, but significant, factors of legitimation.[38] Jurin's ability to utilize the prestige and patronage of the leading scientific society of England at that time – whose president was the formidable Sir Isaac Newton – gave credence and authority to a practice that initially occasioned much hostility and doubt. Even in this world of pre–state bureaucratic statistics, some sort of institutional affiliation served to guarantee the accuracy and truthfulness of the numbers produced.

Correspondents, too, profited from participating in Jurin's project, primarily through connection with the Royal Society. Thomas Nettleton, for example, wrote that it was "the greatest of my ambitions that my letter may be inserted" in the *Philosophical Transactions*.[39] And in a subsequent letter, he confessed: "The Approbation of that Illustrious Body [the Royal Society] will far overballance all the hard censures, & injurious reflections, which every man must expect to meet with, who endeavours to promote a thing so uncommon, & so disagreable to the general Humour of the People, as this has hitherto been."[40]

From the numerous letters he received, it is evident that Jurin had a wealth of information at hand. Some of his respondents delighted in detail: Dr. Henry Jones of Kings College, Cambridge, penned a 12-page report of four sisters who had been inoculated, which in his words, was "a Minute & Impartial Account of all the Particulars that occurred during the time of the Distemper."[41] Dr. William Oliver contributed an 8-page description of the inoculation of two children in Plymouth.[42] Reports of this length took the form of medical case histories. Details concerning the health of each inoculated individual were recorded, from the initial incision until the last pock dried and flaked off the skin. Each day symptoms were noted, including changes in urine, stools, and temperature. The incisions were watched closely and often kept open in order to ascertain if the smallpox graft had taken, a process generally conceived in humoral terms: "[T]he running of Incisions may probably be of great Service, the matter issuing from them being of the same nature with what fills the Pocks."[43] The outbreak

---

[38] The Journal Books of the Royal Society recorded many accounts of inoculation presented at their meetings. See, for example, RS Journal Books XII, pp. 371, 392–393.

[39] Nettleton to Jurin, 5 May 1722, RS Early Letters N.1.92; published in *The Correspondence of James Jurin*, pp. 98–99.

[40] Nettleton to Jurin, 24 January 1723, RS Early Letters N.1.95; published in *The Correspondence of James Jurin*, pp. 125–127.

[41] Henry Jones to Jurin, 25 April 1724, RS *Classified Papers*, XXIII.

[42] William Oliver to Jurin, 16 February 1725, RS *Classified Papers*, XXIII.

[43] Jurin to Thomas Fuller, 19 February 1726, RS *Classified Papers*, XXIII; published in *The Correspondence of James Jurin*, pp. 327–328.

of pocks on the seventh or eighth day was generally agreed to be the true sign of whether the inoculation had been successful. The number of pocks was frequently recorded, for it was widely believed that those who had smallpox through inoculation suffered fewer pocks, which led Jurin to conclude: "The Small Pox given by Inoculation are generally fewer in number, and all the symptoms more favourable, than in the natural way."[44]

Many of Jurin's correspondents, however, were not as diligent in reporting case histories as Dr. Jones and Dr. Oliver, and Jurin frequently requested additional information. In a letter to the surgeon Mr. Hepburn of Stamford, Lincolnshire, Jurin appealed to the public good as a means to soften further demands:

I am favoured with yours of Jan: 21st in which you are pleas'd to give me an Account of your Success in Inoculating the small Pox upon the two Sons of Mr. Richards. The same publick Spirit which has moved you to send me that relation will I hope induce you to satisfie me in the following particulars which are not so expressly set down in your Letter, as I could wish.[45]

Correspondents replied promptly to Jurin's additional queries, and one writer even apologized for his negligence: "I shall be more carefull for the future to Transmit Names or any other particulars, that you may not have so troublesome a Correspondent."[46]

Details about names, ages, and place where the inoculation was performed were the most frequent of Jurin's requests.[47] A complete case history needed as its bare essentials precisely these elements along with outcome, and increasingly, only these elements as the typical course of inoculated smallpox became more widely known and agreed upon, and hence standardized. Name and place provided Jurin with the means of securing further information, should any questions arise about a specific case. "I am obliged to you for the Favour of yours of March 18," Jurin wrote to Nehemiah Towgood of Somerset, "but am under a necessity of giving you this trouble to desire the Names of your two Patients. My intention is not to Print those names but only to keep them by me, as I do all the rest in Order to be provided for any dispute that may happen afterwards."[48] In this way, Jurin's register of the names of inoculated individuals served as one means to guarantee for the accuracy of reported inoculations.

[44] Jurin to Thomas Fuller, 19 February 1726, RS *Classified Papers,* XXIII; published in *The Correspondence of James Jurin,* pp. 327–328.

[45] Jurin to Ino. Hepburn, 18 February 1724, RS *Classified Papers,* XXIII.

[46] John Woodhouse to Jurin, 14 February 1726, RS *Classified Papers,* XXIII.

[47] See, e.g., Jurin to John Woodhouse, 12 February 1726; Jurin to William Thorold, 30 March 1727; RS *Classified Papers,* XXIII.

[48] Jurin to Nehemiah Towgood, 6 April 1727, RS *Classified Papers,* XXIII.

TALLYING THE TYPICAL

The next step in Jurin's project was to assemble the case histories and create a numerical account of the state of inoculation within a given year. By reporting only the number of persons successfully inoculated, Jurin skirted the delicate issues of privacy and propriety. As suggested in his letter to Towgood, Jurin had to balance his need for completeness with his correspondents' desire for confidentiality. Many of his correspondents, in fact, requested that the names of their patients not be published. "You are desired by the parents to conceal their Names," wrote the surgeon Hepburn; "the Father desires the Child may not be mentioned in Print," reported the apothecary Brady; and again, James Burges stated, "As you will see by Mr. Grenvill's Letter, Names are not to be printed. . . ."[49] In at least one instance, the propriety of printing women's ages was challenged by the Royal Surgeon Claude Amyand, whose patients were primarily members of the gentry: "T'were to wish the fair sexes Ages did not Stand upon Records."[50] The desire for privacy, particularly among the upper classes, made Jurin's strategy of reporting only the number of persons inoculated all the more appealing. Numbers provided anonymity.

Essential to quantification – broadly conceived as the process of assigning numbers to represent things – is categorization. In order for Jurin to quantify the success of inoculation, he had to develop categories to enumerate. In his pamphlets, Jurin addressed two questions that he regarded as central to evaluating the efficacy of inoculation: first, whether inoculation provided "effectual Security" against natural smallpox; and second, "Whether the Hazard of Inoculation be considerably less than that of the natural Small Pox?"[51] By framing the questions in this way, Jurin negotiated a complex issue by reducing the number of potential objections to inoculation. Throughout his inoculation correspondence, one can find evidence of Jurin's efforts to restrict the enquiry to these two questions.

To answer the first question, he had to rely upon the experience of inoculated individuals – or as Jurin put it:

For tho' many Trials have been purposely made by Physicians and others, both upon Children and grown Persons, who have had the Small Pox by Inoculation, causing them not only to converse with, but to handle, to nurse, and to lie in the same Bed with others Sick of the natural Small Pox; yet there is no Instance as far as I have been able to learn, of any one Person, either in Turky, New England, or here at Home, who has received the Small Pox by Inoculation, that has afterwards had it in the natural Way.[52]

---

[49] Ino. Hepburn to Jurin, 21 January 1724; Samuel Brady to Jurin, 21 February 1724; James Burges to Jurin, 21 April 1726; RS *Classified Papers*, XXIII.

[50] Claude Amyand to Jurin, 16 January 1724, RS *Classified Papers*, XXIII; published in *The Correspondence of James Jurin*, pp. 223–224.

[51] Jurin, *Account* (1724), p. 3.   [52] Jurin, *Account* (1724), p. 4.

The issue of permanent immunity was difficult to prove: Collecting reports of negative results of a form of human experimentation to convince others that inoculation did prevent individuals from later contracting natural smallpox was not an easy task, and although Jurin never explicitly requested information on this score, some individuals did perform and report the experiment. As late as 1730, Jurin received a letter from Dr. Oliver of Plymouth relating the case of two boys who had been inoculated six years earlier and who had just been exposed to a virulent form of smallpox with no ill effects. Dr. Oliver concluded his letter with the following plea: "I find it urg'd as a Strenuous Argument agt. Inoculation that the Inoculated are liable to have the Small Pox again by Infection in the natural Way. Some more Trials of this kind wou'd finally determine that Part of the dispute."[53] Strikingly, Jurin did not solicit instances of such trials, perhaps because of the questionable ethics of exposing inoculated patients to infected individuals.

To answer his second question about the hazard of inoculation, Jurin turned to a numerical approach. Here his task was simpler: He sought to enumerate the number of persons who were inoculated, and of those, how many survived and how many died, for in fact some did die from inoculation. A quick look at his categories, however, suggests that this process was not quite so straightforward. In his account for the year 1723, for example, Jurin listed 34 inoculators (17 surgeons, 7 apothecaries, 6 physicians, 2 ministers, and 2 women) who inoculated 483 persons. Of those 483:

> 440 had the small pox by inoculation,
> 5 had an "imperfect small pox by inoculation,"
> for 29 individuals the procedure had no effect,
> and 9 persons were "suspected to have died of inoculation."[54]

After exhibiting this tally, he subtracted the number of individuals on whom the operation had no effect, leaving the hazard of dying of inoculated smallpox to be 9 in 445, or roughly 1 in 49 or 50.

The category "imperfect small pox by inoculation" immediately leaps out from the above list and raises myriad questions about how individuals identified smallpox, how they distinguished an "imperfect" sort, and so on. A difficulty encountered by all concerned with inoculation stemmed from the vagaries of diagnosis. How did individuals determine whether they had contracted smallpox from inoculation? Were the symptoms of inoculated smallpox similar enough to natural smallpox to facilitate diagnosis? From the various reports it is clear that individuals reacted to inoculation in different ways, and that although a generalized case history could be abstracted (as Jurin and others did), many inoculated persons did not suffer from the typical symptoms. The challenges in

[53] William Oliver to Jurin, 29 July 1730, RS Early Letters O.2.182; published in *The Correspondence of James Jurin*, p. 385.
[54] Jurin, *Account* (1724), p. 17.

diagnosing one of the most externally visible diseases can be illustrated by one of Jurin's most hotly disputed cases.

George Percivall, age three, according to his mother Lady Catherine Percivall, was inoculated by the royal surgeon Claude Amyand on 5 May 1725.[55] Eight days following the operation, several pocks began to appear on his face, and the boy had a slight fever and quicker pulse. Over the next few days, approximately 120 pocks appeared on his body, but his mother wrote that "they were never so bad but that he could Whip a Top or beat a drum." Eleven days after the first pocks appeared, all the pocks had dried and flaked off, and after a few purges, Lady Percivall wrote, "I thank God he is as well as ever he was in his Life."[56] Three weeks later, however, George became ill, and he was attended by several physicians who offered their opinions on the case in letters to Jurin. Most of those who testified in this case agreed that George had 300 or 400 pustules that stayed from two to three days, and 5 or 6 larger pustules, which stayed much longer. Beyond this no one agreed. Dr. Monro, in a letter dated 14 April 1726, indicated that he met Amyand at the boy's house: "It was his [Amyand's] Opinion it was the Chicken pox in which the thickness of the Skin had pent the matter longer than usuall, to which I Answered poynting to that on his right hand, that I beleived we might from that Pimple inoculate the Small Pox."[57] Later in this letter, he stated that he told Lady Percivall that the larger pustules "were in all their Circumstances so like the Small Pox, that I could not tell what else to Call them, that the rest might be the Chicken Pox."[58]

In August of the same year, the surgeon Amyand wrote to Jurin that because "the Case of the honourable Master George Percivall having been differently reported; the Right Honble Lady Percivall his Mother has given me leave to take a Copy of her Journal of that Case, which for the publicks Satisfaction she is pleased to allow to be printed, as well as the Enclosed Letter." Amyand concluded his letter by asserting that George's second eruption was "nothing more than the Chicken Pox."[59] Jurin published selections from the letters written by Monro, Amyand, and Lady Percivall in his *Account* for the year 1725, and concluded: "From these Accounts it plainly appears, that this young Gentlemen had the Small-Pox by Inoculation; and whether the second Eruption deserves to be call'd the true Small-Pox, is left to the Reader's Judgment."[60]

---

[55] Jurin published the letters from Amyand and Lady Percivall in his *Account . . . for 1725* (1726), pp. 36–53.
[56] "A Copy of the Journall of the Right Honble. the Lady Percivall during the Inoculation of Her Son George aged 3 Years," RS *Classified Papers*, XXIII; reprinted in Jurin, *Account . . . for 1725* (1726), pp. 38–46.
[57] James Monro to [Jurin], 14 April 1726, RS *Classified Papers*, XXIII; published in Jurin, *Account . . . for 1725* (1726), pp. 50–53.
[58] James Monro to [Jurin], 14 April 1726, RS *Classified Papers*, XXIII; published in Jurin, *Account . . . for 1725* (1726), pp. 50–53.
[59] Claude Amyand to Jurin, 26 August 1725, RS *Classified Papers*, XXIII; reprinted in Jurin, *Account . . . for 1725* (1726), pp. 37–38.
[60] Jurin, *Account . . . for 1725* (1726), p. 54.

Throughout his published writings and in his correspondence, Jurin tried to downplay these difficulties in diagnosis and classification by rigidly reducing the variety of inoculation experiences to a limited number of categories. For polemical reasons or perhaps simply for reasons of exigency, Jurin selected the binary categories of life and death. "I need not give you the trouble of drawing up an Account of the accidents happening to any of your Inoculated Patients," Jurin wrote to Nettleton. "I think a Comparison between the naturall and inoculated Small Pox, in point of Life or Death will be sufficient. . . ."[61] In Nettleton's case, a young girl had been left deaf and mute after inoculation, but despite these afflictions, which might or might not have been the result of inoculation, Jurin counted the girl's inoculation experience as a success because it had not resulted in death.[62] Any disability that might have resulted from inoculation was thus pushed to the margins. In Jurin's scheme, inoculation failed in only two instances: 1) by causing death; or 2) by failing to protect the inoculated individual from a subsequent attack of smallpox. To be sure, Jurin offered some justification for this position. In his account for 1723, he argued that if accidents other than death resulting from inoculation were to be reported, so too should conditions emanating from natural smallpox.[63]

Jurin also welcomed accounts about natural smallpox mortality. Although he based his initial calculations on the London bills of mortality, he was fully aware of their shortcomings, and he recommended enumeration:

There is another Method, which, if it were put in practice in several large Towns, or Parishes, and for a sufficient Number of Years, would enable us to come at a nearer and still more certain computation of the Proportion between those that recover and those that die of the Small Pox: which is, to send a careful Person once a Year from house to house, to enquire what Persons have had Small Pox, and how many have died of it, the preceding year.[64]

Nettleton and Whitaker had in fact done just this. Others, too, furnished Jurin with natural smallpox mortality figures and assured him of their accuracy. For example, Dr. Thomas Dixon of Bolton Le Moors wrote: "The Account I here send you will I hope be acceptable being carefully and faithfully taken from house to house thro' this Town. The small Pox visited this place in May 1725 and did not leave us till Christmas. The number that have in the time mentioned been seized with the Small Pox is 341. The number that died of the Small Pox is 64."[65]

[61] Jurin to Thomas Nettleton, 31 March 1726, RS *Classified Papers*, XXIII; published in *The Correspondence of James Jurin*, pp. 334–335.

[62] Thomas Nettleton to Jurin, 17 November 1725; Nettleton to Jurin, 26 November 1725; and Nettleton to Jurin, 22 March 1726; RS *Classified Papers*, XXIII; published in *The Correspondence of James Jurin*, pp. 315–319, 331–332.

[63] Jurin, *Account* (1724), p. 29.   [64] Jurin, "A Letter to the Learned Caleb Cotesworth," p. 222.

[65] Thomas Dixon to Jurin, 15 February 1726, RS *Classified Papers*, XXIII.

	Sick of the Small Pox.	Died.
Several Towns in *Yorkſhire* — — 3405	—	636
Chicheſter — — — — — — 994	—	168
Haverford Weſt — — — — 227	—	52
Total 4626	**—**	**856**

2.5 James Jurin's table of smallpox morbidity and mortality outside of London (1722). *Source:* James Jurin, "A Letter to the Learned Dr. Caleb Cotesworth, ..." *Philosophical Transactions* 32, no. 374 (1722–1723): 23. Burndy Library, Dibner Institute for the History of Science and Technology.

A house-to-house survey was the only way to arrive at a precise figure. "This is a faithfull account," testified Dr. George Lynch of Canterbury, "and I believe may be depended upon being taken by a proper person going about from house to house."[66] But as with more general censuses, such enquiries provoked suspicion. Dr. Beard, after reporting smallpox mortality figures for Romsey, added: "I shall do the same for Worcester as soon as I can break thro' that formidable Objection of our Solemn Clarks viz numbering the People."[67] Smallpox was viewed as damaging to a community's image, and hence, some towns did not want mortality figures made public.[68]

When Jurin published this numerical information, he assured his readers that it was "communicated to me by Persons of Credit," and revealed his concern for authority and legitimacy.[69] He summarized their results in a table and stated that "upon a *medium* between these Accounts, there *died of the Small Pox almost 19 per Cent* or *nearly one in five*, of Person of all Ages, that underwent that Distemper."[70] (See Figure 2.5.) What emerged then was that smallpox was much more deadly outside of London. In the conclusions to his pamphlets, Jurin simply reiterated the hazards of dying from inoculated and natural smallpox, thus reinforcing his claim to present only matters of fact.

CHALLENGING THE ATYPICAL

In a letter to Dr. Richard Beard, Jurin made explicit his decision to suppress "typical" case histories: "I have made it a rule to my Self to publish no particular cases out of the great number that are sent me Except upon the death of the

---

[66] George Lynch to Jurin, 20 January 1727, RS *Classified Papers*, XXIII.
[67] Richard Beard to Jurin, 9 November 1726, RS *Classified Papers*, XXIII; published in *The Correspondence of James Jurin*, pp. 341–343.
[68] Perrott Williams wrote Jurin that in Pembroke smallpox "has entirely ceased above a twelvemonth ago, and I perceive some of the Inhabitants of that Town are (for some reasons to 'emselves best known) very unwilling to have the number of such as lost their lives by the Small-Pox discover'd, and consequently very industrious to conceal their Names etc." Perrott Williams to Jurin, 23 April 1724, RS Early Letters W.3.132; published in *The Correspondence of James Jurin*, pp. 243–244.
[69] Jurin, *Account* (1724), p. 7.   [70] Jurin, "A Letter to the Learned Caleb Cotesworth," p. 223.

party, or any dispute about his having the distemper a second time."[71] After his initial publication, the unique and atypical case history became the subject of concern and publication, testimony to the overwhelming power of one case to dissuade individuals from inoculation. "[I]f any thing goes amiss or seems to do so, the world presently sings of it with all the Aggravations imaginable, but on the other hand many Successfull Experiments are I believe buryed in Silence," wrote Edward Edlin to Jurin in 1726.[72] Dr. Bayly, writing from Havant, conveyed similar sentiments when referring to a patient who did not contract smallpox from inoculation: "In two or three Days afterwards the Incisions were quite healed up and the Patient perfectly well in Body but greatly mortifyed at this Disappointment which also discouraged Some others who were resolved to have been Inoculated, if this Case had Succeeded as well as the former. Thus a Stop was put to the Practice of Inoculation in this Place."[73]

Jurin himself, painfully aware of the imbalance between success and failure, acknowledged the limitations of his quantitative approach in his *Account* for the year 1725:

But though the affirmative Side of this Question cannot be fully establish'd under a considerable Length of Time, and a great Number of Experiments; the Negative may indeed admit of an easier Proof: For a small Number of Instances of Persons receiving the Small-Pox by Inoculation, and having them afterwards in the natural Way, will be sufficient to convince the Publick, that Inoculation is no Security from the naturall Small-Pox.[74]

To remedy the disproportionate effects of negative reports, the atypical case became the subject of extensive case histories in Jurin's later pamphlets, while those individuals who suffered no unusual complaints or symptoms in their course of inoculated smallpox were simply added to his list of successful cases. Thus, for his 1725 account, Jurin devoted only 10 pages to a general discussion of inoculation, but 43 pages to three particularly disputed cases.[75] Underlining this change in focus from the positive to the negative, Jurin added two paragraphs to his advertisement asking for detailed reports of any inoculation cases that either produced no illness or resulted in death.[76]

Jurin had to investigate very carefully all reports that called inoculation into doubt, and the majority of his later pamphlets treated eyewitness accounts of contested cases. One colorful example appeared in the account for the year 1725. The disputed case concerned a child who was supposedly inoculated in the town of Oswestry in Shropshire by a surgeon named Mr. Jones. In the appendix

---

[71] Jurin to Richard Beard, 3 December 1726, RS *Classified Papers,* XXIII; published in *The Correspondence of James Jurin,* pp. 343–344.

[72] Edward Edlin to Jurin, 15 September 1726, RS *Classified Papers,* XXIII.

[73] Edward Bayly to Jurin, Feb. 19, 1724, RS *Classified Papers,* XXIII; published in *The Correspondence of James Jurin,* pp. 230–234.

[74] Jurin, *Account . . . for 1725* (1726), pp. 10–11.   [75] Jurin, *Account . . . for 1725* (1726).

[76] Jurin, *Account . . . for 1725* (1726), unnumbered last two pages.

to a pamphlet published in 1725, Dr. William Clinch cited this case as an instance when an inoculated individual later succumbed to natural smallpox.[77] In response to this pamphlet, Jurin sent letters to a local minister, Mr. Parry, and to Jones, in an attempt to assess the veracity of Dr. Clinch's claims. In his letter to Jones, Jurin noted that

> this matter has Occasioned a great deal of Talk here in Town, as some persons have made it a Question of whether the Child was really Inoculated or not. I am Sensible, Sir, how Dear every honest Man must hold his Reputation, & therefore am concerned to tell you how far yours is affected by these disputes: but the Remedy lies in your own hands by clearing up the truth in such a manner as may be satisfactory to the World.[78]

Jurin received a prompt response from the minister Parry, who doubted Jones's claims to have performed the inoculation because Jones would neither show the incision marks on the child nor identify the person from whom he had taken the infectious matter. Parry cast further doubt on Jones's character in a postscript by suggesting that the surgeon had been inspired by greed: "What he says in Answer to yours is, that if you will give him an handsome reward, he will come up to London, and declare to you the whole State of the Case, and will bring witnesses along with him to prove it upon Oath."[79] Jurin agreed with Parry that Jones's credibility had been severely undermined, but nonetheless Jurin asked for further inquiries. In a rather self-righteous tone, Jurin charged that he could not understand "why he [Jones] should expect what he calls a handsome reward from me, who neither have, nor desire any other recompence for the pains I have taken in my Inquiries about Inoculation, than the Satisfaction of doing some Service to my Countrey. . . ."[80]

Almost two weeks later, Jones himself wrote to Jurin and confessed that "I cannot say that I have Inoculated my own Child nor any body else because I do not know what reall Inoculation is."[81] And Parry added his own postscript to the affair: "What Mr. Jones has said concerning Inoculation is all Rodomontade."[82] In a final letter concerning this matter, Mr. Tomkies, a surgeon in Oswestry, stated that Jones was "a fellow of no Consideration nor ought to be allowed of the profession, he was brought up a weaver & followed that Occupation till I know not by what Inspiration he undertook the Healing Faculty of Physick and

---

[77] William Clinch, *An Historical Essay on the Rise and Progress of the Small-Pox. To Which Is Added, a Short Appendix, to Prove, That Inoculation Is No Security from Natural Small-Pox* (London, 1725).

[78] Jurin to David Jones, 22 February 1726, RS *Classified Papers,* XXIII; also see Jurin, *Account . . . for 1725* (1726).

[79] Edward Parry to Jurin, 1 March 1726, RS *Classified Papers,* XXIII; also see Jurin, *Account . . . for 1725* (1726).

[80] Jurin to Edward Parry, 5 March 1726, RS *Classified Papers,* XXIII; also see Jurin, *Account . . . for 1725* (London, 1726).

[81] David Jones to Edward Parry, 11 March 1726, RS *Classified Papers,* XXIII; also see Jurin, *Account . . . for 1725* (1726).

[82] Edward Parry to Jurin, 13 March 1726, RS *Classified Papers,* XXIII.

Surgery without being able to read English."[83] Jones's report became thoroughly discredited, in part because of his own confession of ignorance regarding inoculation, but also in part through the knowledge of his personal history and family background. In this instance and others, Jurin relied upon social status as a way to guarantee the accuracy of the accounts sent in by unknown correspondents.

From this detailed discussion of a case history, one may conclude that individual case histories continued to be very powerful tools for convincing others. The fact that Jurin devoted considerable effort to challenging those case histories that undermined inoculation, along with the fact that he published the correspondence relating to disputed cases in his annual account, indicates that he was fully aware of the limitations of his numerical approach. Yet at the same time, it is important to stress the vulnerability of case histories as the above instance demonstrates. By their very nature, case histories give rise to questions of authority and testimony. Whose case histories in correspondence are to be regarded as accurate and admitted as evidence? Since Jurin did not know the majority of his correspondents, whose testimony was he to believe, and on whose authority? Part of his correspondence campaign was designed precisely to undermine the testimony of those who presented case histories that purportedly demonstrated the ineffectiveness or danger of inoculation.

Other inoculation pamphlets addressed these same concerns. In 1722, for example, David Neal suggested that stories from Africans concerning inoculation practices should not be accorded full credibility. Neal was referring to an account that originated in New England. "[T]he Truth of this Relation depending chiefly upon the Testimony of *Negroes*," he remarked, should make it "worth while to consult some of our English Traders to those Parts, before we give entire Credit to it."[84] On the other extreme, one pamphleteer stated that the testimony "given by *Gentlemen* of *Learning* to such a Body as that of the *Royal Society*" concerning inoculation left him no choice but to "give Credit to their *Testimony*, in a Matter of Fact whereof they were Eye-Witnesses."[85] Somewhere in between Africans and the gentlemen of the Royal Society, but probably nearer to the latter, lay the testimonies of doctors, surgeons, and apothecaries. Jurin's correspondence reveals these processes of weighing, judging, and legitimating testimony in the form of case histories.

THE APPEAL OF CALCULATION

Jurin received many testimonials to the persuasiveness of his approach of comparing the mortality of inoculated and natural smallpox. Dr. John Woodhouse

---

[83] Mr. Tomkies to Claudius Amyand, 5 September 1726, RS *Classified Papers*, XXIII.
[84] David Neal, *A Narrative of the Method and Success of Inoculating the Small Pox in New England*, (London, 1722), p. 6.
[85] Benjamin Colman, *Some Observations on the New Method of Receiving the Small-Pox by Ingrafting or Inoculating* (Boston, 1721), p. 1.

of Nottingham, for example, gave Jurin "hearty thanks for your good Intentions to the Publick by continuing This Annuall Account which will I doubt not soon Convince all Enemys to this Practice and Establish it for the great benefit of Mankind."[86] Others, such as Dr. Dixon, focused specifically on the advantages of Jurin's numerical method: "I think the Method you pursue of convincing the World by matter of Fact is fair & Just & prejudices in reference to Inoculation can I think, be removed by no other means."[87] Likewise, Dr. Perrott Williams of Haverfordwest in Wales praised Jurin's method. "Yet I doubt not," he declared, "but posterity will hold 'emselves obliged to you for the pains you have taken in drawing up yr accurate Calculations, together with the undeniable Conclusions, necessarily flowing from 'em."[88]

Jurin's faithful friend Nettleton remarked on the impartiality of the numbers: "Your Pieces have been every where well received so far as I can learn, & the more because of the strict Neutrality you observe between the contending Partys. The less you appear to favour the side of Inoculation & the more weight your impartial Representation of it will have with the generality of Mankind who are very much prejudiced against it."[89] And most telling of all, at least one individual declared that Jurin's numerical arguments had persuaded him to inoculate his only daughter. Mr. Edlin of Holborn in London stated that "the disproportion between the Chance of death in the small Pox by naturall Infection & by Inoculation as it appears in your Books be such as makes me entertain thoughts of Inoculating the only Child I have as soon as she is able to give so distinct an Account of what she ails to enable us to apply proper Remedyes."[90]

Physicians writing in midcentury accorded Jurin's work a prominent place in the eventual acceptance of inoculation. James Burges, in *An Account of the Preparation and Management Necessary to Inoculation* (1754), perceived that quantitative arguments were very persuasive, and he provided a brief history of the acceptance of inoculation to illustrate their role. Those who opposed inoculation, Burges wrote, did so "with all the arguments their wit and prejudices could furnish." Those who supported the practice, on the other hand, had "recourse to calculation, by comparing the numbers of those that died in the natural ways, with that of the persons that miscarried under the inoculation, by demonstrating how small the chance was of escaping the distemper, and how little the hazard incurred from this new method of contracting it." Burges concluded that Jurin's approach "carried such conviction with it, as soon confounded their opposers,

---

[86] John Woodhouse to Jurin, 9 February 1726, RS *Classified Papers,* XXIII.

[87] Thomas Dixon to Jurin, 15 February 1726, RS *Classified Papers,* XXIII.

[88] Perrott Williams to Jurin, 19 March 1723, RS Early Letters W.3.131; published in *The Correspondence of James Jurin,* pp. 139–140.

[89] Thomas Nettleton to Jurin, 31 May 1725, RS Early Letters N.1.98; published in *The Correspondence of James Jurin,* pp. 304–306.

[90] Edward Edlin to Jurin, 15 September 1726, RS *Classified Papers,* XXIII.

and established the practice."[91] Others highlighted the role that royal patronage played, but at the same time stressed the importance of Jurin's work. In 1760, Dr. Davies of Bath attributed the acceptance of inoculation to two events: "to the countenance it received from the Royal Family, and to the abilities and integrity of Dr. Jurin, who undertook the office of a candid historian, putting that practice to the fair test of experience."[92]

Among those who objected to Jurin's approach, only a few questioned the relevancy of calculations to medicine. Jurin's most prominent opponent, Dr. William Wagstaffe, summarily dismissed Jurin's figures by describing them as "some obscure and improper Calculations, scarcely intelligible to any body, or if intelligible, altogether foreign to the Purpose."[93] Mathematics, in the mind of this respected physician, had no place in medical theory or practice. This conservative reaction, which drew clear boundaries between the pursuit of mathematics and the pursuit of medicine, was echoed faintly throughout the century by physicians who desired to maintain traditional approaches to medicine.

More typical criticisms addressed the adequacy of Jurin's calculations and figures. Two apothecaries, Francis Howgrave and Isaac Massey, for example, challenged Jurin's work by concentrating on what they saw as fundamental differences between the two groups of people, those with natural smallpox and those with inoculated smallpox, that were being explicitly compared. Howgrave's argument focused on the fact that inoculators recommended that only the strong get inoculated. This initial choice therefore biased the results since natural smallpox struck strong and weak alike. The healthier an individual, the more likely he or she would survive inoculated or natural smallpox.[94]

Massey's critique was even more sophisticated and incorporated health and economic considerations. Massey disputed Jurin's use of the bills of mortality, "wherein no Account is made or supposed of those who die of that Distemper for want of proper Necessaries, and by the ignorance of practising Nurses...."[95] He continued:

The Use I would make of this Observation, is, to shew how insufficient and improper any comparison must needs be between such indigent sick, and the *Inoculated*, who have all imaginable Care and Help afforded them, and for any Person to estimate and compare the success between Patients, *under such unequal Circumstances*, is what, I believe, you did *not well attend to*, or will hereafter *think pertinent to the case in Hand*.[96]

---

[91] James Burges, *An Account of the Preparation and Management Necessary to Inoculation* (London, 1754), pp. vi–vii.

[92] Quoted in James Mackenzie, *The History of Health and the Art of Preserving It* (Edinburgh, 1760), p. 430.

[93] Wagstaffe, *A Letter to Dr. Freind*, p. 48. Wagstaffe's objections were directed against Arbuthnot's pamphlet, but one can assume he felt similarly about Jurin's approach.

[94] Francis Howgrave, *Reasons against the Inoculating the Small-Pox* (London, 1724), p. 69.

[95] Isaac Massey, *A Short and Plain Account of Inoculation*, 2d ed. (London, 1723), postscript, p. 2.

[96] Massey, *Short and Plain Account*, postscript, p. 3.

Only the healthy and wealthy were inoculated, while the deaths attributed to smallpox recorded in the bills of mortality generally referred to the poor and frequently unhealthy. Massey put his point succinctly: "[T]o form a just comparison, and calculate right in this case, the Circumstances of the Patients, must and ought to be as near as may be on a Par."[97] Arguments such as these focused not on the relevancy of numerical arguments in medicine but on the representativeness and accuracy of calculations. At the heart of quantification is classification: Numbers cannot be compared unless and until the things represented by the numbers are the same, or are made to be equivalent.

The numerical arguments introduced by Jurin and Arbuthnot were in large part a direct response to the heated and unresolved controversy surrounding inoculation. "I have no Inclination to enter into this Controversy; it is in better and abler Hands," Jurin asserted,

> but, as the Point in Dispute is of the utmost Importance to Mankind, I heartily wish, that without Passion, Prejudice, or private Views, it may be fairly and maturely examin'd. In order to which, if the following Extracts and Computations, concerning the comparative Danger of the Inoculated and Natural Small Pox, may be of any Use to your self, or to other impartial and disinterested Judges, I shall think my Labour well bestowed.[98]

A comparison of the risks of inoculated and natural smallpox expressed numerically allowed a particular audience, in Jurin's words "impartial and disinterested Judges," to evaluate the safety of the procedure without considering its religious, moral, or ethical dimensions.

Nettleton had a more telling phrase to describe this approach. He called it "the merchants logick" and defined it as follows: "[S]tate the Account of Profitt & Loss to find on which side the Ballance lyes with respect to the Publick, & form a Judgement accordingly."[99] This approach balanced public benefit with personal risk and asked the physician to weigh the welfare of a population against the health of the individual patient. Merchant's logic argued that physicians should calculate the utility of particular practices by summing up the costs and benefits among a population of patients. This definition of reasonableness as economic self-interest, of course, was not limited to medical matters; historians and philosophers have noted its emergence in a variety of contexts over the course of the seventeenth century.[100]

The appeal of numerical arguments in times of protracted, heated controversy is telling. Numerical arguments, at least those constructed by Jurin, Arbuthnot,

---

[97] Massey, *Short and Plain Account,* postscript, p. 5.
[98] James Jurin, "A Letter to the Learned Caleb Cotesworth," p. 214.
[99] Thomas Nettleton to James Jurin, 24 January 1723, RS Early Letters N.1.95; published in *The Correspondence of James Jurin,* p. 126.
[100] Lorraine Daston has summarized the literature on this topic; see Daston, *Classical Probability in the Enlightenment* (Princeton, N. J.: Princeton University Press, 1988), pp. 58–67.

and Nettleton, led to a single conclusion, in this case that the risks of inoculation were substantially less than those of natural smallpox. By defining the issue in this way, anyone could look at the calculations, make the numerical comparison, and draw the intended conclusion. All three men expressed their belief in the transparency of their arguments. This form of argument was not considered mechanical, as it would later be in the machine age of the nineteenth century. Instead, it was considered indicative of reason, of rationality, and hence was part of the dominant discourse of Enlightenment thought. All reasonable men, the argument went, would think along similar lines and draw the same conclusions.[101]

[101] Daston discussed this view of the *homme éclairé*. See Daston, *Classical Probability,* pp. 49–58.

3

The Limits of Calculation: French Debates over Inoculation in the 1760s

> It is not therefore a question here of moral philosophy or theology, it is a matter of calculation: let us avoid making a case of conscience out of a problem of arithmetic.
>
> Charles-Marie de La Condamine (1754)

> In vain the *savants* persuade themselves of the utility of inoculation. There must be a general conviction for this method to be established.
>
> Jean-Antoine Butini (1752)[1]

In his letter on inoculation (1733), Voltaire noted that the "Christian countries of *Europe*" considered the English "Fools and Madmen. Fools, because they give their Children the small-pox to prevent their catching it; and Mad-men, because they wantonly communicate a certain and dreadful Distemper to their Children, merely to prevent an uncertain Evil." The English, on the other hand, he continued, "call the rest of the *Europeans* cowardly and unnatural. Cowardly, because they are afraid of putting their Children to a little Pain; un-natural, because they expose them to die one Time or other of the Small-pox."[2] This wide gulf separating English and French views of inoculation was not bridged until late in the eighteenth century, when the death of Louis XV from smallpox in 1774 silenced most opponents. This is not to say that there were no individuals who promoted inoculation in France – many of the *philosophes* were outspoken advocates. Voltaire's letter on inoculation, wedged between his letters on English government and the English philosophers Bacon, Newton, and Locke, literally placed inoculation on the agenda of enlightened subjects and, at the same time, cemented its association with the English. But unlike

---

[1] Charles-Marie de La Condamine, "Mémoire sur l'inoculation de la petite vérole," *Mémoires de l'Académie Royale des Sciences* 1754 (Paris, 1759), p. 655; Jean-Antoine Butini, *Traité de la petite vérole, communiquée par l'inoculation* (Paris, 1752), p. 4. All translations are by the author unless otherwise noted.

[2] Voltaire, Letter XI, "On Inoculation," *Letters Concerning the English Nation*, ed. with and Introduction and Notes by Nicholas Cronk (Oxford: Oxford University Press, 1994), p. 44.

their English counterparts, French favorers of inoculation were largely unable to convince the public and, more specifically, physicians.[3]

The French debates over inoculation were in many ways similar to those in England. Religious objections, for instance, centered on the question of whether inoculation interfered with divine providence. Likewise, medical opponents considered whether a preventive measure such as inoculation fell within the scope of medical practice, or if medicine should remain primarily curative. In other ways, the debates were very different. The French, for instance, considered the *legal* aspects of inoculation far more thoroughly than did their English counterparts. In particular, they wrestled over issues of liability: Who was to be responsible for the death of an inoculated person? Other cultural differences came to the fore. Many believed that an individual could have smallpox more than once, thus making inoculation a useless practice. Some even held that smallpox was less lethal in France than England and, hence, there was less urgency to be inoculated.

In France, the role of numerical arguments in the inoculation debates was constrained by the social and professional location of those who picked them up. Mathematicians and natural philosophers crafted highly sophisticated numerical arguments in support of inoculation. French physicians did not want to touch these arguments, and more significantly they rejected, out of hand, the basic idea that mathematics had a place in medicine. There were no individuals like Jurin and Arbuthnot, who were practicing physicians *and* mathematicians. The result was a bifurcated controversy: One branch took place at the Paris Faculté de Médecine and the other in the Paris Académie des Sciences.

THE PARIS FACULTÉ DE MÉDECINE

The inoculations performed in London in the 1720s, especially of the royal princesses, were closely followed by the French elite through personal reports and news items in *Journal de Trévoux* and *Journal des Savants*.[4] A few English pamphlets were translated, including William Wagstaffe's *Letter to Dr. Freind* and Jurin's *An Account of the Success of Inoculating the Smallpox in Great Britain*.[5]

---

[3] The French reluctance to practice inoculation has been discussed by several scholars. See Genevieve Miller, *The Adoption of Inoculation for Smallpox in England and France* (Philadelphia: University of Pennsylvania Press, 1957), pp. 180–240; Jean-François de Raymond, *Querelle de l'inoculation ou préhistoire de la vaccination* (Paris: Librairie Philosophique J. Vrin, 1982); Pierre Darmon, *La Longue traque de la vérole: Les pionniers de la médecine préventive*, Collection Pour l'Histoire (Paris: Librairie Académique Perrin, 1986), pp. 75–142; Pierre Darmon, *La variole, les nobles et les princes: La petite vérole mortelle de Louis XV* (Brussels: Éditions Complexe, 1989), pp. 49–81.

[4] Miller, *The Adoption of Inoculation*, p. 180.

[5] The translation of Wagstaffe's pamphlet was published in 1722. Jurin's pamphlet was translated by Pierre Noguez, *Relation du succès de l'inoculation de la petite vérole dans la Grande-Bretagne* (Paris, 1725), and subsequently included in Jean Etienne Montucla, *Recueil de pièces concernant l'inoculation de la petite vérole, et propres à en prouver la sécurité et l'utilité* (Paris, 1756), pp. 80–117.

Correspondence provides further clues about the reception of inoculation in Paris during this time. The Parisian physician Jean Delacoste, for instance, asked Sir Hans Sloane, one of the central figures in the Newgate inoculations, for guidance on how to persuade fellow French physicians to take up the practice.[6] Delacoste had had "a very serious conversation with the King's [Louis XV] first Physician, Mr. Doddard [Claude-Jean-Baptiste Dodart], concerning the Inoculation of the Small Pox." Dodart wanted to introduce the practice of inoculation and had even sought a religious ally, "the Bishop of Fréjus the king's preceptor to obviate the clamours of some stiff Divines," as well as a legal ally, "the Attorney General to have his Leave and thereby to prevent being troubled if any shoud die of it, etc." Despite these precautions, Delacoste and Dodart encountered resistance and were anxious to know "through what motives the King of England has been prevailed with to encourage that practice and if you [Sloane] find it taken among the people notwithstanding the argument us'd against it by several physicians and Divines."[7] Delacoste and Dodart had been rebuffed by a hostile review in *Journal des Savants,* which argued that inoculation was "against the views of the Creator."[8] While Delacoste and Dodart received some royal patronage, they did not enjoy the support of any learned societies. On the contrary, the Paris Faculté de Médecine aggressively opposed inoculation.

During the first half of the century, the die-hard conservatives among France's elite medical bodies, most prominently the Paris Faculté de Médecine, quashed inoculation. The institutional structure of French medicine disciplined the activities of individual physicians and circumscribed the legal and cultural space for medical entrepreneurship that flourished in England. French medicine was, in principle, firmly under the control of local corporations, notably faculties of medicine and colleges of medicine.[9] In 1707, the Edict of Marly formalized this arrangement by granting to faculties the sole right to determine who could practice medicine within their territory. A physician who received a degree from a particular faculty would be licensed to practice medicine only where the degree-granting faculty had jurisdiction.[10] Although this corporative

---

[6] Miller, *The Adoption of Inoculation,* pp. 182–183.

[7] Jean Delacoste to Hans Sloane, Paris, 15 June 1723, British Library, Sloane Ms 4047, f. 5.

[8] Cited in Paul Delaunay, *Le monde médical parisien au dix-huitième siècle* (Paris, 1906), p. 281.

[9] For an insightful and detailed analysis of French medicine in this period, see Laurence Brockliss and Colin Jones's comprehensive *The Medical World of Early Modern France* (Oxford: Clarendon Press, 1997), esp. pp. 1–33; and Matthew Ramsey, *Professional and Popular Medicine in France, 1770–1830* (Cambridge: Cambridge University Press, 1988), esp. pp. 17–70.

[10] See *Edit du Roi donné à Marly au mois de mars 1707. Portant règlement générale pour les Facultés de Médecine du royaume* (Paris, 1707). Cited in Matthew Ramsey, *Professional and Popular Medicine,* p. 20; also see Caroline Hannaway, "Medicine, Public Welfare and the State in Eighteenth-Century France: The Société Royale de Médecine of Paris (1776–1793)," (Ph.D. dissertation, Johns Hopkins University, 1974), p. 21. Exceptions existed to this arrangement: Graduates of Paris, Montpellier, and Avignon were in principle granted the right to practice *urbi et orbi* (in the town and in the world) and *hic et ubique terrarum* (here and everywhere on earth). But, in fact, local corporations for the most part required that a physician become an *agregé.* See Ramsey, p. 40.

structure was under sustained attack throughout the eighteenth century (it was only dismantled during the Revolution, when in March 1791 almost all corporate structures were abolished), it effectively discouraged innovation in the day-to-day practice of French medicine.[11]

Most scholars locate the cause for the "regressive" nature of French medicine during the eighteenth century in the Paris Faculté, historically the most powerful medical institution in France.[12] Certainly the Faculté's position on inoculation confirms this interpretation. In December 1723, the medical student Claude de La Vigne de Frécheville presented to a receptive Paris Faculté a thesis entitled "An variolas inoculare nefas?" which argued that inoculation was harmful and contrary to divine will.[13] The following year, Philippe Hecquet, an older, well-established Faculté member and a "sworn enemy to all novelty in medicine," anonymously published an influential pamphlet that likewise condemned inoculation.[14] Hecquet's criticism resembled that of William Wagstaffe: Inoculation could not be explained using contemporary medical theory nor justified by numerical arguments. Together, Frécheville and Hecquet established the position that the Faculté took on inoculation.

The Paris Faculté's rejection of inoculation was not at all out of character. By the eighteenth century they were renowned for their prohibition on the use of the drugs antimony and cinchona, as well as for their dismissal of William Harvey's theory of the circulation of the blood. Although surgeons, apothecaries, and unorthodox healers of all stripes challenged these dictates, the Faculté did not admit any new medical knowledge into its corpus after the mid–seventeenth century.[15]

The sole institution in France powerful enough to sustain alternative approaches to medicine (in particular, vitalism) was the medical school at Montpellier. Its exceptionalism stemmed from the patronage of the French royalty, who traditionally appointed Montpellier graduates as royal physicians.[16]

---

[11] See Brockliss and Jones, *The Medical World of Early Modern France,* esp. Chapters 8, 9, and 10.
[12] The French medical historian Paul Delaunay has commented, "A cette époque la vieille Faculté de médecine était en pleine décadence." Delaunay, *Le monde médical parisien,* p. 22. Also see J.C. Sabatier, *Recherches historiques sur la Faculté de Médecine de Paris* (Paris, 1835), chap. 5, pp. 76–90.
[13] See Miller, *The Adoption of Inoculation,* pp. 185–189.
[14] Quotation from Théodore Tronchin, "L'Inoculation," *Encyclopédie ou Dictionnaire Raisonné des Sciences, des Arts et des Métiers,* 1st ed., (Neufchastel, 1765), vol. 8, p. 756. [Hecquet, Philippe], *Observations sur la saignée du pied, et sur la purgation au commencement de la petite vérole, des fièvres malignes & des grandes maladies. Preuves de décadence dans la pratique de médecine, confirmées par de justes raisons de doute contre l'inoculation* (Paris, 1724). For a discussion of Hecquet, see Miller, *The Adoption of Inoculation,* pp. 191–192.
[15] Maurice Raynaud, *Les Médecins au Temps de Molière* (Paris, 1863), p. 19; cited in Miller, *The Adoption of Inoculation,* p. 187; also see Brockliss and Jones, *The Medical World of Early Modern France,* pp. 470–473 and passim.
[16] The medical school of Montpellier has a long tradition dating back to the late Middle Ages, when many of the rich medical collections of the Arabic world were translated into Latin at Montpellier. During the eighteenth century, the physicians at Montpellier developed a distinctive strain of medical thought that stressed vitalistic forces. See Louis Dulieu, *La Médecine à Montpellier,* 2 vols. (Paris: Les

Royal physicians were allowed to practice anywhere in France, including Paris, without being members of the particular local faculty of medicine. Their royal status conferred upon them considerable power over the practice of medicine throughout France.[17] Not surprisingly, antagonism often flared between the royal physicians and the members of the Paris Faculté, most of whom had received their degrees in Paris.[18] While the Montpellier Faculté did not formally embrace inoculation, several of its graduates, such as Jean-Antoine Butini, did advocate its adoption.

INOCULATION À LA MODE

The early advocates of inoculation were not French physicians: Pro-inoculators were either physicians who were not French, or French who were not physicians. The former included the Italian Angelo Gatti and the Swiss Théodore Tronchin.[19] The latter were the *philosophes,* among whom Voltaire was the most prominent. He launched the philosophes' campaign with his essay "On Inoculation," which appeared first in English in 1733 and one year later in French in his *Lettres philosophiques.*[20] Voltaire's fondness for the English was well known, and this included an affection for one of their leading philosophical physicians, James Jurin. "Who loves liberty must live in England," Voltaire decided, and "who loves truth ought to read your good authors especially Mr. Jurin."[21]

Théodore Tronchin held an equally high regard for Jurin. "The account of the success of the new method by M. Jurin was the best response that one could make against the rantings of M. Hecquet," Tronchin asserted.[22] In his

Presses Universelles, 1972); and Colin Jones, "La Vie et les revendications des étudiants en médecine à Montpellier au XVIIIe siècle," *Actes du 110e Congrès National des Sociétés Savantes* (Montpellier, 1985), pp. 117–128; Brockliss and Jones, *The Medical World of Early Modern France,* passim; and Elizabeth Williams, *The Physical and the Moral: Anthropology, Physiology, and Philosophical Medicine in France, 1750–1850* (Cambridge: Cambridge University Press, 1994).

[17] Miller, *The Adoption of Inoculation,* p. 188.

[18] See Brockliss and Jones, *The Medical World of Early Modern France,* pp. 330–333; Caroline Hannaway, "Medicine, Public Welfare and the State," pp. 26–28. Also see Charles C. Gillispie, *Science and Polity in France at the End of the Old Regime* (Princeton, N.J.: Princeton University Press, 1980), pp. 216–218; A. Courlieu, *L'Ancienne Faculté de Médecine de Paris* (Paris, 1877), pp. 199–200. For an account of the royal physicians during the eighteenth century and their privileges, see Delaunay, *Le monde médical parisien,* chap. 4, pp. 93–165.

[19] Arnold H. Rowbotham, "The 'Philosophes' and the Propaganda for Inoculation of Smallpox in Eighteenth-Century France," *University of California Publications in Modern Philology* 18 (1935): 265–290; on Gatti and Tronchin, see Miller, *The Adoption of Inoculation,* chap. 8. Brockliss and Jones argue that French physicians embraced inoculation after 1750; Brockliss and Jones, *The Medical World of Early Modern France,* pp. 470–472.

[20] Voltaire, "Sur l'insertion de la Petite Vérole," *Lettres philosophiques* (1734). Following Louis XV's death from smallpox, Voltaire again argued for inoculation in *De la Mort de Louis XV et de la fatalité.* See Rowbotham, "The 'Philosophes' and the Propaganda for Inoculation," p. 280.

[21] Voltaire to James Jurin, [1741], Wellcome MS photocopy 6146; reprinted in *The Correspondence of James Jurin,* pp. 431–432.

[22] Théodore Tronchin, "L'Inoculation," *Encyclopédie ou Dictionnaire Raisonné des Sciences, des Arts et des Métiers,* 1st ed., Vol. 8 (Neufchastel, 1765), p. 756.

lengthy article on inoculation for the *Encyclopédie,* Tronchin cited Jurin's figures regarding the mortality of inoculated and natural smallpox, and calculated how many people would be saved annually in Paris if everyone were inoculated. "It is therefore demonstrated," Tronchin asserted, "that the establishment of inoculation would save the life of twelve or thirteen hundred citizens each year in the city of Paris alone."[23]

Tronchin, along with Angelo Gatti, became the leading inoculators in France during the 1750s and 1760s. Among the Parisian aristocracy, they were known as the "variolateurs à la mode."[24] According to the historian Paul Delaunay, Tronchin's popularity was so great that

all the women of quality went to consult him, the carriages formed a queue at his door as they do at the entrance to the Comedy. It was a craze [*engouement*], the shop-windows displayed bonnets *à l'inoculation,* ample gowns *à la Tronchin* or *tronchines. . . .*[25]

The practice of inoculation, however, never became popular outside aristocratic circles in France as it had in England.[26]

The fad for inoculation among the aristocracy did provoke a pamphlet war. In 1752, the Montpellier physician Jean-Antoine Butini reopened the controversy among physicians with his *Traité de la petite vérole, communiquée par l'inoculation* that discussed in detail the operation of inoculation and how it differed from natural smallpox. Butini was motivated to write the pamphlet in the hope that a physician's voice would add credence to the philosophes' campaign. "In vain the *savants* persuade themselves of the utility of inoculation," he remarked. "There must be a general conviction for this method to be established."[27] To this end, Butini cited the figures and calculations made by Jurin and reported the numbers of inoculations performed in Geneva. "The strongest proof of the justness of reasonings in physical matters," Butini remarked, "is their confirmation by experience; it seals the matter and completes persuasion."[28]

Widely admired for their impartiality, Jurin's tables, ratios, and numerical arguments were often the only quantitative information found in French

---

[23] Tronchin, "L'Inoculation," p. 767.   [24] Delaunay, *Le monde médical parisien,* p. 291.

[25] Delaunay, *Le monde médical parisien,* p. 283.

[26] There are a few exceptions. See, for example, "Tableau des inoculations faites en Franche-Comté pendant les années, 1776 & 1777," *Histoire de la Société Royale de Médecine,* 1777/1778 (Paris, 1780), pp. 187–193. Jean-Pierre Goubert's detailed study of medicine in eighteenth-century Brittany indicated that parish priests hampered efforts to inoculate, and of those medical men who did practice inoculation, they did so on a much smaller scale than inoculators in England. For example, a Dr. Bagot from Brittany reported 50 inoculations that he performed from 1774 to 1784; compare this with the Sutton family's claim that they inoculated 300,000 people in 30 years. See Jean-Pierre Goubert, *Malades et médecins en Bretagne, 1770–1790* (Rennes: Institut Armoricain de Recherches Historiques, 1974), pp. 323–328; and Peter Razzell, *The Conquest of Smallpox: The Impact of Inoculation on Smallpox Mortality in Eighteenth Century Britain* (Sussex: Caliban Books, 1977), p. 67. See Chapter 4 for more on Sutton.

[27] Jean-Antoine Butini, *Traité de la petite vérole, communiquée par l'inoculation* (Paris, 1752), p. 4.

[28] Butini, *Traité de la petite vérole,* p. 39.

pamphlets. The Parisian physician Louis-Charles-Henri Macquart, for example, urged his readers to examine and listen to "legitimate and weighty judges: Mr. Jurin, Doctor of Medicine and Secretary to the Royal Society, followed this operation exactly without taking sides."[29] Even opponents of inoculation referred favorably to Jurin's writings. Jean Astruc, a prominent member of the Paris Faculté de Médecine, considered inoculation a dangerous practice, but nonetheless held high regard for Jurin's work. "Among those [works on inoculation] that seem to me to be the most solidly written, I think the first rank must be given to the treatise by M. Jurin, Doctor of Medicine, entitled 'A Letter to the Learned Caleb Cotesworth.'"[30]

The Swiss physician Samuel Tissot took the further step of arguing that not only the numbers but the English texts needed to be made available to the French. In his *L'Inoculation justifiée* (1754), Tissot wanted to publicize "the works that are available on inoculation . . . written in Latin or English" that were unknown "in the country where only French is spoken." What was "astonishing" to Tissot was that no one had bothered to translate these works, a fact that proved the "strong national prejudices that blind everyone."[31] Two years later, Tissot's complaints were answered when the mathematician Jean-Etienne Montucla published a translation of Jurin's *Account of the Success of Inoculating the Smallpox,* along with other essays on inoculation.[32]

In all of these instances, physicians cited already published figures, but they did not develop numerical arguments of their own. This was not the case for several mathematicians who embraced and expanded the quantitative approach initially developed in England. Much like the Royal Society in the 1720s, the Paris Académie Royale des Sciences in the 1750s and 1760s proved to be an important venue for these developments.[33]

LA CONDAMINE'S LOTTERY

Charles-Marie de la Condamine, natural philosopher and member of the Académie Royale des Sciences, was one of the most prominent French advocates of inoculation. Famous for his participation in the expedition to Peru to measure the shape of the earth and his subsequent exploration of the Amazon, La Condamine, upon his return to Paris, took up the cause of inoculation, which he tirelessly promoted through public addresses and numerous published

[29] Louis-Charles-Henri Macquart, *Extrait d'une question sur l'inoculation de la petite vérole,* inserted in *Journal de Médecine* du mois de Février 1755, pp. 10–11.
[30] [Jean Astruc], *Doutes sur l'inoculation de la petite vérole, proposés à la Faculté de Médecine de Paris* (n.p., 1756), p. 13.
[31] Samuel August André David Tissot, *L'Inoculation justifiée ou dissertation pratique et apologétique sur cette méthode* (Lausanne, 1754), p. xi.
[32] Jean-Etienne Montucla, *Recueil de pièces concernant l'inoculation de la petite vérole, et propres à prouver la sécurité et l'utilité* (Paris, 1756), pp. 80–117.
[33] Miller, *The Adoption of Inoculation,* p. 238.

works.[34] He first presented the topic to an assembly of the Académie on 24 April 1754. Included in the audience were several members of the general public who warmly received his remarks.[35]

La Condamine opened his address with a review of the history of inoculation. He then briefly discussed the benefits of inoculation to the state, namely, a larger and healthier population.[36] The main thrust of his argument, however, was aimed at French fathers. "Can one ever persuade a tender father to make a wound on his only son, deliberately," La Condamine asked, "in order to communicate a disease to him that he might never have and that could cause him to die?"[37] He assumed that the hypothetical father was, like himself, an *homme éclairé*, "already convinced that neither religion nor moral philosophy can prohibit what reason and good sense advise." And here reason meant mathematics. "It is not therefore a question here of moral philosophy or theology, it is a matter of calculation," La Condamine asserted; "let us avoid making a case of conscience out of a problem of arithmetic." Much like Jurin in the 1720s, who had called for inoculation to be "fairly and maturely examin'd" through calculation, La Condamine explicitly equated good sense with good math. After stating the odds of dying from inoculated and natural smallpox (1 of 100 vs. 1 of 10), La Condamine concluded, "It is therefore *demonstrated,* in all the rigor of that term, that whoever does not inoculate his son, under the pretext of not hazarding his life, risks at least ten times more than by inoculating him."[38] The certainty of mathematics justified an individual's decision to inoculate his child.

Unlike the British physicians Arbuthnot and Jurin, La Condamine did not rely upon tables of mortality figures to make his point. Instead, he focused on comparing the risks to the individual of dying from inoculation and dying from natural smallpox. He made only one reference to an empirical basis for these figures: Jurin's compilation of smallpox mortality figures from the London bills of mortality. La Condamine adjusted Jurin's ratio of 1 of 7 to 1 of 10 because of perceived differences between the severity of smallpox in England and France;

---

[34] Charles-Marie de La Condamine, "Mémoire sur l'inoculation de la petite vérole," *Mémoires de l'Académie Royale des Sciences,* 1754 (Paris, 1759), pp. 615–670; La Condamine, "Second mémoire sur l'inoculation de la petite vérole, contenant la suite de l'histoire de cette méthode & de ses progrès, de 1754 à 1758," *Mémoires de l'Académie Royale des Sciences,* 1758 (1763), pp. 439–482; La Condamine, "Suite de l'histoire de l'inoculation de la petite vérole depuis 1758 jusqu'en 1765," *Mémoires de l'Académie Royale des Sciences,* 1765 (1768), pp. 505–532; *Lettres . . . à M. de Dr Maty sur l'état présent de l'inoculation en France* (Paris, 1764); and *Histoire de l'inoculation de la petite vérole,* 2 vols. (Amsterdam, 1773).

[35] Miller, *The Adoption of Inoculation,* p. 208.

[36] La Condamine, "Mémoire sur l'inoculation," p. 666: "Il est donc démontré que l'établissement de l'Inoculation sauveroit la vie à douze ou treize cens citoyens par an dans la seule ville de Paris & à plus de vingt-cinq mille personnes dans le royaume, supposé, comme on le présume, que la capitale contienne le vingtième des habitans de la France."

[37] La Condamine, "Mémoire sur l'inoculation," p. 649.

[38] La Condamine's emphasis; La Condamine, "Mémoire sur l'inoculation," p. 655.

in France, according to La Condamine and others, smallpox was less deadly ("*moins meurtrière*") than in England.[39] La Condamine took his ratio of 1 of 10 from Geneva, probably from the writings of the Swiss Tronchin. Even given this concession, "the risk of inoculation is still ten times less than that of smallpox," La Condamine concluded, and then challenged his audience to answer the question: "Would you risk ten on this very precious life, in order to avoid risking one?" The answer, of course, was that no rational individual would risk a tenfold increase in the chance of dying.

La Condamine extended his argument by comparing inoculation with another set of risks: dying in childbirth. He pointed out that fathers already took greater risks with their daughters when they allowed them to marry: "It has been proven, by enumerations, that of sixty women in childbirth, one will die, and all girls who marry expose themselves many times to running this risk."[40] Since fathers already exposed their daughters to a greater risk, they should not fear exposing their sons to the lesser risk of inoculation.

La Condamine's argument reveals distinctive characteristics of French public culture. He elected not to include numerical tables and concentrated instead on the comparison of risks. Near the end of his paper, he left his audience with an indelible image. Inoculation provided a person with the chance to affect life's lottery, the wheel of fortune:

It is a powerful lottery [*loterie forcée*], in which we find ourselves engaged despite ourselves; each of us has a lottery ticket; the more one delays getting off the wheel, the more the danger increases. In Paris there are, in an ordinary year [*année commune*], fourteen hundred black lottery tickets, for which the lot is death. What does one do in practicing inoculation? One changes the conditions of this lottery; one reduces the number of fatal lottery tickets.[41]

La Condamine continued to promote inoculation and published two subsequent reports in the *Mémoires* of the Paris Académie des Sciences in 1758 and 1765. He discussed and refuted arguments made by those who opposed inoculation, and included a report of the number of inoculations performed in Paris and other French cities by the "variolateurs à la mode," Gatti and Tronchin. Gatti had inoculated almost 100 individuals in 1763 and almost 200 by 1765. "It is time," La Condamine charged, "that these facts buried in silence become known to the public."[42]

La Condamine, however, never put this numerical information in a table; the figures were presented in the text. In fact, his only table appeared in the last of the three essays published in the Académie's *Mémoires,* and it addressed

---

[39] La Condamine, "Mémoire sur l'inoculation," pp. 652–655.
[40] La Condamine, "Mémoire sur l'inoculation," p. 657.
[41] La Condamine, "Mémoire sur l'inoculation," p. 658.
[42] La Condamine, "Second mémoire sur l'inoculation"; La Condamine, "Suite de l'histoire de l'inoculation." The report of inoculations is found in La Condamine, "Suite de l'histoire de l'inoculation," pp. 513–514.

532 MÉMOIRES DE L'ACADÉMIE ROYALE

TABLE *de la mortalité commune de la petite vérole, dans les différentes suppositions qu'on peut faire sur le nombre des exemts ; en partageant la totalité des hommes en treize parts, dont une est destinée à mourir de la petite vérole.*

Si, de treize individus qui naissent, on en suppose

exemts de la petite vérole, il en restera

12 11 10 9 8 7 6 5 4 3 2 1 0

qui auront cette maladie, & de ce nombre il en mourra un.

1 2 3 4 5 6 7 8 9 10 11 12 13

On voit d'abord, en considérant le premier nombre des deux colonnes de cette table, que si de treize personnes qui naissent, il y en avoit douze exemtes de la petite vérole, le seul des treize qui l'auroit, en mourroit infailliblement, & qu'ainsi elle seroit toujours mortelle; ce qui est visiblement faux.

On voit pareillement, en comparant l'un à l'autre le dernier nombre de chaque colonne, que pour qu'il ne mourût qu'un varioleux sur treize, il faudroit qu'aucun des treize ne fût exemt de cette maladie & que tout le monde eût la petite vérole : ce qui est aussi faux que la première supposition, & en parcourant toutes les suppositions intermédiaires représentées par la table, on verra que comme sur treize personnes on ne peut en supposer plus de cinq ou six exemtes de la petite vérole, il s'ensuit que des sept ou huit autres, il en mourra une : savoir une de sept, comme je le suppose, en portant le nombre des exemts à six, & une de huit en bornant le nombre des exemts à cinq sur treize : ce qui est l'hypothèse de M. *Bernoulli*.

3.1 Charles-Marie de la Condamine's table of hypothetical smallpox mortality (1765). *Source:* Charles Marie de la Condamine, "Suite de l'histoire de l'inoculation de la petite vérole depuis 1758 jusqu'en 1765," *Mémoires de l'Académie Royale des Sciences* 1765 (1768), p. 532. Burndy Library, Dibner Institute for the History of Science and Technology.

the objection raised by many French physicians that some individuals might never contract the smallpox, hence, making inoculation an unnecessary risk. (See Figure 3.1.) The table was designed to illustrate a logical argument. It was not a display of actual mortality figures. Basing his table on Daniel Bernoulli's ratio that 1 of 13 individuals will die from natural smallpox (discussed in the next section), La Condamine constructed the first column to show that of 13 individuals born, at least 1 will die of smallpox and some number of individuals ranging from 12 to 0 will be exempt from the disease. Of those not exempt, (the second column, ranging from 1 to 13), at least 1 will die from smallpox

(Bernoulli's ratio, again). He then logically examined various scenarios concerning the other 12 individuals. If all 12 were exempt (the top of the first column), then only 1 individual would contract and die from smallpox (the top of the second column). At the other extreme (the bottom of the second column), if all 13 individuals contracted the smallpox, then only 1 would die. Both of these scenarios were "visibly false." In reviewing the intermediary numbers, La Condamine "supposed" that not more than 5 or 6 individuals could be exempt from smallpox. From this supposition, it logically followed that of the 7 or 8 remaining individuals, 1 would die from smallpox. This ratio confirmed Bernoulli's hypothesis, as well as Jurin's, that 1 of 7 individuals who *contracted* the natural smallpox died.

La Condamine's table was a thought experiment. He reasoned that some portion of the population would be exempt from natural smallpox (5 or 6 of 13), unlike Jurin and Arbuthnot, who assumed in their calculations that everyone would contract the smallpox at some point in life. The point of his table was to show that the chances of dying from smallpox were still considerable, even though some individuals would never catch the disease.

In all of his writings, La Condamine spoke "for everyone, and less to the mathematicians." He tried to make his calculations acceptable to as wide an audience as possible by taking "the most favorable proportions to the enemies of inoculation."[43] This was not the case for Daniel Bernoulli and Jean d'Alembert.

BERNOULLI AND D'ALEMBERT

La Condamine was a close friend of the natural philosopher and fellow member of the Académie des Sciences Pierre-Louis Moreau de Maupertuis, who had also participated in the expeditions to measure the shape of the earth (Maupertuis surveyed Lapland instead of Peru). In 1759, Maupertuis traveled to Basel to visit his friend, the Swiss mathematician and physician Daniel Bernoulli, and he suggested that Bernoulli take a close look at inoculation. Bernoulli, too, was an advocate of the practice and expressed his dismay over the criticism La Condamine's memoir had received among physicians. "[I]t is to be hoped that the doctors," he remarked, "instead of thwarting him [La Condamine] in his enthusiasm, which is as pious as it is enlightened, would wish to help him to perfect the method of inoculation instead of rejecting it without having, perhaps, adequately weighed up the importance of his objective."[44]

The result of Maupertuis's encouragement was Bernoulli's memoir entitled "Essai d'une nouvelle analyse de la mortalité causée par la petite vérole," read

---

[43] La Condamine, "Mémoire sur l'inoculation," pp. 649, 655.
[44] Daniel Bernoulli, "Essai d'un nouvelle analyse de la mortalité causée par la petite vérole et des avantages de l'inoculation pour la prévenir," *Mémoires de l'Académie Royale des Sciences*, 1760 (Paris, 1765), p. 29; trans. L. Bradley, *Smallpox Inoculation: An Eighteenth Century Mathematical Controversy* (Nottingham: University of Nottingham, 1971), p. 42.

to the Paris Académie on 13 April 1760. Bernoulli sought to demonstrate the advantages of inoculation through calculation, and the result was a very sophisticated mathematical analysis of mortality. He calculated the life expectancies for inoculated and noninoculated individuals using the calculus of probabilities, and he incorporated these figures into a table that included calculations of the impact of inoculation and smallpox mortality on the population. He thus developed the types of population arguments that had been made on a more limited scale by Arbuthnot, La Condamine, and others. These earlier authors had not taken age into account in their calculations; they had simply calculated the net gain in population if everyone were inoculated. Bernoulli looked at the advantages of inoculation in terms of population at each year of life.

"In this memoir," Bernoulli explained, "my intention is simply to make a comparison between the condition of mankind as it is without inoculation and what it would be if this salutary operation were either generally admitted or simply followed with certain rules."[45] Bernoulli made two assumptions: (1) The danger of contracting smallpox was the same at every age; and (2) the danger of dying from smallpox once contracted was the same at every age. In his calculus, he relied on the ratio that 1 of 13 deaths was attributable to smallpox, a figure taken from the voluminous work of the Prussian minister Johann Peter Süssmilch (1707–1767).[46] Using these assumptions, Bernoulli created an equation to calculate the number of persons who had not had smallpox at a given age and generated a complex mortality table that included the following information: (1) age; (2) number of individuals still alive out of every 1,300 born (extrapolated from Edmond Halley's mortality table);[47] (3) number at each age who had not yet had smallpox; (4) number who had contracted smallpox and recovered; (5) number who had contracted smallpox the previous year; (6) number of category 5 who had died from smallpox; (7) total number of all who had died from smallpox from birth to age x; and (8) total number of deaths not due to smallpox for that year.[48] (See Figures 3.2 and 3.3.)

The virtues of the table – conciseness, the ability to facilitate comparison – were clearly extolled by Bernoulli. "In composing this Memoir," he wrote, "I was above all concerned to display in a single Table the two conditions of mankind, the one as it actually is and the other as it would be if we were able to rid the whole human race of smallpox." Such a table would allow the "comparisons of these two conditions" and "explain the difference and the

[45] Bernoulli, "Essai," pp. 7–8; trans. Bradley, *Smallpox Inoculation*, p. 26.
[46] Bernoulli, "Essai," pp. 8–10; trans. Bradley, *Smallpox Inoculation*, pp. 27–28. Johann Peter Süssmilch (1707–1767), *Die Göttliche Ordnung*, 1st ed. (Berlin, 1741).
[47] Edmond Halley's mortality table is discussed in Chapter 7.
[48] Bernoulli, "Essai," pp. 14–15; trans. Bradley, *Smallpox Inoculation*, pp. 31–32.

44   MÉMOIRES DE L'ACADÉMIE ROYALE

TABLE I.

AGES par années.	Survivans selon M. Halley.	N'ayant pas eu la pet. vérole.	Ayant eu la pet. vérol.	Prenant la pet. vérole pendant ch. année.	MORTS de la pet. vérole pendant chaq. ann.	SOMME des morts de la pet. vérole.	MORTS par d'autres maladies pend. chaq. année.
0	1300	1300	0				
1	1000	896	104	137	17,1	17,1	283
2	855	685	170	99	12,4	29,5	133
3	798	571	227	78	9,7	39,2	47
4	760	485	275	66	8,3	47,5	30
5	732	416	316	56	7,0	54,5	21
6	710	359	351	48	6,0	60,5	16
7	692	311	381	42	5,2	65,7	12,8
8	680	272	408	36	4,5	70,2	7,5
9	670	237	433	32	4,0	74,2	6
10	661	208	453	28	3,5	77,7	5,5
11	653	182	471	24,4	3,0	80,7	5
12	646	160	486	21,4	2,7	83,4	4,3
13	640	140	500	18,7	2,3	85,7	3,7
14	634	123	511	16,6	2,1	87,8	3,9
15	628	108	520	14,4	1,8	89,6	4,2
16	622	94	528	12,6	1,6	91,2	4,4
17	616	83	533	11,0	1,4	92,6	4,6
18	610	72	538	9,7	1,2	93,8	4,8
19	604	63	541	8,4	1,0	94,8	5
20	598	56	542	7,4	0,9	95,7	5,1
21	592	48,5	543	6,5	0,8	96,5	5,2
22	586	42,5	543	5,6	0,7	97,2	5,3
23	579	37	542	5,0	0,6	97,8	6,4
24	572	32,4	540	4,4	0,5	98,3	6,5

3.2 Daniel Bernoulli's table combining Halley's life table with smallpox mortality figures by age (1760). *Source:* Daniel Bernoulli, "Essai d'une nouvelle analyse de la mortalité causée par la petite vérole," *Mémoires de l'Académie Royale des Sciences* 1760 (1765), p. 44. Burndy Library, Dibner Institute for the History of Science and Technology.

contrast between them better than the most ample commentary."[49] Bernoulli's methodological innovation amounted to the combination of a life table with a table of mortality figures, and he ascribed significant evidentiary weight to the resulting table.

[49] Bernoulli, "Essai," p. 2; trans. Bradley, *Smallpox Inoculation*, p. 22.

DES SCIENCES.   45

TABLE II.

Ages par années.	État naturel & variolique.	État non-varioliq.	Differ. ou gains.	Ages par années.	État naturel & variolique.	État non-varioliq.	Differ. ou gains.
0	1300	1300	0	13	640	741,1	74,1
1	1000	1017,1	17,1	14	634	709,7	75,7
2	855	881,8	26,8	15	628	705,0	77,0
3	798	833,3	35,3	16	622	700,1	78,1
4	760	802,0	42,0	17	616	695,0	79,0
5	732	779,8	47,8	18	610	689,6	79,6
6	710	762,8	52,8	19	604	684,0	80,0
7	692	749,1	57,2	20	598	678,2	80,2
8	680	740,9	60,9	21	592	672,3	80,3
9	670	734,4	64,4	22	586	666,3	80,3
10	661	728,4	67,4	23	579	659,0	80,0
11	653	722,9	69,9	24	572	651,7	79,7
12	646	718,2	72,2	25	565	644,3	79,3

Cette Table fait voir d'un coup d'œil, combien sur 1300 enfans, supposés nés en même temps, il en resteroit de vivans d'année en année jusqu'à l'âge de vingt-cinq ans, en les supposant tous sujets à la petite vérole; & combien il en resteroit s'ils étoient tous exempts de cette maladie, avec la comparaison & la différence des deux états.

3.3 Daniel Bernoulli's table comparing life expectancy with and without smallpox (1760). *Source:* Daniel Bernoulli, "Essai d'une nouvelle analyse de la mortalité causée par la petite vérole," *Mémoires de l'Académie Royale des Sciences* 1760 (1765), p. 45. Burndy Library, Dibner Institute for the History of Science and Technology.

One conclusion Bernoulli drew from this table was that inoculation was advantageous to society, even if a substantial number of inoculated children died from smallpox. "So, however we look at the matter it will always be *geometrically true* that the interest of Princes is to favour and protect inoculation by all possible means; likewise the father of a family with regard to his children."[50] Bernoulli's claim of geometrical truthfulness echoed La Condamine's claim to numerical demonstration. Both men regarded the application of mathematics to questions of medical practice and policy as a way to provide certainty, and Bernoulli reaffirmed La Condamine's assertion that "all reasonable men" would act the

[50] Emphasis added; Bernoulli, "Essai," p. 34; trans. Bradley, *Smallpox Inoculation,* p. 46.

same, given the equivalent information. "A complete theory of the risks of smallpox," Bernoulli argued, "would dictate the rules which every reasonable man should follow."[51] Bernoulli also assumed, much like Arbuthnot, that the interests of the state and the interests of the individual (namely, the father of the family) coincided.

Bernoulli's and La Condamine's arguments reflected the contemporary view of probability where no distinction was made between description and prescription.[52] It was precisely this assumption that Jean d'Alembert challenged at a public meeting of the Académie six months later on 12 November 1760.[53] While he supported the practice of inoculation, d'Alembert rejected the application of the calculus of probabilities to assessing its risks.[54] "My objections attack only those mathematicians who may be in too much of a hurry to reduce the matter to equations and formulae," d'Alembert declared, "but I would regard myself as culpable against society if my aim had been to dissuade my fellow citizens from a practice which I believe to be useful."[55] D'Alembert's argument rested on the impossibility of comparing a proximate risk with a future risk; there existed no way to calculate a future risk:

[T]he man who has himself inoculated is in the position of a gambler, who risks one chance in 200 of losing all his fortune in one day for the hope of adding to his fortune an unknown and probably quite small sum at the end of a very distant number of years, and when he will be much less alive to the enjoyment of this increase in his fortune. But how can we compare this present risk to this unknown and distant advantage?[56]

Bernoulli had argued that if inoculation were practiced by everyone, the average length of life ("la vie moyenne") would increase by about two years. Adding two years, however, would not tempt an individual who must risk imminent death in order to gain those two years. It is just this kind of reasoning, d'Alembert argued, that made most people, "above all so many mothers," not favor inoculation. "They make the reasoning, which we have just developed, implicitly." Here d'Alembert challenged the classical theory of probability, which viewed probability as descriptive of psychological processes, and he, too,

---

[51] Bernoulli, "Essai," pp. 8–9; trans. Bradley, *Smallpox Inoculation*, pp. 27–28.

[52] Lorraine Daston, *Classical Probability in the Enlightenment* (Princeton, N.J.: Princeton University Press, 1988), esp. chap. 2, on the "reasonable man" model and mathematics.

[53] Bernoulli's paper did not appear in print until 1765 when the *Histoire de l'Académie Royale des Sciences* for 1760 was published. D'Alembert preempted Bernoulli by publishing his paper privately in 1761 in his *Opuscules mathématiques*.

[54] For discussions of d'Alembert's notion of probability, see Bradley, *Smallpox Inoculation*, pp. 11–13; Daston, *Classical Probability*, pp. 78–90; Thomas L. Hankins, *Jean d'Alembert – Science and the Enlightenment* (Oxford: Clarendon Press, 1970), pp. 146–149; and Karl Pearson, *The History of Statistics in the 17th and 18th Centuries against the Changing Background of Intellectual, Scientific and Religious Thought*, ed. E. S. Pearson (London: Charles Griffin, 1978), pp. 506–573.

[55] D'Alembert, *Opuscules mathématiques*, vol. 2, p. 45; trans. Bradley, *Smallpox Inoculation*, p. 67.

[56] D'Alembert, *Opuscules mathématiques*, vol. 2, p. 33; trans. L. Bradley, *Smallpox Inoculation*, p. 61.

did so in gendered terms. Whereas La Condamine had invoked the image of a "tender father" and linked him to all reasonable men and Bernoulli had appealed to reasonable men, d'Alembert, by contrast, raised the issue of how mothers regarded the risks of inoculation.[57] He noted that "[w]ithout being able to compare exactly their fear to their hopes, they [mothers] act, if one may so put it, on the confession of the inoculators that one can die of artificial smallpox."[58] He went on to link the reasoning of mothers to that of the crowd: "[We] know how heavily the proximity of a feared danger, or of a hoped-for advantage, weighs in deciding the crowd."[59] D'Alembert undermined the "reasonable man" model by invoking the psychology of two groups that generally were not considered reasonable: women and the crowd.

D'Alembert, thus, challenged the use of mathematical arguments in determining the issue of inoculation. He thought that the type of comparison made between risks was invalid because the risks were insufficiently defined. He also pointed out that the interests of the state and the individual were not identical. Arithmetical arguments, which demonstrated the advantage of inoculation for the state (namely, a larger population), were not at all persuasive to the individual who must risk death.[60] But, he cautioned, "if the advantages of inoculation cannot by their nature be appreciated mathematically, they do not appear less real."[61]

PHYSICIANS RESPOND

The responses of the medical community to the arguments advanced by d'Alembert, Bernoulli, and La Condamine were generally negative. The whole idea of comparing the risks of dying from inoculated versus natural smallpox was questioned on grounds that the different populations – the French, the English, the inoculated, or those who contracted smallpox the natural way – were not comparable. Death from smallpox, some physicians argued, was not simply the result of the deadliness of the disease. More importantly, mathematicians and other philosophes did not have sufficient knowledge or training to evaluate a medical practice. Numerical arguments were not particularly persuasive to a medical audience.

The best example of this attitude can be found in the writings of Dr. LeHoc, a physician to Hôtel Dieu in Paris for thirty years. Physicians should reject inoculation because "the methods that are used to establish inoculation are founded

[57] D'Alembert, *Opuscules mathématiques,* vol. 2, p. 43; trans. Bradley, *Smallpox Inoculation,* p. 66.
[58] D'Alembert, *Opuscules mathématiques,* vol. 2, p. 34; trans. Bradley, *Smallpox Inoculation,* p. 61.
[59] D'Alembert, *Opuscules mathématiques,* vol. 2, p. 34; trans. Bradley, *Smallpox Inoculation,* p. 61.
[60] On this point see Miller, *The Adoption of Inoculation,* p. 228; Pearson, *The History of Statistics,* p. 548.
[61] Jean d'Alembert, "Réflexions sur l'Inoculation," *Oeuvres philosophique, historiques et littéraires* (Paris, 1805), vol. 4, p. 417.

on infidel calculations and false principles."[62] Moreover, it was improper to compare inoculated and natural smallpox, a point that echoed Howgrave's and Massey's objections raised in England in the 1720s. "On one side the subjects were chosen, examined, prepared," LeHoc wrote in his 1764 pamphlet *L'Inoculation de la petite vérole renvoyée à Londres,* "and on the other taken at hazard, without an exam, without regard to age, temperament, actual disposition, &c."[63] According to LeHoc, mathematics and medicine were separate enterprises. He was not at all persuaded by the numerical demonstrations offered by pro-inoculators since "their infidel calculations announce the ignorance of a profession that they scorn because they do not know it, have not studied it, and have not fathomed it."[64]

Other physicians did not reject mathematics entirely, but focused instead on specific facets of the numerical arguments. Pierre DeBaux, Médecin Aggregé at the medical college of Marseille, reviewed Jurin's work and did not find it applicable to France. "This disease," DeBaux asserted, "leaves greater ravages in England than in France, such that the calculations can never serve as a guide for our country."[65] To correct for these national differences, DeBaux, who supported inoculation, advocated the collection of reports of inoculations in France, much as Jurin had done in England during the 1720s. At the end of his pamphlet, DeBaux himself included such a list of 11 people whom he had inoculated successfully, and he appealed to the interests of the state: "The French Government is so enlightened, and so attentive to the conservation and augmentation of the number of subjects of the state, that it will not neglect to favor a method so useful to the population."[66]

Louis-Charles-Henri Macquart reviewed La Condamine's papers in the *Journal de Médecine.* Macquart supported La Condamine's conclusions but challenged his methods and claims to certain knowledge. La Condamine "evaluated the number of subjects that we will save through inoculation." But, Macquart wondered, "are we in a state to make this evaluation with precision? Do we have all the necessary observations?"[67] He regarded La Condamine as a "zealous partisan" in his arguments and equated his calculations with "specious arguments and false imputations" made by enemies of inoculation.[68] Despite these strong reservations, Macquart felt that "the introduction of inoculation will preserve a large number of subjects, put calm in the well-off families, and assure the leaders, to whom is often attached the welfare of the Citizens, of the security

---

[62] [LeHoc], *L'Inoculation de la petite vérole renvoyée à Londres* (A La Haye, 1764), p. 116.
[63] [LeHoc], *L'Inoculation,* pp. 71–72.   [64] [LeHoc], *L'Inoculation,* pp. 48–49.
[65] Pierre DeBaux, *Parallèle de la petite vérole naturelle, avec l'artificielle, ou inoculée, avec un traité intermédiare de la petite vérole fausse, volante, ou adultérine* (Avignon, 1761), p. 48.
[66] DeBaux, *Parallèle de la petite vérole naturelle,* pp. 112–115 (lists of inoculated persons); pp. 111–112 (quotation).
[67] Macquart, *Extrait,* p. 15.   [68] Macquart, *Extrait,* pp. 10–11.

and tranquility of the state."[69] Macquart did not see the tension between benefits to the population and to the individual that troubled d'Alembert.

Against DeBaux and Macquart stood the Dutch physician Anton DeHaen. He questioned the general convention among pro-inoculators to factor out deaths under the age of two in their calculations of the proportion of deaths attributable to smallpox.[70] (This convention had been established by Arbuthnot and Jurin, but came under increased scrutiny during the second half of the eighteenth century.) He also argued that smallpox was "infinitely less fatal" than indicated by those who advocated inoculation.[71] Further, he asserted that inoculation increased the incidence of smallpox. After examining the London bills of mortality for the first half of the eighteenth century, DeHaen concluded "that inoculation had considerably increased the contagion."[72] This last observation became the subject of heated debate in England during the 1770s and 1780s (discussed in Chapter 4).

A PLEA FOR REGISTERS

Whatever the impact of their mathematical arguments, La Condamine, Bernoulli, and d'Alembert supported the collection and use of numerical information about the population. "Let us not, then, stifle the seed of an analysis," Bernoulli pleaded, "which, making use of good lists of sickness, mortality, baptisms and marriages, could be applied to a number of interesting questions, physical as well as moral and political, concerning the various conditions and classes which divide mankind."[73] While they did not agree on the adequacy and persuasiveness of mathematical arguments in the inoculation controversy, they did agree upon the desirability of collecting quantitative information about smallpox incidence and mortality. Each, however, proposed different methods.

La Condamine looked to medical institutions. "If the hospitals are ordered to carefully distinguish, in their annual lists, the number of sick and the number of deaths from each type of disease, as is the practice in England," La Condamine wrote, "the practice will be recognized over time of increasing utility."[74] This was perhaps the most realistic of the proposals, given the experience in England. Hospitals did provide an institutional framework for the recording of morbidity

[69] Macquart, *Extrait*, pp. 15–16.
[70] Anton DeHaen, *Réfutation de l'inoculation servant de réponse à deux pièces qui ont paru cette année 1759. Dont la première est une dissertation lue dans la société de l'académie royale des sciences de Paris par M. De La Condamine, et la seconde, une lettre de M. Tyssot* (Vienne, 1759), pp. 62–63.
[71] DeHaen, *Réfutation de l'inoculation*, p. 76.   [72] DeHaen, *Réfutation de l'inoculation*, pp. 138–139.
[73] Bernoulli, "Essai," p. 6; trans. Bradley, *Smallpox Inoculation*, p. 25.
[74] La Condamine, "Mémoire sur l'inoculation," p. 669.

and mortality information, which could be supervised by physicians, surgeons, and other medical personnel.

D'Alembert turned to more traditional methods of record keeping and advocated the collection of two sets of data, one specifically on smallpox, the other on diseases more generally, by individual physicians and parish priests. "In each country and in each town," d'Alembert hoped that "the doctors keep with all the accuracy and good faith possible, exact registers of the patients whom they treat for smallpox, their temperament, their age, and the fate of those who had this disease."[75] In addition, d'Alembert wished for "the government to order that it be marked in the registers, as far as will be possible, at which age each citizen has died, of what disease he perished, if he had the natural or inoculated smallpox, and at what age he had it; finally, if it is the same place as where he was born!"[76] He did not specify how physicians' records would be collected and analyzed.

For his part, Bernoulli complained that there were no registers that listed the age at death from smallpox, but he anticipated "that we shall soon have such lists from London."[77] Like d'Alembert, he called for doctors to keep registers of their smallpox patients but added the further specification that the registers be sent to the Dean of the Paris Faculté de Médecine. "From a large number of such registers," Bernoulli explained, "the results of which would be communicated to the Dean of the Faculty, we would deduce exactly, for each age at which smallpox was contracted, the risk of dying of it."[78] And finally, Bernoulli hoped "that some parish priests would take the trouble to make enumerations" in order to have accurate accounts of population and mortality.[79] Thus, Bernoulli too hoped that individual doctors would collect quantitative information, but instead of envisioning a new state structure to collect information, he looked to the older tradition of parish priests and individual physicians supervised by the Paris Faculté de Médecine.

Two years after the exchange between Bernoulli and d'Alembert, a severe smallpox epidemic swept through Paris in the fall and winter of 1762. Inoculation was blamed for spreading the disease, and in June 1763 the Paris Parlement issued a ban on inoculation in Paris.[80] This action exacerbated an already charged atmosphere, and the debates surrounding inoculation became even more rancorous. As a result, in 1764, the Paris Faculté de Médecine began an investigation into the practice of inoculation that stretched over several years. The Faculté issued a questionnaire with the following questions:

---

[75] D'Alembert, "Réflexions sur l'inoculation," p. 369.
[76] D'Alembert, "Réflexions sur l'inoculation," p. 414.
[77] Bernoulli, "Essai," p. 4; trans. Bradley, *Smallpox Inoculation*, p. 23.
[78] Bernoulli, "Essai," p. 9; trans. Bradley, *Smallpox Inoculation*, p. 27.
[79] Bernoulli, "Essai," p. 22; trans. Bradley, *Smallpox Inoculation*, p. 37.
[80] Miller, *The Adoption of Inoculation*, p. 231.

1. Has inoculation been long practiced in your country? and with what success?
2. Did some of the inoculated die?
3. Did some who had undergone inoculation take the natural smallpox afterwards, and at what time?
4. Do you know that other diseases have been ingrafted with the smallpox by inoculation?
5. Whether did many, after inoculation, labour under various diseases which seemed to be owing to this operation? and whether did this happen more frequently or seldomer than from the natural smallpox?[81]

Influential physicians throughout Europe responded to this questionnaire, including the British physicians John Huxham, John Pringle, and Alexander Monro *primus*. Their replies provided substantial information about the extent and nature of the practice of inoculation. Despite the overwhelming support of inoculation expressed in these replies, the Paris Faculté remained divided in opinion about the safety of inoculation, and no resolution was ever reached.[82]

Although the medical faculty could not agree, the popularity of the inoculators Tronchin and Gatti continued to grow among members of the nobility. Even the French state began to recognize the benefits of inoculation: In 1769, following the Duke of Choiseul's orders, Gatti inoculated students attending the École Royale Militaire. For many others, the death of Louis XV in 1774 from smallpox proved far more crucial to the acceptance of inoculation in France than the exchanges between the mathematicians and medics. "Gatti is to arrive here perhaps tomorrow in order to inoculate the royal family," wrote Abbé Galiani to Mme de Belzunce of Naples in 1777. "One death caused by smallpox is worth more than the dissertations of La Condamine."[83] The French royal family finally agreed to be inoculated, "thus removing the last reigning house in Europe which had not admitted the operation."[84]

The historian Genevieve Miller argued that the role of the Paris Académie Royale des Sciences, like that of the Royal Society in London, was crucial to the acceptance of inoculation in France.[85] Certainly the Paris Académie provided a forum for discussion and overall was more supportive of the practice than was the Paris Faculté de Médecine. But the impact of the French academicians on public opinion is more difficult to gauge. The review of pamphlet literature suggests that the academicians had minimal effect on the French medical community, and this points to a significant difference between France and England. In England, the natural philosophers who advanced numerical arguments were also practicing physicians, obviating the problem of professional boundaries.

[81] Alexander Monro, *An Account of the Inoculation of Small Pox in Scotland* (Edinburgh, 1765), pp. 2, 23, 26, 41, 43, 45.
[82] Miller, *The Adoption of Inoculation*, pp. 234–237.
[83] Galiani to Mme de Belzunce, of Naples, 27 September 1777. L'Abbé Ferdinand Galiani, *Correspondance* (Paris, 1889), vol. 2, p. 256; quoted in Delaunay, *Le monde médical parisien*, p. 292.
[84] Miller, *The Adoption of Inoculation*, p. 237.   [85] Miller, *The Adoption of Inoculation*, p. 238.

This difference in social and professional location marked the character of quantification found in each national debate. While British physicians made do with basic arithmetic and accounting principles, French academicians created numerical arguments of such complexity that they contributed far more to the development of probability theory than to the cause of inoculation.[86]

---

[86] In her comparative study of the role of science in the industrial revolution, Margaret Jacob noted that the French academicians' "oftentimes theoretical approach brought to industry a social and cultural style best described as aristocratic and hierarchical." Margaret Jacob, *Scientific Culture and the Making of the Industrial West* (Oxford: Oxford University Press, 1997), p. 168.

4

Charitable Calculations: English Debates over the Inoculation of the Urban Poor, 1750–1800

> Every life saved by this practice is so much solid treasure and strength added to the nation.
>
> William Black (1781)[1]

During the 1750s and 1760s in the county of Suffolk, the English surgeon Robert Sutton developed a new inoculation technique that produced a milder case of smallpox and greatly reduced the risks of dying. Instead of a making a deep incision, Sutton made a very slight puncture. His son, Daniel Sutton, followed his father's practice and popularized the new procedure. "The lancet being charged with the smallest perceivable quantity (and the smaller the better) of unripe, crude or watery matter," Daniel Sutton explained, "immediately introduce it by puncture, obliquely, between the scarf [epidermis] and true skin [dermis], barely sufficient to draw blood."[2] Daniel Sutton became a prolific inoculator and cultivated the practice of general inoculations, where all the inhabitants of a small town or village would be treated at once. He and his partners claimed to have inoculated 55,000 persons between 1760 and 1767, "of which number six only died."[3]

When inoculation was first introduced in England, physicians and surgeons had interpreted the practice in humoral terms and deemed it necessary to prepare an individual for the procedure. For up to a month prior to the actual incision, the patient would be bled, purged, and put on a low diet.[4] This

[1] William Black, *Observations Medical and Political: On the Small-Pox and Inoculation: And on the Decrease of Mankind at Every Age, with a Comparative View of the Diseases Most Fatal to London during Ninety Years. Including an Attempt to Demonstrate in What Manner London May Save Near Two Thousand . . . Lives Annually . . .* (London: J. Johnson, 1781), p. 91.

[2] Daniel Sutton, *The Inoculator, or Suttonian System of Inoculation* (1796), p. 77; quoted in Peter Razzell, *The Conquest of Smallpox: The Impact of Inoculation on Smallpox Mortality in Eighteenth Century Britain* (Sussex: Caliban Books, 1977), p. 10.

[3] Robert Houlton, *A Sermon . . . in Defence of Inoculation* (1767), p. 41; quoted in Razzell, *The Conquest of Smallpox*, p. 22.

[4] Genevieve Miller, *The Adoption of Inoculation for Smallpox in England and France* (Philadelphia: University of Pennsylvania Press, 1957), pp. 41–42, 163–165; Razzell, *The Conquest of Smallpox*, pp. 12–15.

rigorous preparation had two direct consequences: It made inoculation much too costly in terms of time and money for the majority of the population; and it increased the chances that the patient would be exposed to natural smallpox during this preparation period. This danger of exposure was especially pressing during smallpox epidemics, precisely when the demand for inoculation increased. In consequence, many practitioners, foremost Robert and Daniel Sutton, decided to dispense with the lengthy preparation during the 1760s.[5]

These changes in procedure made inoculation safer and cheaper and, as Sutton's figures suggest, much more widely practiced. And here was precisely the problem: An individual with inoculated smallpox was potentially contagious. Even in the debates during the 1720s, the possibility that inoculated smallpox might be contagious was recognized, but because the practice was generally limited to the elite who could afford to seclude themselves for a three- to four-week period following inoculation, this potentially hazardous effect was generally ignored or downplayed. With an increase in the number of inoculations during the 1760s and 1770s, the matter of contagion became urgent.

But how to evaluate the risks of contagion? After 1750, most English physicians and surgeons believed that it was in the individual's interest to get inoculated, but they did not agree whether it was in the community's interest. No one denied the benefits of general inoculations in villages, when all individuals who had not had natural smallpox (including the poor) could be inoculated at the same time. But in large cities, where general inoculations were not feasible, opinion was strongly divided on whether the benefits of inoculating the poor outweighed the hazards of contagion.

As in the earlier debates about the relative risks of death to the individual by inoculation, physicians and surgeons turned to numerical arguments to evaluate the risks of contagion. One of the most common numerical arguments against inoculating the poor charged that deaths in London attributed to smallpox had *increased* over the course of the eighteenth century. This observation, taken from the London bills of mortality, suggested that inoculation actually spread, rather than prevented, smallpox. In particular, it was the practice of inoculating the poor in their homes or at a dispensary that was blamed for this alleged increase. Those who supported the inoculation of the urban poor questioned whether the increase in smallpox deaths recorded in the London bills had anything to do with inoculation at all; they suggested alternative explanations to account for the numbers.

Both opponents and supporters relied on tables to make their arguments. Participants raised new and larger questions about population growth, the influence of other diseases on smallpox mortality, and whether smallpox primarily

---

[5] For an account of the change in practice associated with inoculation, see Deborah Brunton, "'Pox Britannica': Smallpox Inoculation in Britain, 1721–1830," Ph.D. thesis, University of Pennsylvania, 1990), chaps. 4 and 5, pp. 98–182.

affected children. In the process they developed more complex tables to represent these ancillary considerations.

THE LONDON SMALLPOX HOSPITAL

The debate over the desirability of inoculating the poor dated back to the establishment of the Smallpox Hospital of London in 1746. This charitable institution provided free inoculations for the poor, as well as care for those who had contracted natural smallpox.[6] Inoculations were carried out in a separate building in another part of the city in order to prevent the possibility of contagion. Once the pocks appeared on an individual who had been inoculated, he or she would be transferred to the building where patients with natural smallpox were treated.

Because the Smallpox Hospital relied on charitable donations, the governors were keenly aware of public opinion. They supported inoculation, but acknowledged that potential contributors might not share their opinion, so they provided the option either to donate to the care of the already afflicted or to cover the expenses of inoculation. They also issued public reports to convince potential subscribers of the worthiness of the institution. They included an account of the hospital's expenses and the number of patients admitted. From 26 January 1746 to 31 December 1752, 1,352 persons were treated for natural smallpox, of whom 1,033 were cured. During the same period, 131 individuals were inoculated, of whom 2 died.[7]

A subsequent report, entitled *A Representation from the Governors of the Hospital for the Small-Pox and for Inoculation,* indicated that 593 persons were inoculated during the four-year period between December 1751 and December 1755. "That out of this large number of 593," the governors reported, "only *one* has died; while this terrible Distemper taken by the common unperceived Infection (usually called the *Natural* way) destroys, *at least,* one in Seven (perhaps in a greater Proportion) of those who are seized with it."[8] Here the governors produced the same ratios that Jurin had calculated 30 years earlier, only they based their figures on evidence drawn from their own patients. When the governors courted additional benefactors, they prominently displayed their commendable accounts. They also described the inoculation procedure and detailed the precautions taken to prevent contagion. This example is straightforward in its connection between financial accounts and the evaluation of a medical procedure. Yet it bears repeating that fiscal imperatives encouraged numerical accounts of patients.[9]

---

[6] For an account of the establishment of the London Smallpox Hospital, see Miller, *The Adoption of Inoculation,* pp. 146–156.

[7] *An Account of the Rise, Progress and State of the Hospital, for Relieving Poor People Afflicted with the Small Pox, and for Inoculation,* n.p., n.d. [1754].

[8] *A Representation from the Governors of the Hospital for the Small-Pox and for Inoculation,* n.p., n.d. [1756].

[9] Anne Borsay examined these connections in her "An Example of Political Arithmetic: The Evaluation of Spa Therapy at the Georgian Bath Infirmary, 1742–1830," *Medical History* 45 (2000): 149–172.

Throughout the 1750s, the Smallpox Hospital remained the only place in London where the poor could be inoculated for free, until the Foundling Hospital began to inoculate children in its care in the 1760s.[10] As their reports revealed, only a small portion of London's poor could be inoculated at the Smallpox Hospital. Moreover, the Hospital would only inoculate persons over the age of seven. Smallpox was endemic in London, and it was rare indeed for a child not to have encountered the disease before the age of seven. (Some historians have speculated that the Smallpox Hospital primarily inoculated servants who moved to London as adults.)[11]

According to one critic, the Smallpox Hospital fell short in both its design and practice. The Hospital could admit only a very limited number of poor each year, and even those few were fearful of putting themselves in the care of nurses, rather than family. The air was often impure, and the Hospital did not allow the popular cold-air treatment advocated by the well-respected physician Thomas Sydenham. "To obviate these objections and to render the practice of Inoculation more general," this critic continued, "it has been thought expedient to establish a Dispensary for Inoculating the Poor."[12] The anonymous critic reported the number of London inhabitants who had perished from smallpox during the previous 50 years (a figure taken from the London bills of mortality). If these individuals had been inoculated, "the number of lives which would have been thereby redeemed, together with the probable encrease from them, must have made a very considerable addition to the strength of the state."[13]

The argument for extending medical benefits to the poor was frequently cast in mercantile terms. This is not to say that humanitarian motives were absent: Many regarded philanthropic and state interests as complementary. The above-mentioned critic understood this. "As the strength of a nation is in some measure proportionate to the number of its inhabitants," he stated in his opening paragraph, "every attempt to encrease population, by preserving life has a just claim to the regard both of Patriotism and Humanity." This critic, much like Arbuthnot, La Condamine, and Bernoulli, linked public health with common wealth.

DISPENSARIES AND HOME INOCULATIONS IN LONDON

Inoculation of the poor became one of the foremost causes among England's religious Dissenters, and influential dissenting physicians took the lead in promoting ambitious plans concerning inoculation. In 1775 the Quaker physician John Coakley Lettsom established the Society for the General Inoculation of

---

[10] On inoculation at the Foundling Hospital, see William Watson, *An Account of a Series of Experiments, Instituted with a View of Ascertaining the Most Successful Method of Inoculating the Small-Pox* (London: J. Nourse, 1768).
[11] Razzell, *The Conquest of Smallpox*, p. 70.   [12] *Plan of a Dispensary for Inoculating the Poor*, n.p., n.d.
[13] *Plan of a Dispensary for Inoculating the Poor*, n.p., n.d.

the Poor in London, which promoted inoculation in individuals' homes.[14] Two years later, the Dispensary for General Inoculation where the poor were treated as outpatients was established, with Lettsom as a consulting physician.[15] Similar dispensaries were proposed in Manchester, Liverpool, and Chester.

The Dispensary encountered stiff opposition, primarily from the physician Baron Thomas Dimsdale.[16] A Quaker by birth, Dimsdale had received his title and the prodigious sum of £10,000 for inoculating the empress of Russia – a sensational event that brought him fame and standing among the elite. In 1776, Dimsdale issued his *Thoughts on General and Partial Inoculations*. Addressing Parliament, Dimsdale declared that the "mischief arising from the practice of inoculation by the illiterate and ignorant is beyond conception."[17] He argued that inoculation should be a regulated practice and that hospitals should provide adequate supervision of both the physicians and the patients.

Dimsdale supported inoculation, but he was firmly convinced that inoculating the poor in their homes or in a dispensary would spread the contagion. To prove his point, he extended Jurin's tables of natural smallpox mortality for the years 1734 through 1767, inclusive, excepting two years for which he could not locate the London bills of mortality. His table had four columns: year, total number of deaths, number of deaths due to smallpox, and the number of infant deaths. (Figure 4.1; compare Figures 2.2 and 2.3.) Like Jurin, Dimsdale adjusted total mortality by subtracting the number of infant deaths, and he calculated the ratio that 1 of 8 deaths were due to natural smallpox, nearly the same ratio Jurin had calculated more than 50 years earlier, a useful consistency that Dimsdale himself pointed out.[18] For the period 1768 to 1775, however, the ratio had increased to 1 of 6 deaths, which Dimsdale attributed to imprudent and indiscrimate inoculation of London's poor. (Figure 4.2.)

Dr. John Watkinson, founding member of the Society for the Inoculation of the Poor, physician to the Dispensary for General Inoculation, and Lettsom's close friend, disagreed. A fierce partisan of inoculating the poor (he was also physician to the Middlesex Dispensary established in 1778), Watkinson marshaled an impressive array of numerical arguments in support of his position.[19] He began with the obvious fact that London's population was continually fluctuating. "No certain conclusion can possibly be drawn, with respect to the increase or decrease of the mortality of the smallpox," he reasoned, "from the *absolute* number of deaths by that disease in one period, compared with the

---

[14] See James Johnston Abraham, *Lettsom – His Life, Times, Friends and Descendants* (London: William Heinemann, 1933), pp. 196–197.
[15] *The Medical Register for the Year 1779* (London: J. Murray, 1779), p. 45.
[16] Abraham, *Lettsom*, pp. 196–197; and Razzell, *The Conquest of Smallpox*, p. 71.
[17] Thomas Dimsdale, *Thoughts on General and Partial Inoculations* (London, 1776), p. 9.
[18] Dimsdale, *Thoughts on General and Partial Inoculations*, pp. 14–15.
[19] *Medical Register for the Year 1779*, p. 45.

Years.	General List of Deaths.	Deaths from Small Pox.	Under two Years of Age.
1734	26062	2688	10752
35	23538	1594	9672
36	27581	3014	10580
37	27823	2084	10054
38	25825	1590	9600
39			
1740	30811	2725	10765
41	32169	1977	10456
42	27483	1429	9030
43	25200	2029	8621
44	20606	1633	7394
45	21296	1206	7689
46	28157	3236	9503
47	25494	1380	8741
48	23869	1789	7637
49	25516	2625	8504
1750	23727	1229	8204
51	21028	998	7483
52	20485	3538	8239
53	19276	774	7892
54	22696	2359	8115
55	21917	1988	7803
56	20872	1608	7466
57	21313	3296	7095
58	17576	1273	5971
59	19604	2596	6905
1760	19830	2187	6838
61	21063	1525	7699
62	26326	2743	8372
63			
64	23202	2382	7637
65	23230	2498	8073
66	23911	2334	8035
67	22612	2188	7668
	760098	66515	268529

4.1 Thomas Dimsdale's table of smallpox deaths from the London bills (1734–1767). *Source:* Thomas Dimsdale, *Thoughts on General and Partial Inoculations* (London, 1776), p. 19. Yale University, Harvey Cushing/John Hay Whitney Medical Library.

absolute number of deaths by the same disease in another period."[20] Instead, Watkinson favored the approach found in the work of Dr. Richard Price, the prominent dissenting minister. Price had "endeavoured to trace the variations in the mortality of this distemper [smallpox], not from the *absolute*, but the

[20] John Watkinson, *An Examination of a Charge Brought against Inoculation, by DeHaen, Rast, Dimsdale, and Other Writers* (London, 1778), p. 4.

Extract from the Bills of Mortality, and a continuation of the estimate from page 19.

	Total of Deaths.	Small Pox.	Under 2 Years.			
1768	23639	3028	8229	Total Deaths		178807
69	21847	1968	8016	Under 2 Years		63056
70	22434	1986	7994			
71	21780	1660	7617		18821)	115751 (6
72	26053	3992	9112			2825
73	21656	1039	6850			
74	20884	2479	7742			
75	20514	2669	7496			
	178807	18821	63056	Totals.		

By the above table it will be found, that with respect to the proportion of infants to the total number of deaths, there is still a surprising agreement with both the former estimates; the number of those under two years of age remains to be somewhat more than one-third of the whole.

But if we pursue the same method as before by subtracting the infants,

$$178807$$
$$63056$$

the number will be $$115751$$

which now amounts to somewhat more than one in six; whereas before it was about one in eight.

4.2 Thomas Dimsdale's table of smallpox deaths from the London bills (1768–1775). *Source*: Thomas Dimsdale, *Thoughts on General and Partial Inoculations* (London, 1776), p. 22. Yale University, Harvey Cushing/John Hay Whitney Medical Library.

relative number of its victims, that is, from the proportion which they bore to those of all the other diseases at one time, compared with the proportion which they bore them at another."[21] Very few disagreed with Watkinson on this point; even Dimsdale had compared the relative proportion of smallpox mortality to total mortality, as he pointed out in a subsequent pamphlet.[22]

To challenge Dimsdale's argument that the ratio of smallpox deaths to total deaths had increased from 1 of 8 to 1 of 6, however, Watkinson had to break

[21] John Watkinson, *An Examination*, p. 5.

[22] Thomas Dimsdale, *Observations on the Introduction to the Plan of the Dispensary for General Inoculation, with Remarks on a Pamphlet Entitled 'An Examination of a Charge Brought against Inoculation by DeHaen, Rast, Dimsdale, and Other Writers, by John Watkinson, M.D.'* (London: William Richardson, 1778), p. 22.

the assumed association between inoculation and increased smallpox mortality. He did so by demonstrating that there was no regular numerical relationship between the two. The following table shows the proportions of "the mean annual number of deaths by the smallpox, compared with the mean annual number of deaths by all the other diseases," for a series of 7-year periods.[23]

1714–1720	1 to 11	before inoculation
1721–1727	1 to 11	after inoculation
1728–1734	1 to 12	
1735–1741	1 to 13	
1742–1748	1 to 13	
1749–1755	1 to 11	
1756–1762	1 to 9	

Before inoculation (that is, prior to 1721), roughly 1 of 11 burials was attributed to smallpox. After the introduction of inoculation, the proportion varied from 1 of 9 (1756–1762) to 1 of 13 burials (1735–1741 and 1742–1748). "That the prevalence of inoculation, and the increased mortality of the smallpox, have in no point of time coincided, I do not mean to insinuate," Watkinson conceded. "By the laws of chance, this must sometimes have happened. But I contend, that the great irregularity of their coincidence may be considered as a fresh proof, that the one, is not the cause of the other."[24] Watkinson could see no connection between inoculation and increased smallpox mortality because of the variation in these ratios.

Watkinson's second criticism focused on Dimsdale's periodization. Dimsdale had calculated the proportion of natural smallpox deaths to total deaths for two unequal periods: 1734–1767 (34 years) and 1768–1775 (8 years). The latter period revealed a significant increase: 1 of 6 deaths due to smallpox, compared to 1 of 8. Watkinson questioned this seemingly ad hoc approach by analyzing the London bills of mortality from 1629 through 1776 in 4-year, 8-year, 12-year, and 24-year periods. For each of these periodizations, Watkinson identified the same kind of variation in natural smallpox mortality that he had found using the 7-year periods. Natural smallpox mortality had been steadily increasing since 1629, long before inoculation was practiced. "The body of evidence now adduced in favour of inoculation," Watkinson ambitiously claimed, "amounts I may venture to say to a demonstration, that the charge which has been preferred against it, of spreading the contagion, and increasing the mortality of the smallpox cannot possibly be true."[25]

Dimsdale responded to Watkinson's attack by dissecting his arguments. Dimsdale noted that any consideration of changes in natural smallpox mortality

---

[23] Various editions of Watkinson's pamphlet exist; in the first edition, the ratios are embedded in text and not displayed in tabular form. Watkinson, *An Examination,* p. 27.
[24] Watkinson, *An Examination,* p. 29. [25] Watkinson, *An Examination,* p. 43.

had to begin in 1700. Prior to that time, smallpox deaths were often counted with other diseases in the bills (a confusion Jurin had remarked upon). Moreover, plague mortality was so great in the seventeenth century that it distorted severely the reporting of all other diseases. "This destructive disorder, less known to later times," Dimsdale pronounced, "must certainly disturb the proportion of deaths as compared in different periods, and to this must be added the desolating calamities of Civil War."[26] For Dimsdale, there was no way to identify the small fluctuations in smallpox mortality against the backdrop of large and often catastrophic mortalities associated with plague and political upheaval.

The Irish physician William Black further complicated the picture by pointing out that smallpox itself was an epidemical disease and that its fluctuations were not consistent from year to year. Black, a firm advocate of inoculation, had received his MD from Leiden in 1772 and was associated with the General Dispensary for Poor Married Women in London. In his 1781 essay *Observations Medical and Political: On Smallpox and Inoculation,* he noted that "there is an ebb and flow in natural Small-pox as in all other diseases, especially of the febrile class." Further, "epidemical and particularly contagious diseases cannot be expected to keep upon an annual equality."[27] Black calculated that between 12,000 and 15,000 individuals fell ill with smallpox in London annually, and he asserted that inoculation could not contribute substantially to these numbers.[28]

The most sophisticted and articulate analysis of the problem of periodization was made by the Scots physician Alexander Monro *primus.* Monro was one of the respondents to the questionnaire on inoculation issued by the Paris Faculté de Médecine, and he published his answers in *An Account of the Inoculation of Small Pox in Scotland* in 1765. In this essay, he presented his own table showing figures for the total number of deaths and the number of deaths due to smallpox in Edinburgh for two 10-year periods, 1744–1753 and 1754–1763. In the first period, inoculation was little practiced; in the second, inoculation was "more frequently, but far from being generally, performed."[29] From this table, Monro calculated that 1 of 10 died from smallpox in both periods. He then carefully delineated the other factors that affected mortality in Edinburgh during these years, including the high number of casualties at the battle of Preston (1745) and the malignant putrid fever that spread in the wake of the battle. Such observations, Monro noted, "shew how necessary it is to consider the different circumstances in calculations."[30] He included such factors as "whether more inhabitants have resorted to the place, or retired from it; – whether there have been more or fewer dangerous epidemical diseases; – whether the provisions

[26] Dimsdale, *Observations,* p. 100.   [27] Black, *Observations Medical and Political,* p. 65.
[28] Black, *Observations Medical and Political,* pp. 78–79.
[29] Alexander Monro, *An Account of the Inoculation of Small Pox in Scotland* (Edinburgh, 1765), p. 11.
[30] Monro, *An Account of the Inoculation,* p. 14.

have been equally good in the years when comparisons are made, &c."[31] In short, Monro argued that to measure smallpox mortality required consideration of fluctuations in the size and health of the population.

These considerations suggest the development of more nuanced views of mortality patterns and represent the incorporation of dynamic factors in discussions of population and mortality. Monro's careful and cautious use of numerical arguments stands in marked contrast to those put forth in the controversy over inoculating the poor. "Tedious tables of calculations, formed on the bills of mortality," one critic complained, "have been repeatedly produced; but by them nothing has been proved decisive to the point in question."[32] In the debate over whether to inoculate the poor of London, physicians wrestled with ways to represent changes in mortality and the kinds of conclusions to be drawn. The tables constructed to demonstrate changes in mortality failed; instead, they revealed that contradictory figures could be calculated from the same data set (in this case, the London bills of mortality). The malleability of the numbers and the tables undermined any claim to authority by anyone participating in the controversy.

INOCULATION OUTSIDE LONDON

Physicians and surgeons generally had more success in inoculating the poor of smaller communities.[33] Dimsdale, who had campaigned vigorously against the London efforts, actively supported general inoculations among inhabitants of villages and towns outside London. He could do this because he firmly believed that in smaller communities, all the inhabitants could be inoculated at the same time and thus prevent any chance of contagion. In Hertford, where his family held property, he oversaw three general inoculations in 1766, 1770, and 1774. Inoculations in the latter two years were almost entirely of young children. The result, Dimsdale wrote, was "that within these ten years not six persons have died in Hertford of this disease."[34] Based on his experiences, he published *Tracts on Inoculation* in 1781, which outlined how general inoculations should be carried out.

During the second half of the eighteenth century, many small villages held general inoculations, and figures were collected and published to demonstrate

---

[31] Monro, *An Account of the Inoculation*, p. 10.
[32] *A Letter to J.C. Lettsom, M.D. FRS, SAS &c. Occasioned by Baron Dimsdale's Remarks on Dr. Lettsom's Letter to Sir Robert Barker, and G. Stacpoole, Esq. upon General Inoculation, by an Uninterested Spectator of the Controversy between Baron Dimsdale and Dr. Watkinson* (London: J. Murray, 1779), p. 8.
[33] Maisie May has recently suggested that the success of the dispensary movement in regards to inoculation be reevaluated by focusing on the motives of the dispensary physicians. See Maisie May, "Inoculating the Urban Poor in the Late Eighteenth Century," *British Journal for the History of Science* 30 (1997): 291–305.
[34] Dimsdale, *Thoughts on General and Partial Inoculations*, pp. 32–33; quoted in Razzell, *The Conquest of Smallpox*, p. 84.

the benefits.[35] The Reverend John Howlett, for example, examined the history of smallpox mortality for the town of Maidstone, and he discovered that every 5 or 6 years mortality doubled because of smallpox epidemics. From 1734, Howlett concluded "that in the short space of 30 years it [smallpox] deprived the town of between 5 and 600 of its inhabitants; whereas in the 15 or 16 years that have elapsed since the general inoculation it has occasioned the death of only about 60. Ample and satisfactory evidence of the vast benefit the town has received from this salutary invention!"[36]

The physician John Haygarth, who practiced in Chester in northwest England, also took an active interest in inoculation and in the use of mortality figures to guide medical policy. From his school days (especially medical studies at Edinburgh), he maintained friendships with several dissenting physicians and shared many of their philanthropic goals. He was, as his most recent biographer has described him, "a physician working with the conviction of the 'philanthropic' responsibility of the 'wealthy and opulent' in society for the 'poor and ignorant.'"[37] During the 1770s and 1780s, Haygarth maintained close correspondence with the Unitarian Thomas Percival, a Manchester physician who established the Manchester Literary and Philosophical Society in 1781, one of the numerous societies created during the second half of the eighteenth century that was devoted to fostering inquiry and exchange on a range of topics, including science and medicine.[38] Percival and Haygarth were also Fellows of the Royal Society. They were keenly interested in issues concerning population, especially the links between manufacturing and population growth.

Percival and Haygarth each compiled accounts from the bills of mortality of their respective cities, which were published in the *Philosophical Transactions*.[39] Haygarth calculated the "proportional fatality of the natural small-pox, in order to demonstrate the advantages of inoculation, and to discover at what age this operation should be performed that it may become the most extensively

---

[35] Razzell provided an extensive account of general inoculations in eighteenth-century England. Razzell, *The Conquest of Smallpox*, pp. 73–92.

[36] [John Howlett], *Observations on the Increased Population, Healthiness, etc. of Maidstone* [Maidstone], 1782, pp. 7–8 (quotation on p. 8); reprinted in D.V. Glass, *The Development of Population Statistics* (Farnborough, Hants, Eng.: Gregg International Publishers Limited, 1973).

[37] Francis M. Lobo, "John Haygarth, Smallpox and Religious Dissent in Eighteenth-Century England," in *The Medical Enlightenment of the Eighteenth Century*, ed. Andrew Cunningham and Roger French (Cambridge: Cambridge University Press, 1990), p. 217.

[38] Robert Kargon, *Science in Victorian Manchester: Expertise and Enterprise* (Baltimore: Johns Hopkins University Press, 1977); A.E. Musson and Eric Robinson, *Science and Technology in the Industrial Revolution* (Manchester: University of Manchester Press, 1968).

[39] John Haygarth, "Observations on the Bill of Mortality, in Chester, for the Year 1772," *Philosophical Transactions* 64 (1774): 67–78; Haygarth, "Bill of Mortality for Chester for the Year 1773," *Philosophical Transactions* 65 (1775): 85–90; Haygarth, "Observations on the Population and Diseases of Chester, in the Year 1774," *Philosophical Transactions* 68 (1778): 131–154; Thomas Percival, "Observations on the State of Population in Manchester, and Other Adjacent Places," *Philosophical Transactions* 64 (1774): 54–66; Percival, "Observations on the State of Population in Manchester, and Other Adjacent Places Concluded," *Philosophical Transactions* 65 (1775): 322–335.

beneficial to society."[40] The dramatic impact of smallpox epidemics on total mortality in Chester emerged clearly. According to Haygarth, 16 persons died from smallpox in 1772, but only 1 in 1773, and a staggering 202 in 1774. The proportion of smallpox mortality to total mortality for this last year was 1 to 2.7 – much greater than the figures for London.[41]

Percival, too, investigated the relationship between age and smallpox mortality. He compiled two tables that recorded information on age of death due to smallpox in two different locales. (Figures 4.3 and 4.4.) "The risque of receiving the natural smallpox by infection appears to be very great during the second year of life; and the fatality of the disease at this period is highly alarming," Percival concluded. "To avert such impending danger, the inoculation of healthy and vigorous children, at the *age of two or three months*, seems to be advisable, especially in large towns."[42] This marked a significant departure from earlier ideas and practices. Arbuthnot, Jurin, and even Dimsdale had subtracted the number of deaths under the age of two from the total number of deaths in order to calculate the proportion of smallpox mortality to total mortality. They reasoned that infants died of other diseases and conditions, and hence the impact of smallpox on this age group was negligible. Percival's tables revealed otherwise.

Haygarth acted on his calculations and established the Small-Pox Society at Chester in 1778, a charitable organization financed by private subscription, which began to carry out the general inoculation of poor children in 1780. Its success led others towns to do the same: Leeds in 1781 and Liverpool in 1781 and 1782.[43] Haygarth kept careful accounts of smallpox mortality and the number of inoculations performed. In Chester from 1778 to 1784, 378 persons died from smallpox. "Inoculation, since its late improvements, according to the most unfavourable computation is not fatal to *one* in 100; consequently, if the whole number had been inoculated, only 27 would have died," he argued, "therefore 351 lives would have been saved by this art, that have perished by the natural small-pox, or above 58 annually."[44]

It was bitterly ironic that Haygarth's publication of *An Inquiry How to Prevent the Small-Pox and Proceedings of a Society* (1784) coincided with the end of the success of his program in Chester. That year, only 1 child was inoculated in Chester (213 had been inoculated in 1783), and the Society collapsed for unknown reasons. Haygarth, however, remained convinced of the benefits of

---

[40] Haygarth, "Observations on the Population...1774," p. 142; quoted in Lobo, "John Haygarth," p. 234.

[41] Haygarth, "Observations on the Population...1774," p. 142.

[42] Emphasis in original; Thomas Percival, "Essay on the Small-Pox and Measles," *Medical Observations and Inquiries*, vol. 5 (1776), p. 281; reprinted in D.V. Glass, *Population and Disease in Early Industrial England* (Farnborough, Hants, Eng.: Gregg International Publishers Limited, 1973).

[43] John Haygarth, *An Inquiry How to Prevent the Small-Pox and Proceedings of a Society* (Chester: J. Monk, 1785), p. 207.

[44] Haygarth, *An Inquiry*, p. 154.

272   *Medical Obſervations and Inquiries.*

An Account of Deaths by the Small-pox, *during ſix Years, viz. from* 1768 *to* 1774, *collected from the Regiſter of the Collegiate Church at* Mancheſter.

T A B L E I.

Ages.	Males.	Females.	Annual Deaths by the Small-pox.		Deaths by all Diſeaſes.
From birth to 3 mcnths.	2	2	A. D.		
From 3 to 6 months.	9	8	1769	74	549
			1770	41	689
From 6 months to 1 year.	51	68	1771	182	678
2	103	113	1772	66	608
3	55	55	1773	139	648
4	33	26	1774	87	635
5	18	16			
10	17	12			
20	1	0			
30	0	0			
Total	289	300		589*	3807

* This account of the *annual deaths* by the Small-pox, from 1768 to 1774, differs from the printed bills of mortality, which make the number amount to 586, and not to 589. But it has been extracted from the church regiſter, with a degree of care and attention not uſually beſtowed upon the printed bills; and the accuracy of it may, I believe, be relied on.

4.3 Thomas Percival's table of smallpox deaths by age and sex in Manchester (1768–1774). *Source:* Thomas Percival, "Essay on the Small-Pox and Measles," in *Medical Observations and Inquiries* 5 (1776), p. 272. Yale University, Harvey Cushing/John Hay Whitney Medical Library.

general inoculation and proposed an ambitious plan to inoculate every individual in Britain. In this plan, "civil regulation" played a prominent role. In his first proposal, fines and rewards served as the mechanisms to encourage the public to get inoculated and to follow his health rules; in his next proposal, Haygarth outlined a formal organization of government officials to oversee and carry out the inoculations and the adherence to his health rules. Fitting such a

Deaths from the Small-pox *at* Warrington *in* 1773.

TABLE II.

Ages.				Numbers.
Under 1 month	-	-		0
From 1 to 3 months		-		4
3	6	-	-	4
6	12	-	-	39
From 1 to 2 years			-	84
2	3	-	-	33
3	4	-	-	18
4	5	-	-	15
5	6	-	-	4
6	7	-	-	2
7	8	-	-	2
8	9	-	-	4
None above		Total		211

4.4 Thomas Percival's table of smallpox deaths by age in Manchester. *Source:* Thomas Percival, "Essay on the Small-Pox and Measles," in *Medical Observations and Inquiries* 5 (1776), p. 275. Yale University, Harvey Cushing/John Hay Whitney Medical Library.

state-directed approach, Haygarth included a political arithmetic calculation made by his friend John Dawson. Dawson, a dissenting mathematician and surgeon, announced that Britain's population would increase by 1 million if Haygarth's plans were adopted.[45] "The plague has been completely exterminated from this country, for above a century, by civil regulations," Haygarth wrote. "There seems to be little doubt that the small-pox is propagated on principles similar to the plague, and that it might be as certainly exterminated from the island."[46]

In 1788, the physician William Black presented a lecture entitled *An Arithmetical and Medical Analysis of the Diseases and Mortality of the Human Species* to the Medical Society of London, founded by Lettsom in 1773. Black subsequently published his lecture, and it enjoyed immediate recognition as the only work to include a numerical account of insanity, a disease of utmost importance

---

[45] On Haygarth's two plans, see Lobo, "John Haygarth," pp. 238–253, and May, "Inoculating the Urban Poor," pp. 301–304.

[46] John Haygarth, *A Sketch of a Plan to Exterminate the Casual Small-Pox from Great Britain; and to Introduce General Inoculation,* vol. 1 [vol. 2 was never published] (London: J. Johnson, 1793), p. 155.

because of George III's illness. Parliament examined numerous physicians on the state of the king's disease. "Throughout that examination, numerical data, in preference to the opinions, professional doctrines, and jarring aphorisms of auguries and oracles, were repeatedly called for: but it so happened," Black continued, "that mine ... were the only data of this description ever published on the disease."[47] Black, much like Petty before him, was not a timid fan of his own accomplishments. And, like Petty, he coined a catchy name for the numerical approach, medical arithmetic. Black ascribed a prominent place to Jurin in his history of medical arithmetic:

> I believe the first dawn of medical arithmetick will be found in Dr. Jurin, and was the last resource in support of inoculation, then in its infancy, but vilified in print by physicians and divines. It was by demonstrating in numbers the comparative success under inoculation, and the natural disease, that this inveterate conspiracy against the practice could be defeated.[48]

Smallpox inoculation served as a lightening rod for the uses of numerical arguments in eighteenth-century medicine. "There never was in my opinion since the origin of physick," Black wrote, "a medical controversy agitated of more consequence to mankind. It is not only a medical, but also a political, and a great national question."[49] Black might have overstated the case; nonetheless, inoculation had been widely accepted by the end of the eighteenth century, and the numerical arguments used to persuade and demonstrate its benefits encouraged a similar approach in other areas of medicine, the subject of the following two chapters.[50]

---

[47] William Black, *An Arithmetical and Medical Analysis of the Diseases and Mortality of the Human Species* (1789), p. iii; reprinted with an introduction by D.V. Glass, (Farnborough, Hants, Eng.: Gregg International Publishers Limited, 1973).
[48] Black, *An Arithmetical and Medical Analysis*, p. i.   [49] Black, *Observations Medical and Political*, p. 52.
[50] Miller, *The Adoption of Inoculation*, p. 26.

PART TWO

Medical Arithmetic and Environmental Medicine

5

Medical Meteorology: Accounting for the Weather and Disease

The fear of epidemics inspired physicians, natural philosophers, and government officials to study the effects of weather on health, or, in other words, medical meteorology.[1] These individuals were strongly influenced by prevalent Hippocratic ideas about the link between the environment and the incidence and mortality of different diseases. Medical meteorologists took a passionate interest in recording weather and disease observations often over a period of several years, and most of their accounts included quantitative information.

The motivation for this quantitative approach came in part from the relatively new belief that numbers, the tabular display of numbers, and the comparison of numbers would yield new knowledge about the causes and courses of epidemics and other diseases. Two developments undergirded this trust in numbers. First, the creation of techniques to analyze mortality numerically (initiated by John Graunt and successfully deployed by James Jurin in the inoculation debates) had set a new model for medicine. Second, the invention of instruments to measure temperature, air pressure, and humidity had transformed the study of meteorology. Developed over the course of the seventeenth century by many natural philosophers, including Galileo, Torricelli, Huygens, Hooke, and Wren, these instruments frequently incorporated numerical scales into their design, thus allowing for the quantification of weather phenomena.

[1] For a recent overview of medical meteorology see Caroline Hannaway, "Environment and Miasmata," in *Companion Encyclopedia of the History of Medicine,* ed. W.F. Bynum and Roy Porter (London and New York: Routledge, 1993), vol. 1, pp. 292–308, esp. pp. 296–300. Medical meteorology was part of environmental medicine, a term dubbed by Ludmilla Jordanova; see L.J. Jordanova, "Earth Science and Environmental Medicine: The Synthesis of the Late Enlightenment," in *Images of the Earth: Essays in the History of the Environmental Sciences,* ed. L.J. Jordanova and Roy Porter (British Society for the History of Science, 1979), pp. 119–146. Also see Mary J. Dobson, *Contours of Death and Disease in Early Modern England* (Cambridge: Cambridge University Press, 1997), esp. chap. 1; James C. Riley, *The Eighteenth-Century Campaign to Avoid Disease* (London: Macmillan, 1987); James C. Riley, *Population Thought in the Age of the Demographic Revolution* (Durham, N.C.: Carolina Academic Press, 1985), esp. chap. 5, pp. 83–103; and Clarence J. Glacken, *Traces on the Rhodian Shore: Nature and Culture in Western Thought from Ancient Times to the End of the Eighteenth Century* (Berkeley and Los Angeles: University of California Press, 1967), chaps. 12 and 13.

Medical and scientific societies provided critical support for the pursuit of medical meteorology, much as they had done for the study of inoculation. This was especially important because observing and noting the temperature and weight of the air (a barometric reading) on a daily basis required not only a certain temperament and a significant degree of self-discipline but, more importantly, a faith in the usefulness of such observations, a faith that was boosted by participation in various organized, institutionally based projects to collect meteorological and disease observations. Thus, individuals located outside metropolitan areas viewed correspondence with established societies as intellectually and socially rewarding. The memoirs and transactions of the societies provided a venue for publishing proposals, suggestions, and observations, and in general served to promote further contributions. Finally, societies frequently offered material support: Some sent meteorological instruments to observers who did not have access to the latest equipment, others provided preprinted forms, while others covered postage costs.

Generally speaking, those individuals interested in demonstrating numerically the links between health and environment faced two central problems: (1) how to ensure the consistent and reliable collection of numerical information, and (2) how to make use of that information. Tables were often heralded as the solution to the first problem, but tables, as a method to understand weather, disease, and the links between them, had only limited success in answering the second. A study of medical meteorology thus shows the strengths and weaknesses of numerical tables as a scientific method.

NUMERICAL NATURAL HISTORIES OF THE WEATHER

By 1700, meterology had become so well established that the keeping of weather diaries was a common hobby among educated Europeans. In these diaries, descriptive accounts of the weather became increasingly replaced by tables consisting of columns of numbers for the date, time, temperature, air pressure, and so on. During the eighteenth century, significant improvements in instrumentation and record keeping further encouraged systematic weather observations.[2] The format of these diaries, however, was by no means uniform. Contemporaries wrestled with a way to construct tables that would be comprehensive, readable, and easy to use.

---

[2] For histories of meteorology, see Theodore S. Feldman, "Late Enlightenment Meteorology," in *The Quantifying Spirit in the 18th Century,* ed. Tore Frängsmyr, J.L. Heilbron, and Robin E. Rider (Berkeley: University of California Press, 1990), pp. 143–178; H. Howard Frisinger, *The History of Meteorology to 1800* (New York: Science History Publications, 1977); Jan Golinski, "Barometers of Change: Meteorological Instruments as Machines of the Enlightenment," in *The Sciences in Enlightened Europe,* ed. William Clark, Jan Golinski, and Simon Schaffer (Chicago and London: University of Chicago Press, 1999), pp. 69–93; and Gordon Manley, "The Weather and Diseases: Some 18th-Century Contributions to Observational Meteorology," *Notes and Records of the Royal Society of London* 9 (1952): 300–307.

The changes in the construction of tables between the mid-seventeenth and the late eighteenth centuries can be analyzed by juxtaposing three proposals for improving meteorological observations: two made to the Royal Society of London and the third to the Société Royale de Médecine in Paris. The first was Robert Hooke's "Method for Making a History of the Weather," (1663); the second was James Jurin's "Invitatio ad Observationes Meteorologicas communi consilio instituendas" issued exactly sixty years later in 1723; and the final example was Félix Vicq d'Azyr's *Mémoire instructif sur l'établissement fait par le Roi d'une commission ou société et correspondance de médecine* of 1776.

England

Robert Hooke was one of the founders of the Royal Society and one of its most active members. He invented and improved numerous instruments, including the first device to use the freezing point of water as a fixed point on a thermometric scale.[3] His seven-page proposal for making a history of the weather, written in English and included in Thomas Sprat's *History of the Royal Society* (1667), called for observations using new instruments, such as the thermometer, hygroscope, and barometer, as well as for notes on the state of the sky, tides, and the varied effects "produc'd upon other bodies: As what Aches and Distempers in the bodies of men: what Diseases are most rife, as Colds, Fevours, Agues, &c. What putrefactions or other changes are produc'd in other bodies; As the sweating of Marble, the burning blew of a Candle, the blasting of Trees and corn."[4] It was common knowledge that the weather affected animate and inanimate bodies and, likewise, that changes in these bodies were clues to understanding the weather.

Hooke advocated the use of the table for explicitly methodological reasons that he framed in Baconian terms. "Now that these and some other [observations] . . . may be registered so as to be most convenient for the making of comparisons, requisite for the raising *Axioms*, whereby the Cause or Laws of Weather may be found out," Hooke reasoned, "[i]t will be desirable to order them so, that the Scheme of a whole Moneth, may at one view be presented to the Eye."[5] (See Figure 5.1.) Hooke's scheme facilitated comparison among observations that led to the formulation of general axioms – critical steps in the Baconian method. Hooke gave careful and precise instructions on how to construct a table for making a history of weather. He specified the paper size (folio); how many columns to draw (nine); the width of the columns (the first six should be $\frac{1}{2}''$); the headings for each column; and, finally, what abbreviations to use. Such detail highlights the novelty of the form.

[3] Frisinger, *The History of Meteorology to 1800*, p. 57.
[4] Robert Hooke, "Method for Making a History of the Weather," in Thomas Sprat, *History of the Royal Society* (1667; reprint edition with critical apparatus by Jackson I. Cope and Harold Whitmore Jones, St. Louis: Washington University Studies, 1959), pp. 174–175.
[5] Hooke, "Method for Making a History of the Weather," p. 175.

ROYAL SOCIETY.   179

A
SCHEME

At one View reprefenting to the Eye the Obfervations of the Weather for a Month.

Days of the Month and place of the Sun. Remarkable houfe.	Age and fign of the Moon at Noon.	The Quarters of the Wind and its ftrength.	The Degrees of Heat and Cold.	The Degrees of Drynefs and Moyfture.	The Degrees of Preffure.	The Faces or vifible appearances of the Sky.	The Notableft Effects.	General Deductions to be made after the fide is fitted with Obfervations: As,
4 8 14 II 12.46	27 12 ☿ 9. 46. 8 Perigeü.	W. 2. 3 3½ 10 W.SW.1	9 12 16 7	¾2 ½2 ⅛ ½2	5|29 1c 8 2 9 29 ⅛ 29 ⅜	Clear blew, but yellowifh in the N. E. Clowded to-ward the S. Checker'd blew.	A great dew. Thunder, far to fhe South. A very great Tide.	From the laft quar:of theMoon o the changethe weather was ve-·y temperate but cold for the fea-fon; the Wind pretty conftant between N. and W.
8 15 II 13.40	28 6 ♂ 24.51.N.	N.W. 3 4 2 8 1	4 7	½ 7	2 8½ 29 ¼ 2 9 2 1029	A clear Sky all day, but a little chec-ker'd at 4. P.M. at Sun-fet red and hazy.	Not by much fo big a Tide as yefterday. Thunder in the North.	A little before the laft great Wind, and till the Wind rofe at its higheft, the Quickfilver con-tinued defcend-ing till it came ·ery low; after which it began o reafcend,
10 N.Moon. S. 16 II 14.37	at 7. 25' A.M. II 10. 8.	1 10	1	1 10 28 ½		Overcaft and very lowr-ing.	No dew upon the ground, but very much upon Marble ftones, &c.	
&c.	&c.	&c.	&c.	&c.	&c.	&c.		&c

5.1 Robert Hooke's proposed table to record meteorological observations (1667). *Source:* Thomas Sprat, *History of the Royal Society* (London, 1667), p. 179.

Despite such detailed instructions, Hooke's proposal was not taken up on a wide-scale basis. Some individuals might have adopted his rules and guidelines, but there was not a systematic effort to collect and collate these diaries at the Royal Society or elsewhere. Hooke's proposal, while complete in form, was thus not effective in practice. Neither he nor anyone else collected the individual accounts.

Dies & Hora 1723. Nov. St. V.	Barom. alt. dig.dec	Therm alt. gr. dec	Vent.	Tempestas.	Pluvia. dig.dec
1. 8 *a. m.*	29.75	49 . 6	S. W. 1	Cœlum nubibus obduct. Imbres interrupti.	0.035
4 *p. m.*	29.56	47 . 3	S. W. 2	Sol pervices inter- currens	0.043
2. 7 ½ *a. m.*	29.24	48 . 5	S. 1	Pluviæ fere perpetua	0.725
3. 9 *a. m.*	29.95	49 . 7	N. 1	Cœlum fudum	0.032
5 *p. m.*	30. 4	49 . 2	N. 1	Cœlum fudum	0.000
4. 7 *a. m.*	29. 9	47 . 0	S. W. 1	Nubes fparfæ	0.000
10	29. 7	46 . 2	S. W. 2	Imbres intercurrentes	0.103
12	29. 4	45 . 0	S. 3	Cœlum nubibus un- dique fere tectum	0.050
3 *p. m.*	28. 8	46 . 0	S. 4	Nubes fparfæ	0.000
5	28. 6	47 . 2	S. W. 4	Eadem Cœli facies	0.000
7	28. 9	48 . 0	S. W. 2	Pluit	0.000
9	28. 9	48 . 2	0	Pluvia fere perpetua	0.305
5. 7 *a. m.*	29. 7	53 . 4	N. E. 1	Sudum. Gelu.	0.250

5.2 James Jurin's proposed table to record meteorological observations (1723). *Source:* James Jurin, "Invitatio ad Observationes Meteorologicas communi consilio instituendas," *Philosophical Transactions* 32, no. 379 (1722–1723): 427. Burndy Library, Dibner Institute for the History of Science and Technology.

Some 50 years later, James Jurin proposed to do just that. Under the auspices of the Royal Society, Jurin launched a project to collect meteorological records from observers in Europe and North America. At a meeting in December 1723, at roughly the same time he began his project to gather information on inoculation, he "set forth the great advantages which would accrue to Mankind from having a compleat Theory of the Weather, and that especially in the improvement in the Medicinal art."[6] He subsequently published an invitation in the *Philosophical Transactions* addressed to "men of learning."[7] Writing in Latin, Jurin aimed to create an international network of observers, and to this end, he printed his proposal separately and sent it to British diplomatic secretaries and Englishmen living abroad for distributution.[8]

Jurin, like Hooke, gave specific instructions for collecting and recording observations, and he included a sample table. (See Figure 5.2.) Several signif- icant features distinguish Jurin's table from Hooke's. Jurin replaced astronom- ical markings of time, found in the first two columns of Hooke's proposal,

[6] 12 December 1723, RS *Journal Book* XII.

[7] This phrase appears in a letter Jurin wrote to Zollman, 28 January 1724, Bodleian, MS Rawl. D.871; published in *The Correspondence of James Jurin (1684–1750), Physician and Secretary to the Royal Society,* ed. Andrea Rusnock (Amsterdam and Atlanta: Rodopi Press, 1996), p. 226.

[8] James Jurin, "Invitatio ad Observationes Meteorologicas communi consilio instituendas," *Philosophical Transactions* 32, no. 379 (1722–1723): 422–427.

with simply the date and hour of observation. Jurin employed decimals, where Hooke relied on fractions. Jurin designed a column for precipitation; Hooke recorded humidity. Jurin omitted the last two columns of Hooke's table that included observations on the tides, diseases, dew, and so on, as well as the "General Deductions." In sum, Jurin pared down the number of words to a minimum and instead wrote numbers in most of the columns. The result was a neater and more concise table, but one with fewer unique details.

Correspondents as far away as Uppsala, St. Petersburg, Berlin, Leiden, Naples, Lunéville, and Boston, as well as many towns in Great Britain and Ireland, embraced Jurin's proposal.[9] But in spite of such international enthusiasm, Jurin encountered many obstacles in executing his project. The lack of standardized measurements proved especially troublesome. Jurin urged his correspondents to construct conversion tables between their local measures and London measures (e.g., the Neapolitan palm and the London foot), but the actual work of converting measurements remained Jurin's. Even worse, the instruments used to make the measurements varied tremendously. Acknowledging the incompatability of observations made with idiosyncratic instruments, the Royal Society Council granted Jurin permission to send thermometers made by the London instrument maker Francis Hauksbee "at their expense as gifts to particular Observers, especially in more distant Regions."[10] One year later, Jurin informed the Royal Society Council that the distribution of the thermometers had improved the quality of observations and requested permission to distribute additional ones. The Council granted this request and disbursed funds for six more instruments in 1726, and another six in 1727.[11]

Along with conformable instruments and measures came the problem of uniform and consistent entries in weather journals. Jurin was often disappointed by his correspondents' sloppy record-keeping habits. "Please be so good as to write the time, along with the date, of each observation," he pleaded with Niccolò Cyrillo of Naples. "Please enter the actual numbers everywhere; short transverse lines, which occur in various entries, leave me in doubt whether an observation has been omitted or the numbers written by the previous observation are to be understood."[12] On occasion, Jurin had to instruct his correspondents on the use of decimal numbers.[13] Trickier still was the issue of dates; Britain did not use the same calendar as many countries on the Continent. Jurin repeatedly requested that his correspondents use the Julian calendar, even though

[9] The Royal Society Archives contain 18 weather diaries, spanning one or more years dating from Jurin's tenure, and many more from the following years. See Royal Society, Meteorological Archives.

[10] Jurin to Eric Benzel, 21 May 1725, Wellcome MS 6146; published in *The Correspondence of James Jurin*, pp. 302–303; RS Council Minutes, 15 April 1725.

[11] RS Council Minutes, 12 May 1726; RS Council Minutes, 20 April 1727.

[12] Jurin to Niccolò Cyrillo, 1 April 1727, Wellcome MS 6146.

[13] See, for example, Jurin to Eric Burman, 16 December 1726, Wellcome MS 6146; published in *The Correspondence of James Jurin*, pp. 346–347.

he conceded that the new style was "nearer the truth, if we are considering astronomical exactitude."[14]

Beyond the technological and metrological problems, Jurin faced the delicate task of recruiting observers and ensuring their continued contributions. The voluntary recording of detailed meteorological observations on a regular basis took self-discipline and/or at least some sense of greater reward. Jurin relied upon the prestige of the Royal Society to motivate observers, as well as flattery and guilt. "I must hope you, or some of your Friends will be so good as to furnish me with some Observations on ye Weather," he wrote to Robert Simson, professor of mathematics at Glasgow University. "I should be concern'd that a Country, which has always, & still continues to produce so many Curious and Learned Men, should contribute nothing to a design, in which almost all ye rest of Europe readily concurr."[15] With continental Europeans, Jurin frequently resorted to blandishment. In one case, he sought the advice of an English nobleman residing in Italy, who responded with explicit directions concerning an observer in Naples: "[P]uff him up a little in order to encourage him the more to proceed in his work, for he is of a Nation, that loves excessively to be flatter'd, & as he will certainly spread all over Italy your answer, it may serve to animate others of his temper to contribute the sooner to the accomplishment of the great undertaking."[16]

Some correspondents exceeded Jurin's requests. A Dutch engineer, Nicolaas Cruquius, designed a beautiful graph that incorporated his observations on temperature, air pressure, phases of the moon, wind strength, and humidity into a single form.[17] The Royal Society, at least in Jurin's words, seemed almost dumbstruck by such an innovation. "It is impossible to express, my dear Sir," Jurin wrote to Cruquius, "with what amazement everyone observed such a succinct conclusion of so much work. When they saw so many different facts compressed into so small a space; nevertheless all was so splendidly and suitably arranged that no item blocked any other or caused even the least difficulty in seeing any other."[18] Despite the Society's admiration, none of the Fellows attempted to replicate Cruquius's graph; it remained a marvel, and unlike the table, was not adopted as a useful form of representation.

From the very beginning of the meteorological project, Jurin had planned to summarize his correspondents' observations into a natural history of the air. He confidently wrote to a fellow physician:

---

[14] Jurin to Niccolò Cyrillo, 26 March 1725, Wellcome MS 6146; published in *The Correspondence of James Jurin*, p. 291.

[15] Jurin to Robert Simson, 29 January 1726, Wellcome MS 6146; published in *The Correspondence of James Jurin*, pp. 323–324.

[16] Thomas Dereham to Jurin, 16 February 1725, RS Early Letters D.2.21; published in *The Correspondence of James Jurin*, p. 287.

[17] See Royal Society, Meteorological Archives, 54.

[18] Jurin to Nicolaas Cruquius, 5 March 1726, Wellcome MS 6146; published in *The Correspondence of James Jurin*, p. 330.

I hope in a little time to be in a condition to publish ye result of ye Journals I have recd, but must always be a considerable time behind hand, on account of ye foreign Journals, some of wch come in very late. But I find great encouragement to go on in my design, & hope in time to deduce some thing of good, ye number of Observations yearly encreasing.[19]

However, he never compiled his natural history of the air. When Jurin stepped down from his secretaryship of the Royal Society at the end of 1727, his formal involvement with and enthusiasm for the project ended.

His successor as secretary, William Rutty, also found the task too daunting. "The observers seldom follow Dr Jurin's Invitatio," Rutty complained;

they not only each make use of their own Instruments, and generally neglect to put the main sum either to the Year of respective months under the particular head. Whereby the reducing this variety to the mean of our own Instruments, and finding out the Medium of theirs will occasion a great deal of trouble, before we can draw any Corollaries from the whole.[20]

Two of Jurin's contemporaries did, however, make use of the diaries collected by the Royal Society. William Derham, Fellow of the Society and author of the popular *Physico-Theology* and other natural theological works, published in the *Philosophical Transactions* several abstracts of the Society's meteorological diaries from the beginning of Jurin's project through 1728. When Derham died in 1735, the astronomer George Hadley, FRS, took over the arduous task and published an account of the diaries received for the years 1728 through 1730. Hadley referred to Jurin's method of calculating mean temperature and barometric readings by month and year, and included tables of these averages in his account.[21]

Even without a comprehensive natural history of the air, Jurin's meteorological project did have a lasting effect on the recording of weather observations in Britain. In the preface to his book on weather and epidemic diseases, the physician John Huxham noted that his observations had been made "on the Plan, which the celebrated Dr. James Jurin published in Philosoph. Transact. No. 379, which every one now follows, particularly the very highly esteemed Society of Edinburgh."[22] Other publications, especially those found in the *Philosophical Transactions*, showed the influence of Jurin's method on meteorology.[23]

---

[19] Jurin to John Huxham, 24 March 1726, Wellcome MS 6141; reprinted in *The Correspondence of James Jurin*, pp. 332–333.

[20] William Rutty to John Huxham, 21 March 1730, RS Letter Book Copy 19.411.

[21] William Derham, see "An Abstract of the Meteorological Diaries Communicated to the Royal Society," *Philosophical Transactions* 38 (1733–1734): 101–109, 334–344, and 458–470; George Hadley, "An Account and Abstract of the Meteorological Observations Communicated to the Royal Society for the Years 1731, 1732, 1733, 1734 and 1735," *Philosophical Transactions* 42 (1742): 243–263; and George Hadley, *Philosophical Transactions* 40 (1738): 154–175.

[22] The Society for the Improvement of Medical Knowledge of Edinburgh, renamed the Philosophical Society in 1739; John Huxham, *Observationes de aëre et morbis epidemicis . . . 1727–1737, Plymuthi factae. Hic accedit opusculum de morbo colico Damnoniensi* (London: S. Austen, 1739), p. xxxii.

[23] See, for example, "Extracts of Two Letters from Dr. John Lining, Physician at Charles-Town in South Carolina, to James Jurin, M.D. F.R.S. Giving an Account of Statical Experiments Made Several Times

France

The final example of a proposal for recording meteorological observations comes from the Société Royale de Médecine in Paris. Granted its letters patent in 1778, the Société evolved from the Commission for Epidemics, which had been set up by the Comptroller-General of Finances, Anne Robert Jacques Turgot, to monitor both epidemics and epizootics.[24] The Société Royale de Médecine, like the Paris Académie Royale des Sciences, was much more intimately connected with government interests and policies than was the Royal Society of London. The main functions of the Société Royale de Médecine were to regulate patent medicines and mineral waters, monitor and limit epidemics, and suggest and enforce measures to promote public health. The Société Royale de Médecine became the center of a national correspondence network with provincial doctors and *intendants,* and Félix Vicq d'Azyr (1748–1794) was appointed permanent secretary to oversee this correspondence. Well known for his work in comparative anatomy, Vicq d'Azyr was personal physician to Marie Antoinette and a member of both the Académie Royale des Sciences and the Académie Française. Ambitious and energetic, he defined the Société Royale de Médecine's goals. "Of all the functions to which the Société de Médecine was called on being instituted," he wrote, "it has always felt that the most useful was that of gathering by an extensive correspondence observations that could hasten the progress of our art."[25]

Meteorological observations were seen as an integral part of that correspondence. In the first volume of the *Histoire de la Société Royale de Médecine,* Vicq d'Azyr directed future correspondents to record weather observations three times a day following the method recommended by Père Louis Cotte.[26] Cotte, a priest of the Oratory and one of the foremost meteorologists in France, had outlined his method for recording weather observations in his *Traité de météorologie*

in a Day upon Himself, for One Whole Year, Accompanied with Meteorological Observations," *Philosophical Transactions* 42, no. 470 (1743): 491–509.

[24] For a history of the Société Royale de Médecine, see Laurence Brockliss and Colin Jones, *The Medical World of Early Modern France* (Oxford: Clarendon Press, 1997), pp. 760–782; Charles C. Gillispie, *Science and Polity in France at the End of the Old Regime* (Princeton, N.J.: Princeton University Press, 1980), chap. 3, pp. 187–256; Caroline Hannaway, "Medicine, Public Welfare and the State in Eighteenth-Century France: The Société Royale de Médecine (1776–1793)," Ph.D. dissertation, Johns Hopkins University, 1974. For a survey of the archives of the Société, see Jean Meyer, "Une enquête de l'Académie de médecine sur les épidémies (1774–1794)," *Annales – Economies, Sociétés, Civilisations,* 1966, pp. 729–749; and Jean-Pierre Peter, "Disease and the Sick at the End of the Eighteenth Century," in *Biology of Man In History,* ed. Robert Forster and Orest Ranum, trans. Elborg Forster and Patricia Ranum (Baltimore: Johns Hopkins University Press, 1975), pp. 81–124 [originally published in *Annales – Économies, Sociétés, Civilisations,* 1967, pp. 711–751].

[25] Vicq d'Azyr in memo to Legislative Assembly, 1792, Bibliothèque de l'Académie Nationale de Médecine, MS 114, doss. 21; translated and quoted in Gillispie, *Science and Polity,* p. 196.

[26] Vicq d'Azyr, *Histoire de la Société Royale de Médecine,* 1776 [Vol. 1], Preface, p. xi. Much of the information presented here is from Caroline Hannaway, "The Société Royale de Médecine and Epidemics in the Ancien Régime," *Bulletin of the History of Medicine* 46 (1972): 257–273; and Hannaway, "Medicine, Public Welfare and the State," pp. 157–161.

(1774). Cotte advised Vicq d'Azyr and essentially directed the Société Royale de Médecine's meteorological correspondence.[27]

Vicq d'Azyr utilized existing government bureaucracies to create his correspondence network to a much greater degree than had Jurin, who had relied on Fellows of the Royal Society who happened also to be diplomatic secretaries. In a memoir to the intendants, Vicq d'Azyr outlined the meteorological project and instructed them to forward it to local medical faculties and provincial physicians. Vicq d'Azyr's strategy proved the more successful: As secretary to the Société Royale de Médecine, he headed a large network comprised of approximately 150 physicians from most areas of France and from some of France's colonies. In part, this broad reach can be attributed to the benefits that correspondents expected from participation, namely, more government assistance during times of epidemics. Jurin, by contrast, could only offer the warm thanks and hearty commendation of the Royal Society.

Beginning in 1780, the Société Royale de Médecine began to distribute preprinted tabular forms to the intendants.[28] There are several noteworthy features that distinguish this table from Jurin's and Hooke's. Perhaps the most important is that the date and times of observations were printed on the form, in effect forcing the observer to record the requested information three times a day, every day. Numerical readings from a thermometer, hygrometer, and barometer, plus notes on precipitation, winds, and the state of the sky formed the core of the observations. Two other columns were devoted to more qualitative descriptions of astronomical and agricultural observations, such as aurora borealis or when particular plants flowered. Finally, the largest column on the form was designed to accommodate a monthly summary that included both the record high and low readings, plus the numerical averages for temperature, air pressure, and humidity.

The Société Royale de Médecine also recommended that observers use instruments made by the Parisian instrument maker Mossy, which could be purchased from him at the price of 24 livres for a barometer and 9 livres for a thermometer. (Mossy was also the instrument maker of choice for the Académie Royale des Sciences.)[29] These instruments were more precise and dependable than those

---

[27] Cotte published a subsequent work in 1788: *Mémoires sur la météorologie, pour servir de suite et de supplément au Traité de météorologie*, 2 vols. (Paris, 1788). For more on Cotte, see E. Le Roy Ladurie and J.-P. Desaive, "Étude par ordinateur des données météorologiques constituées par les correspondants de la Société Royale de Médecine (1776–1792)," in Jean-Paul Desaive, Jean-Pierre Goubert, Emmanuel Le Roy Ladurie, Jean Meyer, Otto Muller, and Jean-Pierre Peter, *Médecins, climat et épidémies à la fin du XVIIIᵉ siècle* (Paris: Mouton, 1972), pp. 23–134, esp. pp. 25–27; Feldman, "Late Enlightenment Meteorology," pp. 164–177; and Gillispie, *Science and Polity*, pp. 226–229.

[28] See Hannaway, "The Société Royale de Médecine and Epidemics in the Ancien Régime," p. 268, esp. footnote 3. This form is reproduced and discussed in Le Roy Ladurie and Desaive, "Étude par ordinateur," pp. 27–29; also see Harvey Mitchell, "Rationality and Control in French Eighteenth-Century Medical Views of the Peasantry," *Comparative Studies in Society and History* 21 (1979): 82–112.

[29] See *Avis sur la correspondance de la Société Royale de Médecine, et sur les objets dont cette compagnie est chargée* (Paris, n.d.), p. 1, footnote 3; quoted in Hannaway, "Medicine, Public Welfare and the State," p. 160, footnote 17.

available to Jurin during the first half of the century, and they aided in the goal of making observations more comparable.[30] Correspondents were instructed to send in their reports every three months, and Père Cotte produced annual summaries of these observations and published them in the Société's *Mémoires*.

Cotte's annual accounts followed much the same pattern established by the Englishmen William Derham and George Hadley, who had summarized the Royal Society meteorological diaries. Cotte presented figures for the high, low, and average temperature and air pressure in a table for each month at each location.[31] (See Figure 5.3.) On the reverse side of the table he listed general observations about prevailing diseases, but did not include any quantitative information in these remarks. He generally avoided lengthy tables, commenting that "tables are not pleasant for the reader."[32]

Taken together, Hooke's, Jurin's, and Vicq d'Azyr's proposals and the various networks they generated demonstrate an increasing reliance on the new weather technologies – more precise and uniform thermometers, barometers, and hygrometers, as well as carefully and usefully designed tables. Based on the coordination of far-flung observers by a central figure, these projects depended on the resources of national societies or academies. Contributions from observers were either voluntary (Jurin's) or official (Vicq d'Azyr's), and the types of benefits and rewards that accrued to observers certainly affected levels of participation. All, however, recognized the importance of an established and esteemed institution. "Men die," Cotte reminded his readers, "but the academic body always subsists."[33]

LINKING DISEASE AND WEATHER

The problems in creating a quantitative natural history of the weather were compounded when individuals attempted to link meteorological observations with observations on disease.[34] One could either begin with weather observations and tack on comments about disease, or begin with individual case histories of disease and append observations about the weather. The central difficulty lay in the fact that disease and weather have different narrative structures. An individual's experience with illness had its unique course, although some elements of that experience might be shared by others. Respiratory ailments, for example,

---

[30] Feldman, "Late Enlightenment Meteorology," pp. 156–158.
[31] See for example, "Observations Météorologiques," *Histoire de la Société Royale de Médecine,* 1776 (Paris, 1779), pp. 129–184.
[32] Cotte, *Traité de météorologie* (Paris, 1774), p. 517; quoted in Feldman, "Late Enlightenment Meteorology," p. 167.
[33] "Observations Météorologiques," *Histoire de la Société Royale de Médecine,* 1777 and 1778 (Paris, 1780), pp. 92–93.
[34] See Mary Dobson for a discussion of seventeenth- and eighteenth-century English views on the links between disease and weather; Dobson, *Contours of Death and Disease in Early Modern England* (Cambridge: Cambridge University Press, 1997), pp. 19–26.

NOMS DES VILLES.	JOURS		THERMOMÈTRE.		
	de la plus grande chaleur.	du plus grand froid.	Plus grande chaleur.	Plus grand froid.	Chaleur moyenne.
			Degrés.	*Degrés.*	*Degrés.*
Saint-Domingue . . .	21.	16.	21, 0.	17, 0.	19, 5.
Perpignan	26.	4.	28, 0.	10, 0.	15, 9.
Aix	25.	8.	25, 3.	8, 0.	15, 8.
Montpellier.	24. 25.	8.	26, 0.	8, 0.	16, 6.
Sévérac le-Château . .	25.	. . .	23, 5.		
Bordeaux	25.	7.	24, 8.	8, 8.	14, 0.
Villefranche	. . .	. . .	25, 0.	9, 0.	. . .
Briançon	. . .	. . .	. . .	5, 5.	
Padoüé	. . .	. . .	. . .		. . .
Poitiers	21.	7.	23, 3.	6, 0.	13, 2.
Clermont-Ferrand . .	22.	7. 8.	21, 5.	8, 0.	14, 2.
Saint-Maurice-le-Girard .	27.	5.	21, 5.	5, 0.	13, 1.
Chinon	21.	7.	23, 0.	9, 5.	14, 3.
Montargis	3.	. . .	24, 0.	16, 0.	. . .
Nancy	22.	7.	20, 0.	8, 0.	13, 7.
Paris.	21.	7.	22, 0.	9, 0.	14, 7.
Meaux	21.	26.	19, 0.	11, 0.	14, 4.
Montmorenci	21.	7.	24, 0.	5, 2.	13, 7.
Arras	3.	7.	24, 0.	8, 0.	. . .
Bruxelles	2.	7.	24, 0.	8, 5.	15, 3.
La-Haye	3.	8.	23, 5.	10, 0.	14, 8.
Amsterdam	3.	7.	23, 5.	9, 7.	16, 8.
Franeker	2.	8.	24, 8.	8, 3.	15, 2.
Léwarden	2.	7.	26, 3.	8, 0.	17, 2.
Londres.	. . .	. . .	15, 2.	0, 3.	13, 5.

5.3 Louis Cotte's meteorological table for June 1776. *Source: Mémoires de la Société Royale de Médecine* 1776 (1779), p. 170. Yale University, Harvey Cushing/John Hay Whitney Medical Library.

were more common in the winter months. But the specific twists and turns of a case of pneumonia often had little to do with daily variations in temperature or air pressure. Further, it was always a struggle to standardize etiologies, as the case of smallpox had illustrated.

Hist. de la Société Roy. de Méd. année 1776, page 170.

DE JUIN 1776.

JOURS de la plus grande élévation.	de la moindre élévation.	BAROMÈTRE. Plus grande élévation.	Moindre élévation.	Élévation moyenne.	Nombre des jours de pluie.	Quantité de pluie.	Vents dominans.	TEMPÉRATURE.
		Pouc. Lign.	*Pouc. Lign.*	*Pouc. Lign.*		*Pouc. Lign.*		
4.	10.	28. 4, 0.	28. 0, 6.	28. 2, 7.	6.	. . .	. . .	chaude & sèche.
9.	26.	28. 4, 6.	27. 10, 0.	28. 1,10.	8.	. . .	N. O. & E.	*idem.*
9. 22.	12.	27. 8, 6.	27. 3, 0.	27. 6, 2.	6.	1. 4, 9.	N.O. & O.	*idem.*
19.	12.	28. .5, 0.	27. 11, 0.	28. 2, 0.	7.	3. 2, 0.	E. & N.O.	chaude & humide.
19.	. 12.	28. 3,11.	27. 10, 6.	28. 1, 5.	18.	3. 7, 9.	O.	*idem.*
. . .	. . .	27. 9, 0.	27. 6, 0.	. . .	15.	. . .	S. O. & N.	*idem.*
. . .	. . .	. . .	. . .	27. 11, 2.	14.	2. 6, 9.	. . .	*idem.*
19.	26 27.	28. 3, 6.	27. 9, 3.	28. 0, 7.	10.	. . .	S.O. & N.O.	douce & sèche.
19.	12.	27. 1, 0.	26. 7, 6.	26. 10, 6.	17.	. . .	S. O. & S.	douce & humide.
19.	12.	28. 3, 6.	28. 0, 0.	28. 1, 7.	17.	. . .	S. & S. O.	*idem.*
20.	6.	28. 1, 6.	27. 9, 9.	27. 11, 4.	15.	. . .	O. & N.O.	froide & humide.
. . .	. . .	28. 2, 0.	27. 9, 6.	. . .	7.	. . .	N.O & S.O.	
19.	13.	27. 6, 3.	27. 0, 0.	27. 3, 4.	13.	. . .	S. O.	douce & humide.
19.	12.	28. 4, 9.	27. 9, 0.	28. 0, 7.	13.	2. 9, 3.	S. O.	chaude & sèche.
19.	12.	28. 4, 0.	27. 8, 0.	28. 0, 6.				
19.	12.	28. 2, 6.	27. 7, 0.	27. 10, 6.	16.	2. 5, 9.	S.O. & N. E.	*idem.*
19.	6.	28. 0, 6.	27. 5, 0.	. . .	10.	1. 11, 3.	O. & S.O.	
19.	6.	28. 4, 9.	27. 8, 0.	27. 10, 1.	13.	. . .	S.O. & O.	froide, assez sèche.
19.	6.	28. 3, 0.	27. 5, 0.	27. 9, 9.	9.	. . .	N.O.	froide & humide.
19.	. 6.	28. 2, 0.	27. 4, 0.	27. 9, 0.	. . .	. . .		*idem.*
19.	6.	28. 4, 9.	27. 6, 9.	27. 10,10.	11.	3. 5, 6.	N. O.	*idem.*
19.	6.	28. 5, 9.	27. 6, 9.	28. 0, 2.	. . .	. . .		*idem.*
. . .	. . .	28. 4, 1.	17. 5, 8.	27. 10, 4.	. . .	1 9, 0.		

5.3 *(cont.)*

Eighteenth-century physicians were well aware of these difficulties and wrestled with methods to record comparable information about symptoms, weather, climate, and so on, which might prove useful in the evaluation, treatment, or prevention of disease. In England, several physicians independently proposed methods to accomplish these goals, all of which relied on tables. In France, several institutional projects advanced medical meteorology, some of which relied on tables. Whether in England or France, medical meteorologists struggled to create meaningful and comparable accounts of weather and disease.

England

The most popular way to link weather and disease was to append observations on disease to meteorological records. Early in Jurin's project, for example, Edward Bayly, a physician who practiced in Havant, wrote that he "added a Column for Diseases which I extracted from a log [,] in which I keep [,] of all the Distempers wch appear from time to time in & about this Town." Here the individual physician acted as public health official:

I find more difficulty in managing this part then I first imagin'd when I propos'd it to you, but I am still perswaded that notwithstanding the difficulty of reducing the several Species of Diseases to their proper Classes yet by nicely observing those that are most predominant one may be able in time to collect some Observations towards the forming a Natural History of Diseases.[35]

As contemporary debates over nosology attest, defining diseases by their symptoms and properly classifying them posed a formidable challenge. Yet Bayly was convinced it was possible and Jurin wrote in agreement:

Your acct of ye reigning diseases, tho' attended as you Say, with considerable difficulties, may however be of very good service, especially if ye same be done by other Observers in different parts. Upon ye hint you gave me, I inserted that article into a Second Edition of my Invitation & have already had some Observations of that kind Sent me, & hope for more. Perhaps ye comparing them together may give us some light into ye obscure Theory of Epidemical Distempers.[36]

While Jurin did not set guidelines for recording disease observations, one of his contemporaries at the Royal Society did. Francis Clifton, MD from Leiden in 1724, Fellow of the Royal Society in 1727, and Fellow of the Royal College of Physicians in 1729, combined the Hippocratic method of case histories with Bacon's call for natural histories.[37] "The great *Lord Bacon* has judiciously inculcated the *Hippocratical* method of improving Physick, by observation," Clifton asserted.[38] To improve knowledge of diseases, Clifton recommended the use of a table in order to ensure regular collection of case histories. (See Figure 5.4.)

---

[35] Edward Bayly to Jurin, 21 June 1725, RS Early Letters B.2.99.

[36] Jurin to Edward Bayly, 29 January 1726, Wellcome MS 6146; published in *The Correspondence of James Jurin*, p. 323.

[37] For a laudatory, although brief, discussion of Clifton, see E. Ashworth Underwood, *Boerhaave's Men* (Edinburgh: Edinburgh University Press, 1977), p. 43.

[38] Francis Clifton, *Tabular Observations Recommended as the Plainest and Surest Way of Practising and Improving Physick in a Letter to a Friend* (London, 1731), p. 4. Clifton quoted the original Latin passage from Bacon (*de Augment. Scientiar.* Lib. IV. Cap. 2) in a footnote.

TABULA MEDICA GENERALIS.

Sexus, Ætas, Species,Temperies, Occupatio, & Victus Ægri.	Dies Morbi.	Morbi Phænomena.	Dies Mensis.	Remedia.	Eventus.

5.4 Francis Clifton's proposed table to record observations of disease (1731). *Source:* Francis Clifton, *Tabular Observations Recommended as the Plainest and Surest Way of Practicing and Improving Physick in a Letter to a Friend* (London, 1731), p. 19. Yale University, Harvey Cushing/John Hay Whitney Medical Library.

He included two complete examples in his aptly titled *Tabular Observations Recommended as the Plainest and Surest Way of Practising and Improving Physick in a Letter to a Friend* (1731). He assigned a column for meteorological observations in his initial tabular design, but subsequently partitioned those observations into a separate work. "There was another column at first, for the *Weather*," Clifton explained, "but having since got a Book by it self for those observations, in which I every day set down the course of the wind, and the dryness or moistness of the air; I have long left this article out."[39] This move underscored the material constraints of the existing technology for recording information on weather and disease on a single form.

Clifton's book was reviewed at a meeting of the Royal Society in April 1731 by the secretary to the society, Cromwell Mortimer, who flagged the tabular form as a significant break from traditional forms of medical writing: "In order to facilitate the business of Observation the Doctor has invented a new kind of Table wth separate Columns, to contain the several remarkable particulars that can happen in any Distemper. So that the Labour of the Physician is thus greatly eas'd and the Observations at once properly rang'd, or class'd, for Inspection and use."[40] In fact, Mortimer, a physician by training himself, was quite optimistic about the usefulness of such a design: "... upon this footing Disease might possibly, in time be found to be as regular in their Course as any other Phænomena, and are cur'd with as much ease as they are now contracted."[41]

---

[39] Clifton, *Tabular Observations*, p. 18.   [40] Register Book Copy of the Royal Society, RBC.15.344.
[41] Register Book Copy of the Royal Society, RBC.15.344.

Thus, according to Mortimer, using a tabular format fulfilled two purposes: It reduced the labor of the individual physician, and it promoted the nosological goals of classification and comparison.

Both Clifton's and Jurin's proposals depended on the assessment of prevailing disease by individual physicians, who in turn relied upon their private practice. There were obvious shortcomings to this approach, and several suggestions were made to develop alternative means for determining disease incidence. In a later work, Clifton proposed that hospitals might serve as a vehicle to forward medical knowledge:

> [T]hree or four persons of proper qualifications shou'd be employ'd in the *Hospitals* (and that without any ways interfering with the Gentlemen now concern'd) to set down the cases of the patients there from day to day, *candidly* and *judiciously*, without any regard to private opinions or publick systems, and at the year's end publish these facts just as they are, leaving every one to make the best use of 'em he can for himself.... Wou'd not some such method as this let us more into the *Nature* of diseases in a few years, than all the books of *theories*, or even the books of *Observations*, hitherto publish'd?[42]

Clifton's comments were prescient: Physicians who attended the newly established dispensaries and hospitals during the latter half of the eighteenth century published essays drawing on their experience at these places.[43]

Others proposed dispensing with physicians altogether. At a meeting of the Royal Society on 3 May 1744, Roger Pickering presented "A Scheme of a Diary of the Weather; together with Draughts and Descriptions of Machines Subservient Thereunto."[44] Pickering detailed a new method of record keeping, as well as descriptions of several new instruments to measure the force of the wind (the anemoscope), the moisture (his own hygrometer), and the amount of rain (the ombrometer). His method consisted of nine horizontal columns drawn in a diary for date, time, weight of air, temperature, moisture or dryness, wind direction, wind force, weather (rainy, cloudy, clear), and quantity of rain. (See Figure 5.5.) Below this, Pickering added, "the Space between the last Line and the End of the Paper, for the Bill of Mortality."[45] Acute cases were to be written in the record, as they depended upon the "State of the Air."

This last addition distinguished Pickering's proposal from others presented to the Royal Society. Individuals who had added observations on epidemic diseases to their meteorological reports as part of Jurin's project had all been physicians.

---

[42] Francis Clifton, *The State of Physick, Ancient and Modern, Briefly Consider'd: With a Plan for the Improvement of It* (London, 1732), p. 171.

[43] See, for example, the writings associated with the General Infirmary at Bath discussed in Anne Borsay, "An Example of Political Arithmetic: The Evaluation of Spa Therapy at the Georgian Bath Infirmary, 1742–1830," *Medical History* 44 (2000): 149–172.

[44] Roger Pickering, "A Scheme of a Diary of the Weather; Together with Draughts and Descriptions of Machines Subservient Thereunto; Inscribed to the President and Fellows of the Royal Society," *Philosophical Transactions* 43, no. 473 (1744): 1–18.

[45] Pickering, "A Scheme of a Diary of the Weather," pp. 3–4.

APRIL 1744.							
Days of the Month and Week.	1 Sabbath.	2 Monday.	3 Tuesday.	4 Wednesday.	5 Thursday.	6 Friday.	7 Saturday.
Hours of the Day.	8 a.m. 8 p.m.	8 a.m. 8 p.m.	8 a.m. 8 p.m.	8 a.m. 8 p.m.	8 a.m. 11 p.m.	8 a.m. 8 p.m.	8 a.m. 8 p.m.
Barometer.	$29\frac{196}{400}$ $29\frac{192}{400}$	$29\frac{126}{400}$ $29\frac{45}{400}$	$29\frac{144}{400}$ $29\frac{246}{400}$	$29\frac{297}{400}$ $29\frac{305}{400}$	$9\frac{146}{400}$ $29\frac{114}{400}$	$29\frac{132}{400}$ $29\frac{231}{400}$	$29\frac{392}{400}$ $29\frac{378}{400}$
Thermometer.	37 —	36 —	37 35	38 35	40 45	49 34	55 45
Hygrometer.	70 77	— 79	81 80	— 74	91 74	77 74	— 69
Anemoscope { Quarter. / Force.	W. :8	N. W. 30	— 74	— 16	S. E. 20	N. W. 16	W. 0
Weather.	Sleet. Rains	Snow. Sleet.	— Cloudy	— Starlight.	Rain. Cloudy.	Overcast. Starlt.	Fine. Overcast.
Ombrometer.	1:1	13 22	3	1	1 13		
Bill of Mortality.	Buried.	Males — 176 / Females · 217 / Total · 393 / Decreased 76	Died of	Apoplexy — 1 / Asthma — 8 / Colic — 1	Fever — 52 / Gripes — 4 / Lunatic — 2	Small Pox 32 / Suddenly 2	

5.5 Roger Pickering's proposed table of meteorological and acute disease observations (1744). *Source:* Roger Pickering, "A Scheme of a Diary of the Weather, . . ." *Philosophical Transactions* 43, no. 473 (1744): 15. Burndy Library, Dibner Institute for the History of Science and Technology.

Their observations had been based on their own personal experience as healers. Similarly, Clifton's proposal for tabular observations on disease patterns had been directed to physicians. Pickering, by contrast, advocated that mortality figures for acute diseases taken from the bills of mortality be added to the weather reports. He realized that he might encounter professional resistance to this idea:

Perhaps the Ignorance of the Searchers, appointed to inspect dead Bodies, as to the precise Diseases People die of, may lay this Method open to Objection. . . . To which it may be sufficient to answer, That this being obviously a requisite Article for a Diary, we must be content to take our Advices on this Point from such Hands, rather than none; especially, as all Political Arithmetic has always been allowed upon no more certain a Foundation.[46]

For Pickering, more information was better than precise information.

In the event, Pickering got no information. Neither his nor Clifton's scheme was taken up on a systematic basis. Their proposals were presented to the Royal Society, which provided a critical forum for the discussion of how to pursue medical meteorology but little actual support. The Royal Society could only encourage voluntary, cooperative projects. Across the Channel, the French government could actually implement medical meteorological projects on a national scale through various royal societies.

[46] Pickering, "A Scheme of a Diary of the Weather," pp. 4–5.

France

In France, coordinators of official correspondence networks provided some instruction for recording details about health and disease. In 1763, for example, the French army physician François-Marie-Claude Richard de Hautesierck advanced a plan to create a correspondence network among physicians and surgeons employed in military hospitals, with the express aim of the "preservation of the King's troops."[47] The plan was adopted and given official sanction by the Duke of Choiseul, the secretary of state for war, who had also promoted the policy of inoculating military students.

Richard de Hautesierck's work resulted in two published volumes entitled *Recueil d'Observations de Médecine des Hôpitaux Militaires.*[48] In the preface to the first volume, Richard de Hautesierck recommended the Hippocratic treatise *Airs, Waters and Places* as a model for his correspondents.[49] Contributors were urged to submit reports in the following areas: "Topographical and Medical Memoirs," "Meteorological and Clinical Observations," "Human and Animal Epidemics," and "Particularly Extraordinary Cases." Just as Vicq d'Azyr would later encourage contributors to the Société Royale de Médecine to report only the facts, so too did Richard de Hautesierck:

> There is no need to recommend to observers of candour and judgment, an absolute disengagement from systematic opinions, and proscription of all digressions from the subject and from experience. We already have too many imperfect descriptions of disease....[50]

In surveying the contents of the two volumes of the *Recueil,* it is clear that case histories were the preferred form of communicating medical information. Only in the "Topographical and Medical Memoirs" did quantitative information appear, and then only in reference to the number of inhabitants.[51]

An example from the *Recueil* can illustrate the demonstrative status accorded to individual case histories. One Dr. Cousin, physician to the military hospital of Bapaume, submitted a report of a soldier from Limosin whom he successfully treated with quinine for a case of gangrene. After describing the treatment, Cousin concluded: "This observation proves in the most complete manner, how one can count on the antiseptic virtue of quinine." Further, Cousin claimed, "one cannot insist too much on parallel facts, nor make them too public. How many people in fact have been mutilated or led to their graves in order to follow

---

[47] Richard de Hautesierck, *Receuils d'observations de médecine des hôpitaux militaires* 2 vols. (Paris, 1766), vol. 1, p. xvi.

[48] The volumes were published in 1766 and 1782.   [49] Richard de Hautesierck, *Recueil,* vol. 1, p. xi.

[50] Richard de Hautesierck, *Receuil,* vol. 1, p. xxiii.

[51] See for example Renaudin, "Mémoire sur le sol, les habitans et les maladies de la province d'Alsace," in Richard de Hautesierck, *Recueil,* vol. 2 (1782), pp. 6–48. For an overview of eighteenth-century French medical topographies, see Jean-Pierre Peter, "Aux sources de la médicalisation, le regard et le mot; le travail des topographies médicales," in *Populations et cultures: Études réunies en l'honneur de François Lebrun* (Rennes: Université de Rennes 2 Haute-Bretagne and the Institut Culturel de Bretagne, 1989), pp. 103–111.

another method, or to have ignored this one!"[52] Even when the possibility existed for more quantitative approaches to evaluating therapies, case histories remained the predominant form of medical evidence.

The reports sent to the Société Royale de Médecine were similar to those of Richard de Hautesierck's correspondents. The Société Royale de Médecine combined weather and disease observations by asking correspondents to complete two sides of a preprinted form. One side had the well-designed meteorological table, but the other side was simply labeled "Nosology." There was no table; it was a blank form. (This is in marked contrast to the highly structured tables of Clifton and Pickering.) Vicq d'Azyr, however, did provide some guidance: He directed correspondents to write reports that were purely descriptive and without medical theory. "A succinct and methodical account stripped of all system and all explanation," mandated Vicq d'Azyr, "will suffice to preserve the history of the described epidemic and to enable the Society to give useful advice regarding its treatment."[53] But what actually constituted a history of epidemics? For Vicq d'Azyr, a history combined *both* individual case histories and accounts of the numbers sick: "The description of an epidemic is only a statement of results drawn from daily particulars of each individual" – in other words, case histories. "It is desired," Vicq d'Azyr continued, "that if possible a register of the sick who recovered and who died be provided."[54]

The historian Jean-Pierre Peter has examined the correspondence of the Société Royale de Médecine and found that while contributions varied greatly in detail and in frequency, few contained quantified information.[55] Some physicians sent only a yearly report; others sent monthly accounts. Some included descriptions of gout, nosebleeding, and colds, while others restricted their observations to epidemic diseases, such as smallpox. Very few constructed registers. Peter lamented:

What is sadly lacking in all of this material is any kind of effort at measuring. The fact is that we never know *how many* people had red fever, or *how many* children contracted smallpox. . . . The manuscripts sometimes do furnish a few figures of mortality for the most serious epidemics, but fail to relate them in any meaningful way to the number of people affected, or to mention the size of the population as a whole.[56]

Thus, although the Société Royale de Médecine recommended "a register of the sick who recovered and who died," few contributors presented their

[52] Cousin, "Sur la vertu anti-septique du quinquina," in Richard de Hautesierck, *Recueil*, vol. 2, p. 531.
[53] *Histoire de la Société Royale de Médecine*, 1776 (Paris, 1779), p. xxxv.
[54] *Histoire de la Société Royale de Médecine*, 1776 (Paris, 1779), p. xxxii.
[55] This correspondence is preserved in the Archives of the Société Royale de Médecine in the Académie Nationale de Médecine. Some of the reports were printed in the *Histoire de la Société Royale de Médecine*. For analyses of the correspondence see Mitchell, "Rationality and Control"; and Peter, "Disease and the Sick."
[56] Peter, "Disease and the Sick," p. 93.

observations in quantitative form, reflecting the fact that French physicians had little interest, experience, or encouragement in the use of numbers. By design, then, Vicq d'Azyr's blank form could not create uniform or comparable medical observations in the way his detailed meteorological form could.

OBSERVATIONS REDUCED

Despite the difficulties in record keeping, there were numerous publications on medical meteorology. Many of these appeared in the journals of learned societies and a few were published separately as books. The summaries of the weather diaries sent to the Royal Society made by William Derham and George Hadley appeared in the *Philosophical Transactions,* and Père Louis Cotte's annual compilations were published in the *Mémoires* of the Société Royale de Médecine. In the *Mémoires* of the Académie Royale des Sciences, Henri-Louis Duhamel du Monceau published annual tables of meteorological observations taken just south of Paris. For 40 years, he made numerical tables of the temperature (recorded three times daily), air pressure, and wind direction and strength, but like Cotte he also included prose comments on the state of the sky, on agriculture, pests, and reigning diseases.[57]

Weather observations were generally reported in tables, but reports on disease, births, and deaths were put in prose, as illustrated in Cotte's and DuHamel du Monceau's articles. Another example of this pattern is found in Paul-Jacques Malouin's "Histoire des maladies épidémiques, observées à Paris, en même temps que les différentes températures de l'air," published annually from 1746 through 1754 in the *Mémoires* of the Paris Académie Royale des Sciences. For January 1754, for example, Malouin reported the following observations on disease, births, and deaths:

Il y a eu pendant ce mois beaucoup de morts subites & des hémorragies; il y a aussi eu des maux de gorge, des rhumes & des fluxions. M. Fournier a eu occasion d'observer des érésipèles; M. Macquer a fait la même observation.

Il s'est présenté à l'Hôtel-dieu en Janvier 2465 malades; il y en avoit déjà le 1er. de ce mois, 2765.

Il est mort pendant ce temps à Paris, 1847 personnes; 991 hommes & 856 femmes.

Il es né 2189 enfans, savoir, 1120 garçons & 1069 filles: de ces 2189 enfans, on en a parté aux Enfans-trouvés 390, savoirs, 202 garçons & 188 filles.

Il s'est fair dans le cours de Janvier, 406 mariages.[58]

---

[57] See, for example, H.L. Duhamel du Monceau, "Observations botanico-météorologiques, faites au château de Denainvilliers, proche Pluviers en Gâtinois pendant l'année 1753," *Mémoires de l'Académie Royale des Sciences,* 1754 (Paris 1759), pp. 383–412. For a discussion of Duhamel's career and work, see Gillispie, *Science and Polity,* pp. 337–360.

[58] Paul-Jacques Malouin, "Histoire des maladies épidémiques de 1754, Observées à Paris en même temps que les différentes températures de l'air," *Mémoires de l'Académie Royale des Sciences,* 1754 (Paris 1759), p. 499.

For each month, Malouin gave the number of births, deaths, and marriages in Paris, as well as figures for the number of new patients at the Hôtel Dieu and the number of abandoned children. His use of prose, however, made it difficult to compare figures between months; nevertheless it was consistent with Cotte's opinion that prose was easier to read than tables.

The societies of London and Paris were not the only ones that published medical meteorological observations. The Medical Society of Edinburgh, for example, encouraged its correspondents to follow Jurin's proposal for making observations, and it published contributions in its *Medical Essays and Observations* from 1733 through 1744. In France, the *Mémoires* of the Académie Royale des Sciences of Montpellier included the meteorological work of Jacques-Augustin Mourgue, an economist and philanthropist. Mourgue submitted annual meteorological observations for the years 1772 through 1785 made in Montpellier, along with figures for the number of births, deaths, and marriages, and comments on disease and agriculture.[59] Later in the 1790s, he compiled his observations and used them to calculate life expectancy, a result he presented to the Institut de France and issued under the title *Essai de statistique*.[60]

For the most part, journals supplied annual summaries of either individual or collected weather observations. While these provided a public record of numerical information, they did not make the links between weather and disease. In other words, numerical knowledge was being diffused, but the actual theoretical work of linking disease and weather was left to the reader.

Perhaps the best example of this approach is Jean Razoux's unique work, *Tables nosologiques et météorologiques très-étendues dressés à l'Hôtel-Dieu de Nismes depuis le premier juin 1757 jusques au premier janvier 1762*. Razoux, hospital physician to the Hôtel-Dieu in Nîmes, undertook a detailed clinical study of the hospital patients, coupled with daily observations of the weather.[61] The result was a striking set of monthly tables for a period of five years. (See Figures 5.6, 5.7, 5.8, 5.9, and 5.10.)

When the academician La Condamine visited Nîmes, he stayed with Razoux, who showed him the tables. Impressed with Razoux's work, La Condamine took the tables to Montpellier and shared them with the well-known physician and nosologist François Bossier de Sauvages. Both men urged Razoux to

---

[59] Jacques-Augustin Mourgue (1734–1818), "Plan d'observations sur la cause des variations de l'atmosphère," *Mémoires de la Société Royale des Sciences de Montpellier*, 1772. For Mourgue's meteorological observations (1772–1785) see Archives départementale de l'Hérault, D144, ff. 3–118; for his observations on births, deaths, and marriages, see Archives départementale de l'Hérault, D189, ff. 84–112.

[60] Jacques Augustin Mourgue, *Essai de statistique* (Paris, an IX).

[61] For a discussion of the Hôtel-Dieu in Nîmes and an analysis of Razoux's observations, see Colin Jones and Michael Sonenscher, "The Social Functions of the Hospital in Eighteenth-Century France: The Case of the Hôtel-Dieu of Nîmes," in Colin Jones, *The Charitable Imperative: Hospitals and Nursing in Ancien Regime and Revolutionary France* (London and New York: Routledge, 1989), pp. 48–86.

120   1758.   TABLES METEOROLOGIQUES.

Juillet, le	Baro-mètre.	Therm. Mat. à 5 h.	Soir à 3 h.	Vents.	Etat du Ciel.
	pouc. lign.	degr.	degr.		
1	27 - 4	16	23	Sud ✠ N✠Sud.	Dans la nuit pluye, couvert tout le jour, le soir grosse pluye de 2 vents du Nord & du Sud.
2		12	19	Nord-Ouest.	Le mat. beau, à midi nuageux & le reste.
3	27 - 8	12½	19	Nord. - - -	Beau tems serein , vent fort.
4		13	20	N+N. O+O+N.	Tems variable, sur les 3 h. menace d'orage.
5		14	24	N-N-O+ O.+S.	Idem.
6		14	16	Sud- ✠ Est. .	Le mat. couvert, à midi pluye jusqu'au soir.
7		14	21	Nord-N-Ouest.	Le mat. nuageux, à midi beau & le reste du jour.
8		14	20½	idem - -	Beau, nuageux par intervalles.
9		14	20¾	idem - -	Idem.
10		12½	21¼	N·N. O+NN·E.	Le mat. nuageux, à midi beau, & le reste.
11		13	24¾	Nord ✠ Ouest.	Le mat. beau, à midi nuageux, & le reste.
12		16	28	Ouest ✠ Sud.	Tems couvert.
13		18	27	Sud. - -	Tems couvert, pet. pluye par intervalles.
14		17	23	Sud ✠ Nord.	Dans la nuit pluye, le mat. couvert, à 10 h. beau, & le reste.
15		15½	24	No-Ou. ✠ Ou.	Le mat. beau , à 3 h. du soir menace d'orage.
16		14	21	Nord. - -	Beau tems serein.
17		14	21	Nord ✠ Ouest.	Le mat. beau, à 11 h. nuageux, & le reste var.
18	27 - 3	17	15½	Nord ✠Sud.	Pluye tout le jour, de 2 vents N. & S.
19	27 - 2	13	17½	Nord. - - -	Tems nuageux par intervalles, vent fort.
20		14	22	N.✠S. ✠S-Ou.	Le mat. très-beau tems serein, le soir nuageux.
21		15	22	Sud. - -	Pluye tout le jour, dans la nuit grosse pluye.
22		14½	20	Sud ✠ Ouest.	Le mat. pluye, à 10 h. couvert, & le reste.
23		14	20½	Ouest. - -	Beau tems serein.
24		14	26½	Ouest. - -	Le mat. nuageux, le soir couvert, dans la nuit pluye.
25		14	26⅔	Nord. - -	Beau tems serein.
26		14	22	Nord-Est. -	Idem.
27		16	29½	Est✠Sud✠Ou.	Le mat. beau, à 4 h. menace d'orage, le soir beau.
28		18	29	Nord ✠Sud.	Beau tems serein.
29		18	31	Ouest. - -	Idem.
30		18	29½	Ouest. - -	Idem.
31		16	19½	Ouest ✠ Nord.	Le mat. couvert, à 8 h, pluye jusqu'à midi, à 1 h. beau, & le reste.

La plus grande chaleur marquée par le Thermomètre, pendant ce mois, a été de 31 degrés au-dessus du terme de la congelation de l'eau, & la moindre chaleur a été de 12 degrés au-dessus de ce même terme.   La différence entre ces deux points est de 19 degr.   La plus grande hauteur du mercure dans le Baromètre a été de 27 pouces 8 lign. & son plus grand abaissement, de 27 pouces 2 lign. La différence entre ces deux termes est de 5 lignes.

Le vent a soufflé {		Il y a eu {	
14 fois du Nord.		9 jours de tems serein.	
1 fois du Nord-Nord-Est.		9 jours de pluye.	
1 fois du Nord-Est.		4 jours des menaces d'orages.	
5 fois du Nord-Nord-Ou.		8 jours de tems couvert.	
3 fois du Nord-Ouest.		10 jours de tems nuageux par intervalles.	
2 fois de l'Est.		8 jours de tems variable.	
13 fois du Sud.		1 jour de gros vent.	
1 fois du Sud-Ouest.			
13 fois de l'Ouest.			

5.6 Jean Razoux's meteorological table for July 1758. *Source:* Jean Razoux, *Tables nosologiques et météorologiques*... (Basle, 1767), p. 120. Yale University, Harvey Cushing/John Hay Whitney Medical Library.

publish, which he did in 1767, and he dedicated his book to the "Messieurs de l'Académie Royale des Sciences."[62]

Razoux's remarkable tables were arranged by month. In the first table for each month, he recorded a daily account of the weather: barometer and thermometer

[62] Razoux, *Tables nosologiques et météorologiques très-étendues dressés à l'Hôtel-Dieu de Nismes depuis le premier juin 1757 jusques au premier janvier 1762* (Basle, 1767), pp. 13–14.

TABLES NOSOLOGIQUES. 121

| 1758 Juillet. | SALLE DES HOMMES. | | | | Hôtel-Dieu de Nîmes. |

Nom des Maladies.	Nomb. des Malades.	Guér.	Morts	Convalescens	OBSERVATIONS.
Pleuro-pneumonies putrides.	12	7	1	4	Le seul malade, qui nous soit mort pendant ce mois de la pleuropneumonie, avoit commis des fautes essentielles dans le régime, qui lui coutèrent la vie : il mangeoit en cachette, & ne se refusoit pas même les alimens de mauvaise qualité. — J'ai compris dans cet article un malade qui avoit essuyé une fièvre continuë de quelques jours, & quoiqu'il parut très nécessaire de le faire saigner, malgré mes sollicitations il ne voulut jamais y consentir. Il sortit de l'Hôpital, & se crut guéri. Deux jours après il revint avec une vraye peripneumonie. Le crachement de sang fut même très abondant, & c'est ce qui contribua peut-être le plus à sa guérison.
Fièvres putrides avec douleur au côté.	16	9	0	7	J'ai vû de ces malades en qui les douleurs étoient si vagues qu'elles changeoient de lieu presque tous les jours ; elles rouloient d'un côté à l'autre, entre les épaules, sur la poitrine, au bas des fausses-côtes &c. je regarde pour lors ces douleurs comme rheumatismales.
Fièvres ardent.	2	1	0	1	Un de ces malades avoit une chaleur si vive & si ardente qu'après l'avoir touché pendant quelque tems, on se sentoit le bout des doigts comme engourdis. La peau de son corps étoit sèche & aride.
Fièvres contin. simples.	119	97	0	22	Nous n'avions jamais vû tant de fièvres continuës simples ; les malades se succédoient mutuellement, & la maison ne désemplissoit pas. Ces maladies n'étoient point facheuses.
Fièvres contin. putrid.	22	18	0	4	Un Soldat malade d'une fièvre continuë putride avoit des accidens convulsifs toutes les fois qu'il entroit dans un redoublement ; il perdoit connoissance, faisoit des contorsions, des yeux, des lèvres, des bras, des jambes, & restoit ensuite dans une espèce de léthargie pendant quelques heures. Après les saignées au bras & au pied, les émetiques, les purgatifs &c. je fis usage des vésicatoires qui firent un effet au delà de toute esperance. — Lorsque la fièvre fut calmée, je lui fis user pendant 20 jours des apozemes aperitifs, que j'avois soin d'aiguiser, & de rendre purgatifs de 3 en 3 jours ; par ces moyens il recouvra la sante.
Fièvres éphém.	56	52	0	4	
Fièvres interm. quotid. & tierc.	35	33	0	2	
Fièvre occasionée par la peur.	1	1	0	0	Le 28e du mois dernier, le tems avoit été tout le jour bien serein, le vent du Nord soufloit légerement, tout à coup à 5 heures du soir le vent change à l'Oueft, un seul éclair précède la foudre, & tuë une femme enceinte de huit mois qui étoit à côté (*). Le Soldat qui fait le sujet de cette remarque étoit sur le gerbier avec deux de ses camarades ; il fut si saisi de frayeur qu'il se laissa tomber par terre : il perdit connoissance, & ne la reprit que quelques momens après. Il fut

P   fut

(*) . . . Voyez l'Hist. de l'Acad. Roy. des Sciences, année 1761. p. 53.

5.7 Jean Razoux's nosological table for male patients treated at the Hôtel-Dieu of Nîmes (July 1758). *Source:* Jean Razoux, *Tables nosologiques et météorologiques...* (Basle, 1767), p. 121. Yale University, Harvey Cushing/John Hay Whitney Medical Library.

readings, strength and direction of the winds, and brief remarks on the state of the sky. This daily account provided far greater detail than monthly summaries. The next two sets of tables (one for men, the other for women) were divided by disease. Figures were given for the number of patients with

122   **TABLES NOSOLOGIQUES.**

1758. Juillet.   SALLE DES HOMMES.   *Hôtel-Dieu de Nimes.*

Noms des Maladies.	Nomb des M.d.s.	Guéris.	Morts.	Convalescens.	OBSERVATIONS.
					fut faigné le lendemain & ne fut apporté à nôtre Hôpital que trois jours après cet accident, il avoit groffe fièvre, & grand mal de tête, fa maladie n'eut pas cependant de fuite, il fut bientôt guéri; fes deux autres camarades ne reffentirent aucun mal.
Angines	5	5	0	0	On ne trouvera pas hors de propos ce que je vais ajoûter. J'examinai le corps de la femme qui avoit été frappée
Rougeol	6	6	0	0	du tonnèrre, une heure après ce trifte accident : elle n'etoit
Petites veroles	2	2	0	0	point noire, & n'avoit aucunement changé de couleur, fes lèvres étoient feulement un peu livides; il ne paroiffoit ni
Flux au vifage.	6	6	0	0	contufion, ni aucune marque de coup nulle part; elle avoit feulement à la nuque du col deux travers de doigt ou environ
Dyffen-teries.	3	2	0	1	de cheveux brûlés, & la peau de cet endroit étoit un peu ridée, elle étoit debout, & la tête courbée lorfqu'elle reçut le coup. Je lui fis ouvrir devant moi la veine du bras. Le
Diarrh.	5	5	0	0	fang jaillit à un demi pied, & on en tira environ une once.
Coliq.	2	2	0	0	J'étois d'avis de tenter l'opération Céfarienne pour tacher de fauver l'enfant qu'elle portoit dans fon fein, & qui avoit plus
Ictères.	1	1	0	0	de 7 mois : les parens n'y voulurent jamais confentir.
Phtifies.	4	1	1	2	C'étoit un homme vieux qui mourut plûtôt dans le marafme
Cat. rr.	28	27	0	1	que phtifique.
Hydrop.	6	3	0	3	
Ophtal.	3	2	0	1	
Doul. rheum.	10	8	0	2	
Dyfurie.	2	1	0	1	
Artère ouverte.	1	1	0	0	En faifant une faignée un garçon chirurgien ignorant ouvrit l'artère au-lieu de la veine. Ce facheux accident n'eut point cependant de fuite. Mr. *Mitier*, chirurgien de cette maifon, les prévint par fes foins, & guérit en peu de jours ce malade.
Total	347	290	2	55	

RECAPITULATION des Hommes du mois
de Juillet 1758.

Il eft entré pendant ce mois   252 Soldats.
                                   39 Bourgeois.
Il y avoit dans la maifon   56 Convalefcens.
                                   347

Dans la claffe des Guéris   290
Dans celle des Morts   2
Dans celle des Convalefcens   55
                                347

5.8 Jean Razoux's nosological table for male patients, continued. *Source:* Jean Razoux, *Tables nosologiques et météorologiques* ... (Basle, 1767), p. 122. Yale University, Harvey Cushing/John Hay Whitney Medical Library.

particular illnesses (smallpox, flux, etc.), and of those how many were cured, convalescent, or dead. In these tables, Razoux added a column for observations of specific cases. In the table reproduced here in Figure 5.8, he indicated that an apprentice surgeon mistakenly cut open an artery instead of a vein

TABLES NOSOLOGIQUES.   123

| 1 7 5 8. Juillet. | | | | SALLE DES FEMMES. *Hôtel-Dieu de Nîmes.* |

Nom des Mala- dies.	Nomb des Ma- lades.	Gue- ris.	Morts.	Con- vale- scens	OBSERVATIONS.
Pleuro- pneum. putrid.	I	I	0	0	Je mets au nombre des mortes d'une fièvre éphémère une femme qui mourut de vieillesse, sans fièvre & sans aucune es-
Fièvres continu. putrid.	2	I	I	0	pèce de mal. Celle qui est morte d'une dyssenterie, étoit aussi une vieille femme fort épuisée. Les deux malades, qui
Fièvres contin. simples.	5	3	0	2	font marquées à l'article *obstruction des viscères abdominaux*, font deux filles qui avoient fait longtems les pâles-couleurs & qui avoient les viscères obstrués ; elles n'avoient point de
Fièvres interm.	5	4	0	I	fièvre, étoient fort dégoutées, & ne pouvoient remplir leurs fonctions ordinaires à cause de la foiblesse & de l'abbate-
Fièvres éphém.	2	I	I	0	ment qu'elles ressentoient.
Phtisies.	2	0	0	2	
Catarrh.	I	I	0	0	
Dyssent.	3	I	I	I	
Diarrh.	I	I	0	0	
Coliq.	2	2	0	0	
Hydrop.	2	0	0	2	
Angin.	2	2	0	0	
Ophtal.	I	0	0	I	
Eresyp.	I	I	0	0	
Palpita- tion de cœur.	I	I	0	0	
Obstruc- tion des viscères.	2	I	0	I	
Total	33	20	3	10	

RECAPITULATION des Femmes du mois
de Juillet 1758.

Il est entré pendant ce mois   -   28 Malades.
Il y avoit du mois dernier   -   5 Convalescentes.
                                               33

Dans la Classe des Guéries   20
Dans celle des Mortes   3
Dans celle des Convalescentes   10
                                               33

5.9 Jean Razoux's nosological table for female patients treated at the Hôtel-Dieu of Nîmes (July 1758). *Source:* Jean Razoux, *Tables nosologiques et météorologiques . . .* (Basle, 1767), p. 123. Yale University, Harvey Cushing/John Hay Whitney Medical Library.

during a routine bloodletting. The chief surgeon of the hospital quickly intervened to save the patient, who luckily survived.

The final table for each month was in Latin, rather than French, and it summarized the number of patients treated for each disease, with the diseases grouped

124   SUMMA TABULÆ NOSOLOGICÆ
Menfis JULII 1758.

CLASSES.	GENERA.	ÆGRI.	SANATI.	MORTUI.	RESIDUI in alt. menf.
Febres.	trit.exquif.& amph.	26	20	1	5
	Synochus	124	100	0	24
	quot. 3tiana, 4tana	40	37	0	3 }249
	Ephem. extens.	58	53	1	4
	Febris fingul.	1	1	0	0
Phlegma-fiæ.	Pleuropneum.	13	8	1	4
	Pleuritis putris.	16	9	0	7
	Cynanche.	7	7	0	0
	Rubeola.	6	6	0	0 }51
	Variola.	2	2	0	0
	Eryfipelas.	1	1	0	0
	Pfeudo eryfip.	6	6	0	0
Dolores.	Ophtalmia.	4	2	0	2
	Rheumatifmus.	10	8	0	2 }20
	Hepatalg.ac fplenat.	2	1	0	1
	Colica.	4	4	0	0
Convulf.	Cordis palpitatio.	1	1	0	0] 1
Fluxus.	Dyffenteria.	6	3	1	2
	Diarrhæa.	6	6	0	0 }43
	Dyfuria.	2	1	0	1
	Catarrhus.	29	28	0	1
Cachexiæ	Phtifis.	6	1	1	4
	Aurigo.	1	1	0	0 }15
	Hydrops.	8	3	0	5
Vitia.	Arteriotom.	1	1	0	0] 1
CLASSES 7	GENERA 25	ÆGRI 380	SANATI 310	MORTUI 5	RESIDUI 65

Viri - 347
Mulieres 33
380

5.10 Jean Razoux's summary table based on François Boissier de Sauvages's nosology (July 1758). *Source:* Jean Razoux, *Tables nosologiques et météorologiques…* (Basle, 1767), p. 124. Yale University, Harvey Cushing/John Hay Whitney Medical Library.

into larger categories based on the nosology of Boissier de Sauvages. Although meteorological and nosological tables were placed next to each other in the text, Razoux did not draw any specific conclusions connecting the two. Significantly, he left that work to the reader by insisting that the connections between weather and disease could be perceived immediately by looking at his tables:

In consulting these tables one can determine the temperature and the dominant illness of a season; if it was deadly and until what date; the most common illnesses of this climate, if they are fatal or not; the danger one runs if attacked; the cure that was most successful. Other information can be extracted from these tables, on which I do not insist, but which can be observed at first glance [qu'on aperçoit au premier coup d'oeil].[63]

[63] Jean Razoux, *Tables nosologiques et météorologiques*, pp. 12–13.

The medical meteorological conclusions one could draw from the tables, Razoux claimed, were self-evident.

Presenting as much detailed information as possible in a table was not the only strategy adopted by medical meteorologists. Over the course of the eighteenth century, several physicians published books based on observations of both weather and patients over a period of years. Clifton Wintringham, for example, provided temperature and air pressure readings, coupled with an account of reigning diseases in York for the years 1715 through 1730; similarly, William Hillary recorded observations from 1726 through 1734 in Ripon in Yorkshire, and Thomas Short in Sheffield for the years 1711 through 1748.[64] For Plymouth, the renowned physician and Fellow of the Royal Society John Huxham published his *Observations on the Air and Epidemic Diseases from the Year [1727] to [1737] Inclusive.* Huxham had contributed to Jurin's meteorological project and had dedicated his book specifically to Sir Hans Sloane, president of the Royal Society, and more generally to the "illustrious Members" of the Society.[65] The bulk of his book contained monthly and annual meteorological observations, coupled with remarks on the prevailing epidemic diseases during the same periods. Huxham took the further step of trying to explain how various types of air rendered the human body more or less susceptible to certain diseases. John Arbuthnot, who had earlier written on smallpox inoculation, also linked medical meteorology and contemporary physiology in his influential *An Essay Concerning the Effects of Air on Human Bodies* (1733).[66]

An entirely different approach was adopted by John Rutty in his *A Chronological History of the Weather and Seasons, and of the Prevailing Diseases in Dublin. With Their Various Periods, Successions, and Revolutions, during the Space of Forty Years. With a Comparative View of the Difference of the Irish Climate and Diseases, and those of England and Other Countries* (1770). Rutty based his history on observations for the years 1725 through 1761 and was quite forthright about his methods. "The following account has been drawn up from diaries constantly kept both of the weather and diseases," he explained. "I have reduced the diaries of the weather to the form of monthly registries; and greatly contracted the accounts of the

[64] Clifton Wintringham, *Commentarium Nosologicum Morbos Epidemicos et Aeris Variationes in Urbe Eboracensi Locisque Vicinis* (London, 1733); William Hillary, "An Account of the Principal Variations of the Weather and the Concomitant Epidemical Diseases from 1726 to 1734 at Ripon," bound with his *Essay on the Smallpox* (London, 1740); and [Thomas Short], *A General Chronological History of the Air, Weather, Seasons, Meteors &c. in Sundry Places and Different Times* (London, 1749). Caroline Hannaway discussed some of these in her "Environment and Miasmata," pp. 292–308.

[65] John Huxham, *Observations on the Air and Epidemic Diseases from the Year MDCCXXVII to MDCCXXXVII Inclusive; together with a Short Dissertation on Devonshire Colic, Translated from the Latin Original by his Son, John Corham Huxham* (1739; London: J. Hinton, 1759).

[66] John Arbuthnot, *An Essay Concerning the Effects of Air on Human Bodies* (London, 1733). For a discussion of these efforts to link Newtonian physiology and medical meteorology, see Andrea Rusnock, "Hippocrates, Bacon and Medical Meteorology at the Royal Society, 1700 to 1750," in *Reinventing Hippocrates*, ed. David Cantor (Burlington, Vt.: Ashgate, 2001), pp. 144–161.

diseases."[67] Moreover, he had observed mainly "plebians," not the wealthy, a circumstance that "ought to recommend [rather] than disparage the work; inasmuch as these last named persons [plebians] are more exposed to the injuries of the air and weather than the other, who, by means of their warm cloathing, good fires, and the moderate use of wine, are less susceptible thereof."[68]

The actual process of recording and collating case histories is much more visible in Rutty's book than in any other medical meteorological work. At the end of his book, Rutty had a section entitled "A Summary Review of the Diseases above-mentioned, during a Series of above 30 Years, chiefly with regard to the Seasons in which they prevailed," in which he provided figures for the number of patients suffering from particular illnesses in each season. For example:

That agues or intermittent fevers were observed

In Spring	19	
in Summer	4	times
in Autumn	1	
in Winter	0	

Or again:

Diarrhoeas occur

In Spring	1	
in Summer	00	times
in Autumn	9	
in Winter	5	

Corollary. The diarrhoea is plainly an autumnal disease.[69]

In highlighting his method, Rutty could assert that his corollaries were "drawn not by idle and random guesses, but by fair induction from facts, minuted down, and faithfull related, with a sole view to the discovery of truth."[70] Here then was a clear articulation of the Hippocratic-Baconian method – medical meteorologists recorded individual case histories and used tables to summarize and aid in the drawing of conclusions.

---

[67] John Rutty, *A Chronological History of the Weather and Seasons, and of the Prevailing Diseases in Dublin. With Their Various Periods, Successions, and Revolutions, during the Space of Forty Years. With a Comparative View of the Difference of the Irish Climate and Diseases, and Those of England and Other Countries* (London, 1770), p. vi.

[68] Rutty, *A Chronological History*, p. v.   [69] Rutty, *A Chronological History*, p. 232.

[70] Rutty, *A Chronological History*, p. 228.

6

Interrogating Death: Disease, Mortality, and Environment

I propose . . . , in imitation of the geographers, to spread out and to review, in one general Chart, the enormous host of diseases which disgorge their virulence over the earth, and with frightful rapacity, wage incessant hostilities with mankind. By this means, we shall, to use a military phrase, reconnoitre more distinctly our enemies arranged in hostile front; and be warned to make the best disposition and preparation for defence where the greatest danger is apprehended, and the most formidable assaults to be sustained.

William Black (1789)[1]

Death emerged as a topic of quantitative study during the long eighteenth century. Individual mortality had, of course, always been a subject of contemplation as had experiences with epidemics, famine, and war. The plague especially led many to reflect on the causes and repercussions of great mortalities, but there was little systematic inquiry of death prior to the eighteenth century. One reason for this absence might be the fatalism that much of European society attached to death. Death had been tamed in European culture in the sense that society accepted death as a constant and certain companion of life. Cemeteries, for instance, were immediately adjacent to churches and were in themselves social gathering places.[2] During the eighteenth century, however, individuals began efforts to separate the living from the dead; they moved cemeteries to the outskirts of town; they prohibited burials in churches. They increasingly used coffins and embalming to hide, deflect, or distance themselves from the process of physical decomposition.[3]

---

[1] William Black, *An Arithmetical and Medical Analysis of the Diseases and Mortality of the Human Species* (London, 1789), pp. 35–36; reprinted with an introduction by D.V. Glass, (Farnborough, Hants, Eng.: Gregg International Publishers Limited, 1973).

[2] Philippe Ariès, *Western Attitudes toward Death from the Middle Ages to the Present,* trans. Patricia M. Ranum (Baltimore: Johns Hopkins University Press, 1974), pp. 24–25.

[3] Clare Gittings, *Death, Burial and the Individual in Early Modern England* (London & Sydney: Croom Helm, 1984), pp. 13–14; on the French cemeteries, see Laurence Brockliss and Colin Jones, *The Medical World of Early Modern France* (Oxford: Clarendon Press, 1997), pp. 753–754. Also see John McManners, *Death and the Enlightenment: Changing Attitudes to Death among Christians and Unbelievers in Eighteenth-Century France* (Oxford: Clarendon Press, 1981).

These changes reflected a discomfort or anxiety about death and signaled a growing desire to control and understand it. This new attitude had everything to do with rising expectations based on changes in the demographic experience. Investigations of death were one way of responding to this anxiety. Mortality was examined, dissected, described, and classified. Historians are familiar with the pathological anatomy of Giovanni Battista Morgagni and Xavier Bichat, but they are much less informed about classificatory and numerical studies of death.[4]

Eighteenth-century physicians, clergymen, and others were keenly interested in characterizing death. They carefully recorded the sex, age, and status (married, widowed, monk, nun, etc.) of the dead, along with notes on local geography, time of year, and cause of death. This information was collected, quantified, and tabulated into accounts of the dead. Medical men took the lead in interrogating death, although clergymen and government officials made significant contributions to these investigations.[5] New urban medical institutions, such as dispensaries and specialized hospitals, provided physicians and surgeons opportunities to analyze death.[6] Others living in more rural areas sent their individual observations, if in France, to the Société Royale de Médecine in Paris, or, if in Britain, to the Royal Society of London or the Royal Society of Edinburgh, as well as to the various metropolitan and provincial medical and scientific societies established during the last three decades of the eighteenth century.[7] Finally, the military provided a critical arena for the development of studies of mortality.[8] In short, whether metropolitan or provincial, civilian or military, new institutions and their publications played central roles in fostering critical inquiries of mortality.

This chapter focuses on the efforts to classify and quantify death that gave contemporaries, to use a phrase borrowed from the epigraph, the means to

---

[4] This is not to say that there have been no historical accounts of mortality statistics. See, for example, McManners, *Death and the Enlightenment,* chap. 4. For a recent historical account of pathological anatomy, see Russell C. Maulitz, *Morbid Appearances – The Anatomy of Pathology in the Early Nineteenth Century* (Cambridge: Cambridge University Press, 1987).

[5] Mary Dobson has analyzed a wide variety of sources (personal diaries, parish registers, overseer of the poor accounts, etc.) for contemporary assessments of causes of death in her study of early modern southeast England; Dobson, *Contours of Death and Disease in Early Modern England* (Cambridge: Cambridge University Press, 1997), chap. 5, pp. 223–286.

[6] Foucault emphasized the critical role clinics played in the formation of nosological knowledge. Michel Foucault, *The Birth of the Clinic,* trans. A.M. Sheridan Smith (1963; New York: Vintage Books, 1975), especially chap. 4, pp. 54–63. On the London hospitals and dispensaries, see Susan C. Lawrence, *Charitable Knowledge: Hospital Pupils and Practitioners in Eighteenth-Century London* (Cambridge: Cambridge University Press, 1996).

[7] For a list of London societies, see Lawrence, *Charitable Knowledge,* p. 261. For France, see Daniel Roche, *Le Siècle des lumières en province: Académies et académiciens provinciaux, 1680–1789* (Paris: Mouton, 1978).

[8] For example, Richard de Hautesierck's work drawn from the French military (see Chapter 5). For Britain, see Ulrich Tröhler, "Quantification in British Medicine and Surgery," Ph.D. thesis, University College London, 1978, pp. 66–76, and chaps. 4 and 5.

"reconnoitre more distinctly our enemies arranged in hostile front." Black's metaphor was telling: He intended to use the methods of geographers – tables and charts – to interrogate death.

TO IMPROVE THE CLASSIFICATION OF DEATH

The English were the most interested in cataloging different causes of death, in large part because the London bills of mortality provided the curious and creative with extensive records on just this topic.[9] Graunt's *Natural and Political Observations Made upon the Bills of Mortality* (1662) established a tradition of using the London bills to create more detailed and numerical accounts of particular diseases and of variations in mortality according to age. Graunt was also the first to criticize the manner in which the bills were compiled. He cautioned his readers that the information in the bills was not entirely accurate because ill-educated women (the searchers) were responsible for ascribing cause of death. Over the course of the eighteenth century, physicians and others became increasingly concerned about the reliability of the bills. "These searchers are, for the most part, ignorant poor women," the Quaker physician John Fothergill reminded members of the London Society of Collegiate Physicians in 1768,

> who, if they see the body emaciated, immediately enter it in their report as consumption. I need not inform you, how many chronic as well as long-continued acute diseases, in which the lungs are no otherwise affected than as suffering with all the other parts, waste the whole frame, and bring it to the same state as those who died tabid; but these ought not to be ranked under consumptions, but under the several heads to which they belong.[10]

Fothergill believed that the excessive number of burials attributed to consumption gave London an unjust reputation among foreigners as being unhealthy.[11]

And it was not just the London bills of mortality that suffered from these errors of identification. So long as the process of determining cause of death remained in the hands of local parish clerks and searchers, medical arithmeticians questioned the accuracy of conclusions drawn from parish records. John Aikin, a dissenting minister, compiled a bill of mortality for Warrington for the year 1773 in which he wrote:

---

[9] The bills continue to attract attention. See Thomas Forbes, "By What Disease or Casualty: The Changing Face of Death in London," *Health, Medicine and Mortality in the Sixteenth Century*, ed. Charles Webster (Cambridge: Cambridge University Press, 1979), pp. 117–139.

[10] John Fothergill, "Some Remarks on the Bills of Mortality in London," *Works* (London, 1783), vol. 2, pp. 111–112; first published in *Medical Observations and Inquiries*, vol. 4 (1768); reprinted in D.V. Glass, *The Development of Population Statistics* (Farnborough, Hants, Eng.: Gregg International Publishers Limited, 1973).

[11] Fothergill, "Some Remarks on the Bills of Mortality in London," pp. 112–113.

With respect to the general Table of Diseases, the obvious uncertainty and inaccuracy of an enquiry which, in most cases, could only be made by the clerk in the church-yard, made me despair of rendering it in any great degree subservient to the purposes of science. It has not, therefore, been attempted to give it a scientific form; but the articles have for the most part been inserted just as they were given in.[12]

The categories used by the searchers and parish clerks reflected popular ideas of death, but as several historians have noted, the boundary between popular and elite culture was not hard and fast, and disease categories were continually redefined over the course of the eighteenth century.[13] Indeed, Graunt's demonstration that rickets and livergrown were different names for the same condition (discussed in Chapter 1) provides a nice example of this phenomenon. Medical arithmeticians began to adopt the new nosologies of François Boissier de Sauvages and William Cullen in the accounts they constructed.[14] John Heysham, for example, who received an MD from Edinburgh in 1777, used Cullen's categories to organize his observations on mortality taken from the public dispensary he established in Carlisle.[15]

Heysham was not unusual in gathering accounts from a local institution. In Britain during the second half of the eighteenth century, the number of charitable medical institutions – dispensaries and hospitals – increased dramatically, and, at the same time, they became key sources of quantitative information about mortality. Similar to the Smallpox Hospital of London (discussed in Chapter 4), these institutions issued annual reports to subscribers and to the general public, reports usually interspersed with accounts of the number of patients treated and of those, how many had died. The London Dispensary for Sick Children, for instance, released quarterly and annual accounts of mortality between the years 1769 and 1781.[16] Another example is the London General Dispensary in Aldersgate Street where the attending physician, the Quaker John Coakley Lettsom, an avid supporter of inoculation, published numerical accounts of patients. "From the useful hints suggested by my ingenious friend Dr. Percival," Lettsom wrote, "I was induced to keep an exact register of the diseases and

[12] John Aikin, "The Bill of Mortality of the Town of Warrington, for the Year 1773," *Philosophical Transactions* 64 (1774): 440–441.
[13] On the relations of popular and elite cultures, see Brockliss and Jones, *The Medical World of Early Modern France*, pp. 15–16. J.P. Peter provides an eloquent account of the continual redefinition of disease categories in his article on the Société Royale de Médecine. Jean-Pierre Peter, "Disease and the Sick at the End of the Eighteenth Century," *Biology of Man in History – Selections from the Annales Économies, Sociétés, Civilisations,* ed. Robert Forster and Orest Ranum, trans. Elborg Forster and Patricia Ranum (Baltimore: Johns Hopkins University Press, 1975), pp. 81–124.
[14] For a recent overview of nosology, see W.F. Bynum, "Nosology," in *Companion Encyclopedia of the History of Medicine,* ed. W.F. Bynum and Roy Porter (London and New York: Routledge, 1993), vol. 1, pp. 335–356. Also see Margaret DeLacy, "Nosology, Mortality, and Disease Theory in the Eighteenth Century," *Journal of the History of Medicine* 54 (1999): 261–284.
[15] John Heysham, *Collected Bills of Mortality for Carlisle, 1779–1787;* reprinted in Glass, *The Development of Population Statistics.*
[16] Cited in Tröhler, "Quantification in British Medicine," pp. 102–103.

deaths which fell under my observation in the . . . Dispensary, agreeable to the following tables which include a period of twelve months."[17] Here we see the Dissenting network in action. Thomas Percival, a Unitarian physician, had collected numerical accounts of Manchester's population and submitted them to the *Philosophical Transactions*. Owing to these accounts, he had supported inoculation. In general, the accounts collected by physicians such as Lettsom and Percival were regarded by medical arithmeticians as more reliable than the observations recorded in the London bills of mortality.

In France, physicians seldom compiled quantitative accounts, and hospitals kept registers of the names (not the number) of patients. (Razoux was a notable exception.) It was government officials – intendants, local police, and so on – who developed the new numerical forms of record keeping. An episode in the 1780s nicely illustrates this point. In his comprehensive study *Mémoires sur les hôpitaux de Paris* (1788), the surgeon Jacques Tenon evaluated the Paris hospitals. One of his recommendations was the establishment of a specialized hospital for the insane. When Tenon wanted to know how many insane were admitted to Hôtel Dieu, he found that the hospital did not keep such records. Rather, the lieutenant general of the Paris police had the information. The municipal government, not physicians and surgeons, generated numerical information about patients.[18]

French writers recognized the dearth of numerical information about death and disease in France, compared with that available in England. In his chapter on mortality from *Recherches et considérations sur la population de la France* (today considered a masterpiece in early demography),[19] Jean-Baptiste Moheau, secretary to the intendant Antoine Auget, Baron de Montyon,[20] briefly addressed

[17] John Coakley Lettsom, *Medical Memoirs of the General Dispensary in London* (London, 1774), p. 343; quoted in Tröhler, "Quantification in British Medicine," p. 104.
[18] Jacques Tenon, *Memoirs on Paris Hospitals,* trans. with an Introduction, Notes and Appendices by Dora B. Weiner (1788; Science History Publications, 1996), pp. 197–200. This story is told in Jan Goldstein, "Foucault among the Sociologists: The 'Disciplines' and the History of the Professions," *History and Theory* 23 (1984): 185–187.
[19] For evaluations of Montyon's contributions to demography, see the excellent collection of essays appended to the new edition of his book: Jean-Baptiste Moheau, *Recherches et considérations sur la population de la France (1778),* reedition annotated by Eric Vilquin (Paris: Institut National d'Études Démographiques, Presses Universitaires de France, 1994). Also see Jacques and Michel Dupâquier, *Histoire de la démographie* (Paris: Perrin, 1985), p. 171; J.C. Perrot, "Les économistes, les philosophes, et la population," in *Histoire de la population française,* ed. Jacques Dupâquier (Paris: Presses Universitaires de France, 1988), vol. 2, p. 530; and William Coleman, "Inventing Demography: Montyon on Hygiene and the State," in Everett Mendelsohn, ed., *Transformation and Tradition in the Sciences – Essays in Honor of I. Bernard Cohen* (Cambridge: Cambridge University Press, 1984), pp. 215–235.
[20] There is an extended historical debate about the authorship of *Recherches et considérations*. The stated author is Moheau, the secretary to the enlightened bureaucrat Auget de Montyon; the latest historical assessment is that Moheau wrote the first part of the book, and Montyon the second. See Éric Brian, "Moyens de connaître les plumes: Étude lexicométrique," in Moheau, *Recherches et considérations sur la population de la France (1778),* reedition annotated by Eric Vilquin (Paris: Institut National d'Études Démographiques, Presses Universitaires de France, 1994), pp. 383–396. For earlier

the causes of death and readily acknowledged the English work in this area: "These researches have been done in England, and especially in the city of London. . . ."[21] He admitted that he could not say much about the French situation, although he did note that "there is a province where a great number of Curés have promised to make mention in their registers of the causes of death of the people who are buried. . . ."[22] Reflecting his desire for more information about disease, this reform-minded secretary advocated the establishment of bills of mortality in France. Similarly, the Montpellier political economist and philanthropist Jacques-Augustin Mourgue (1734–1818), who published several papers and books on numerical studies of the population, called for the collection of this information in France: "It would be desirable to introduce the custom that I have seen practiced in England where the doctors and surgeons who have seen the patient certify the cause of death: this certificate is then mentioned in the mortuary registers of the parishes."[23] The English did have substantially more numerical information, but Mourgue's description of English customs certainly did not apply to the London bills of mortality.

During the last decades of the eighteenth century, several English physicians proposed new methods of recording information to improve the reliability and usefulness of the bills of mortality. Some focused on the records themselves. John Fothergill, for example, provided a sample form. It was a model of conciseness – deaths were to be recorded and cataloged not only by cause but also by age, sex, and whether the individual was native to London.[24] Other reformers focused their attention on who actually recorded the cause of death. William Black, for instance, argued for the complete medicalization of the bills. He thought that the 147 parish clerks and 294 searchers should be replaced by 28 medical inspectors (surgeons or apothecaries) who would determine cause of death and issue a certificate necessary for interment. These inspectors would be paid from the money saved by not replacing the parish clerks and searchers. The burial certificates would then be deposited at a general hall where monthly and annual bills would be compiled (weekly bills were no longer necessary, given the absence of plague). According to Black: "Instead of appointing a person ignorant of the principles of calculation, and still more so of medicine, to superintend the general hall, to arrange and class diseases, I propose to fill that important office with an able physician, and to allow him the reasonable

discussions, see E. Esmonin, "Montyon, véritable auteur des *Recherches et considérations sur la population*, de Moheau," *Population* 13 (1958): 269–282; J. Lecuir, "Deux siècles après: Montyon, véritable auteur des *Recherches et considérations sur la population de la France*, de Moheau," *Annales de démographie historique*, 1979, pp. 195–249. Also see, Jacques and Michel Dupâquier, *Histoire de la démographie*, pp. 180–181.

[21] Moheau, *Recherches et considérations*, p. 239.   [22] Moheau, *Recherches et considérations*, p. 240.
[23] Jacques-Augustin Mourgue, "Observations sur les naissances, les mariages et les morts de la ville de Montpellier pendant l'année 1777," Archives départementales de l'Hérault D189, f.85.
[24] This form is reproduced in Glass, *The Development of Population Statistics*.

sum of 200 pounds, annual salary."[25] Death needed to be classified "in a much more comprehensive and methodical manner than the present"; the existing bills were "a mere farrago of diseases and mortality."[26]

Perhaps the most interesting facet of Black's proposal was his suggestion to "place this medical and philosophical observatory, or factory if you please, under the controul and direction of the Royal Society, who should chuse the physician and inspectors." The Royal Society would gain much from this arrangement because publishing the bills of mortality and comments thereon in the *Philosophical Transactions* might "excite an avidity for each volume of the Philosophical Transactions amongst the literati of Europe." This in turn would encourage a more coordinated effort in political and medical arithmetic than had hitherto existed in "the shreds, fragments, and meagre essays of unconnected individuals, however learned and assiduous."[27] Harkening back to Bacon's call for the coordination of observations, political and medical arithmetic in Black's hands would become collective enterprises, and the Royal Society would serve as the center for their development, as it had for Graunt and Petty in the 1660s and 1670s and for Jurin in the 1720s.

Unfortunately for Black, his proposal was not taken up. Only in medical institutions – hospitals and dispensaries – did physicians, surgeons, and apothecaries do the collecting and classifying. Outside these institutions, nonmedical persons continued to identify and record cause of death, and popular classifications continued to hold sway.

THE LONDON BILLS OF MORTALITY ANALYZED

Despite complaints about the searchers and the uncertainty of nosology, physicians and others relied upon the bills of mortality to make observations; in particular, they looked for changes over time in cause of death. Three books, one from midcentury and the other two from the end of the century, provide excellent examples of the ways the bills were employed to generate numerical tables.

In 1750, Thomas Short published one of the most ambitious works in political and medical arithmetic, an ambition reflected in its grand title: *New Observations, Natural, Moral, Civil, Political, and Medical on City, Town, and Country Bills of Mortality*. Originally from Scotland, Short (1690?–1772) established his medical practice in Sheffield, where he wrote several works, including *A General Chronological History of the Air* (1749) and *A Comparative History of the Increase*

---

[25] William Black, *Observations Medical and Political, on the Small-Pox, and the Advantages and Disadvantages of General Inoculation, Especially in Cities: And on the Mortality of Mankind at Every Age in City and Country*, 2d ed. (London: J. Johnson, 1781), p. 274.

[26] Black, *Observations Medical and Political*, 2d ed., postscript, p. 276.

[27] Black, *Observations Medical and Political*, 2d. ed. p. 282.

and Decrease of Mankind (1767). Like many philosophically inclined physicians, Short combined interests in meteorology, population, and medical arithmetic. His primary aim was to analyze country bills of mortality (constructed from parish registers) and thus provide a contrast to Graunt's focus on the London bills of mortality. Like many of his contemporaries, Short was convinced that the country was more salubrious than the city, which he sought to demonstrate numerically by designing various tables to display information on burials, christenings, marriages, topography, and meteorology taken from the registers of more than 160 country parishes and dozens of market towns. Short's book, over 500 pages in length, contained 27 tables that ranged considerably in subject and complexity.

In many ways, Short epitomized both the ambitions of eighteenth-century medical and political arithmeticians and their limitations. His work was at once both inspiring and confusing – his intent was clear, but its realization was almost incomprehensible. A quick perusal of one of his tables reveals how difficult it was to extract information from them. Part of the complexity stems from the fact that Short did not label the columns in his table; instead, he placed the description of the table on a separate page, thereby making it practically impossible to remember what the numbers in each column represented. Moreover, he sometimes did not label the rows, thus forcing the reader to consult an earlier table to determine which parish the numbers came from. Following is the description for Short's second table, in which neither the columns nor the rows were labeled. (See Figure 6.1.)

Column 1st of each Period contains the number of Years of each Register; Column 2d Males baptized in that Period; Column 3d Females baptized; Column 4th Total of both; Column 5th Weddings; Column 6th Males buried; Column 7th Females buried; Column 8th Totals of both; Column 9th the Encrease.[28]

Short's prose further complicated the issue: It was simultaneously imprecise and overly detailed. William Black, whose work will be discussed below in this section, could only have had Short in mind when he wrote that "the few authors who have written on bills of mortality, have obscured their works in a cloud of figures and calculation.... [T]hey often tax the memory and patience with a numerical superfluity, even to a nuisance."[29]

Short's ambitions for numerical tables help to explain their complexity. Tables, or what he called registers, measured salubrity and, at the same time, gauged the effects of industry. "Registers are not only the surest Test what Places have the best Air, Situation, and Soil, and enjoy the greatest Health and long Life, or

---

[28] Thomas Short, *New Observations, Natural, Moral, Civil, Political, and Medical on City, Town, and Country Bills of Mortality* (London, 1750), p. 21.

[29] William Black, *An Arithmetical and Medical Analysis*, p. 37.

Period Firſt.   Diviſion Firſt.

68	115	69	184	49	68	42	110	74
138	558	513	1071	220	275	236	511	560
200	307	321	628	200	216	184	400	228
46	193	161	354	141	163	126	289	65
101	426	403	829	201	268	228	496	333
81	400	394	794	181	251	230	481	313
50	151	134	285	61	84	85	169	116
45	246	242	488	95	138	154	292	196
106	332	322	654	169	218	209	427	227
69	305	258	563	114	165	153	318	245
87	288	269	557	194	168	166	334	223
49	147	147	294	90	107	90	197	97
55	453	400	853	238	294	274	568	285
73	473	359	832	166	232	220	452	380
82	2087	1946	4033	937	1184	1150	2334	1700
43	1430	1403	2833	539	973	963	1936	897
91	2236	2241	4477	881	1524	1465	2989	1388
65	362	328	690	178	228	257	485	205
87	288	269	557	149	168	166	334	223
61	338	261	599	99	201	186	387	212
30	425	392	817	168	287	258	545	272
35	405	366	771	200	281	267	548	223
25	192	166	358	126	109	112	221	137
82	309	315	624	150	208	212	420	204
45	395	375	770	234	255	289	544	226
38	108	85	193	30	68	67	135	58
Totals	12969	12139	25108	5810	8133	7789	15922	9087

6.1 Thomas Short's table of baptisms and burials from country parishes (seventeenth century). *Source:* Thomas Short, *New Observations, Natural, Moral, Civil, Political, and Medical on City, Town and Country Bills of Mortality* (London, 1750), p. 22. Yale University, Harvey Cushing/John Hay Whitney Medical Library.

prove most sickly and fatal to the Inhabitants," he explained, "but of the different Effects of several Trades or Manufactures, in the same or like Situations."[30] Short considered the English Civil War a significant turning point in the health of the English people, and his chronology reflected this belief. Many tables were divided into two periods, the first period comprising data taken from parish registers roughly 100 years prior to 1640, and the second period, the 100 years following 1640. Short averred, "I find in the Registers, that sometimes Disturbances of the Body politick, attend Disorders of the natural Body, as from 1556 to 59, 1623–4, 1643–4, 1684, 94 to 7, 1723, 40, 41, &c. As though Religion, Liberty, Property, and Trade declined, sickened and died, or revived, flourished and rejoiced together."[31] He envisioned his registers as a measure of

[30] Thomas Short, *New Observations*, p. 58.   [31] Short, *New Observations*, p. 107.

government: "By comparing our own and foreign Registers together, we find where the Births vastly exceed the Burials, the Country is either very healthy, or it is under an arbitrary Government, or both."[32]

Short conceded that registers had already been profitably used for "several political, civil, arithmetical, and natural" inquires by men such as Graunt and Petty. But, he argued, "none have tried whether they might afford any Hints of medical Uses." (This claim ignored the fact that many of Graunt's and Petty's observations were medical in nature, and it completely overlooked the role that the London bills had played in the debates over smallpox inoculation.) Short then proceeded to catalog the types of medical questions that his registers might be used to answer:

What Soils, Situations, Trades, Manner of Life, &c. are best adapted to health and Long Life, or the contrary. Or if they are unhealthy, whether they are equally fatal as well as sickly; or in what Degree, to what Age, Sex, and Constitution; in what Seasons, Weather, Periods, and at what Distances; and whether by chronic or acute Diseases; Or whether a Mortality moves with a quick, slow, or moderate Pace; whether it proceed chiefly from Epidemics or Endemics, where the fatal Diseases that overrun the Nation begin, which Way they extend and spread, where and how they terminate. . . . [33]

In sum, Short was determined to put medical arithmetical inquiries on the right track, and numerical accounts recorded in registers were the best method for ensuring certain and authoritative knowledge. "These are only a few of the many necessary and useful Things that have hitherto been made only Matter of Speculation and Dispute, but could never otherwise be truly determined, but by the Help of Registers," he concluded.[34] Like Jurin, Short considered numerical tables as an effective method to create consensus and resolve controversy.

To demonstrate the value and relevance of his approach, Short did a detailed analysis of the London bills of mortality from 1629 through 1750. He determined that deaths attributed to falling sickness, gravel, stone, cholera, and childbed were on the decline, and convulsions, smallpox, measles, and jaundice were "gathering fresh Vigour and greater Strength" and were "both more frequent and fatal."[35] He noted that "*Excessive Drinking* had neither Name nor Place in the old Table, now it makes a handsome Article."[36] Short took the further step of dividing the different causes of death listed in the London bills into the following categories: 1) childhood diseases; 2) diseases common to children and adults; 3) diseases of adults and the aged; 4) external diseases; and 5) unnatural, or violent, deaths. (See Figures 6.2, 6.3, 6.4, and 6.5)

Again, the columns were not labeled. Short's description was found in the text following the tables:

---

[32] Short, *New Observations*, pp. 61–62.   [33] Short, *New Observations*, pp. xi–xii.
[34] Short, *New Observations*, p. xiv.   [35] Short, *New Observations*, p. 209.
[36] Short, *New Observations*, p. 211.

TABLE SIXTEENTH.
Of Difeafes and Cafualties of Three Octenaries.

Disease						
Abortives and Still-born	3798	1 of 20	3614	1 of $28\frac{11}{18}$	4780	1 of $45\frac{1}{6}$
Chryfoms and Infants	17730	1 of $4\frac{1}{7}$	9162	1 of $11\frac{13}{43}$		
Convulfions	2232	1 of 35	6584	1 of 15	61567	1 of $3\frac{1}{2}$
Chin-cough					882	1 of $244\frac{9}{22}$
Chicken and Swine Pox	36	1 of $2183\frac{1}{2}$	12	1 of 8631		
Fluxes and Small Pox	2547	1 of $30\frac{2}{15}$	6189	1 of $16\frac{4}{5}$	16062	1 of $13\frac{7}{8}$
Meafles	210	1 of $374\frac{1}{3}$	399	1 of $259\frac{3}{5}$	1927	1 of 112
Rafh					24	1 of $8992\frac{1}{6}$
Head-mold Shot, Horfe-shoe Head					1106	1 of $195\frac{1}{8}$
Rickets	113	1 of $695\frac{1}{2}$	3162	1 of $32\frac{4}{5}$	587	1 of $367\frac{3}{5}$
Scald Head			2	1 of $51785\frac{1}{2}$	16	1 of $13488\frac{1}{4}$
Sore Mouths, Thrufh, and Canker	282	1 of $278\frac{3}{4}$	437	1 of 237	70	1 of 3083
Teething	3382	1 of $23\frac{1}{4}$	7584	1 of $13\frac{24}{37}$	11135	1 of $19\frac{1}{4}$
Thrufh	181	1 of $434\frac{1}{7}$	123	1 of $842\frac{5}{24}$	769	1 of $280\frac{5}{8}$
Worms	179	1 of $439\frac{1}{8}$	53	1 of $1954\frac{1}{6}$	97	1 of 2225
	30690	1 of $2\frac{1}{4}$	37320	of $2\frac{1}{4}$	99022	1 of $2\frac{1}{4}$

6.2 Thomas Short's table of children's deaths listed by disease from the London bills. *Source:* Thomas Short, *New Observations, Natural, Moral, Civil, Political, and Medical on City, Town and Country Bills of Mortality* (London, 1750), p. 199. Yale University, Harvey Cushing/John Hay Whitney Medical Library.

In this 16th Table of *Diseases* and *Casualties,* we have the Numbers that died during three *Octenaries,* at distant and different Periods. The first begins with 1629, and ends with 1636, and will be a kind of Key to the other two. The second begins with 1653 and ends with 1660. The third with 1734, and ends with 1742; 39 and 43 are omitted to make the Number in each equal. In the first Column of the Table we have the Names of the Diseases, in the 2d the Number that died of each Disease; in the 3d the Proportions that such as die in the first Class, bear to the whole that died in that Octenary. After the first Class, or that of Childrens Diseases, the Children buried are not included in the remaining four Classes; but the Sum total that died not of Childrens Diseases, but died of others, is carried through each Article of all the other Classes, and made the constant Dividend of each Octenary. The 4th and 5th Columns are the same for the 2d Octenary, that the 2d and 3d were for the first. The 6th and 7th Columns are for the 3d Octernary, the same as the other two.[37]

Given the complexity of the contents of his columns, it is no wonder that he chose not to label them.

The categories mirrored Short's concerns: The first provided a measure of infant and child mortality, and pointed to the causes for such high mortality. As he indicated in his lengthy description of the table, he followed the precedent set by Graunt (and followed by Arbuthnot and Jurin) and subtracted infant and child

[37] Short, *New Observations*, p. 203.

TABLE Sixteenth, continued.

Died of Diseases common to Children and Adults.						
Ague and Fever	10484	1 of $4\frac{12}{21}$	10466	1 of $6\frac{1}{3}$	31	1 of $3767\frac{2}{3}$
Asthma and Pthisick					4670	1 of 25
Bleach			1			
Blasted	58	1 of 826	25	1 of $2650\frac{1}{25}$		
Bleeding and Hemorrhage	23	1 of 2083	35			
Bloody-flux, Loosenefs, and Flux	3063	1 of $15\frac{18}{30}$	2314	1 of $28\frac{7}{12}$	93	1 of $1255\frac{5}{8}$
Burftings and Ruptures	51	1 of $939\frac{1}{2}$	140	1 of $473\frac{1}{4}$	150	1 of $778\frac{1}{3}$
Calenture	4	1 of $11978\frac{1}{2}$	5	1 of $13250\frac{1}{3}$		
Cholick, Wind, and Iliat	192	1 of $249\frac{1}{2}$	961	1 of $68\frac{4}{8}$	2310	1 of $50\frac{1}{2}$
Cold and Cough	381	1 of $125\frac{4}{5}$	274	1 of $241\frac{11}{14}$		
Confumptions and Cough	15513	1 of $3\frac{1}{13}$	23707	1 of $2\frac{7}{11}$	35650	1 of $3\frac{5}{18}$
Cramp	1					
Dropfy and Tympany	2282	1 of 21	5767	1 of $11\frac{2}{3}$	8294	1 of $14\frac{7}{12}$
Dry-Gripes					12	1 of $9732\frac{1}{2}$
Falling-Sicknefs	48	1 of 998	22	1 of $3011\frac{4}{11}$	3	1 of 3890
Fever and Purples	977	1 of 49	968	1 of $68\frac{1}{2}$	33461	1 of $3\frac{1}{4}$
Gravel, Stones, and Strangury	299	1 of $160\frac{1}{4}$	381	1 of $173\frac{3}{4}$	422	1 of $276\frac{1}{4}$
Head-ach	6	1 of $7985\frac{1}{2}$	90	1 of $736\frac{1}{5}$		
Jaundice	381	1 of $125\frac{9}{19}$	531	1 of $124\frac{3}{4}$	1174	1 of $101\frac{9}{11}$
Jaw-fallen	82	1 of $584\frac{1}{5}$	8	1 of $828\,1\frac{1}{8}$		
Inflammation					309	1 of 378
Lethargy	12	1 of $3992\frac{2}{8}$	44	1 of $1505\frac{1}{4}$	61	1 of $1914\frac{1}{4}$
Liver-grown and Spleen	748	1 of $64\frac{1}{8}$	346	1 of $191\frac{1}{2}$	60	1 of $1946\frac{1}{2}$
Megrim	46	1 of $1041\frac{1}{2}$	51	1 of $1299\frac{3}{8}$		
Mortification					1836	1 of $63\frac{5}{8}$

6.3 Thomas Short's table of deaths common to children and adults from the London bills. *Source:* Thomas Short, *New Observations, Natural, Moral, Civil, Political, and Medical on City, Town and Country Bills of Mortality* (London, 1750), p. 200. Yale University, Harvey Cushing/John Hay Whitney Medical Library.

deaths from the total number of deaths for the remainder of his calculations. The second category essentially became a catalog of acute, contagious diseases that affected all ages. The third category encompassed chronic diseases common among the aged; and the fourth comprised "outward griefs." Into the final category, Short collected deaths classified

accidental, as drowned out of Ships or Boats, or by washing or bathing, starved by Hunger or Cold, scalded to Death, overlaid, bitten by Animals, murthered, smothered, bruised, or having their Bones broken; and such other Accidents as depend on Men's Trade and Employment: Or as the Effect of their own Wickedness, as the *French-Pox,* excessive Drinking, &c. or such as fall by their own bloody Hands immediately, or by common Justice.[38]

This was not simply a catchall category. These deaths were unnatural in the sense that they were the result of human actions, and thus this type of mortality was potentially controllable. Short's frequent admonitions for moral rectitude found ample support in his observations made on these types of deaths. It was

[38] Short, *New Observations,* p. 204.

TABLE Sixteenth, continued.

Palſy	159	1 of $301\frac{1}{4}$	162	1 of 409	322	1 of $362\frac{1}{4}$
Planet-ſtruck					1	
Plague	12000	1 of $3\frac{3}{20}$	105	1 of 631		
Plague in the Guts			1535	1 of $43\frac{1}{6}$		
Pleuriſy	202	1 of $237\frac{1}{5}$	114	1 of $581\frac{1}{7}$	436	1 of $267\frac{19}{22}$
Quinſey	109	1 of $439\frac{3}{5}$	107	1 of $619\frac{1}{6}$	171	1 of 683
Spleen	1		53	1 of $1250\frac{1}{7}$	8	1 of $14598\frac{3}{4}$
Surfeit	1166	1 of $41\frac{1}{11}$	1428	1 of $46\frac{1}{3}$	32	1 of $3649\frac{6}{11}$
Vomiting or Cholera	23	1 of 2083	104	1 of 637	114	1 of $1024\frac{1}{2}$
	37511	1 of $1\frac{2}{7}$	49741	1 of $1\frac{2}{3}$	89593	1 of $1\frac{1}{4}$
Died of Diſeaſes proper to Adults.						
Aged	5458	1 of $8\frac{21}{27}$	6622	1 of 10	15630	1 of $7\frac{1}{2}$
Bed-ridden					78	1 of $1497\frac{3}{5}$
Apoplexies and ſuddenly	169	1 of $283\frac{1}{2}$	807	1 of $82\frac{7}{12}$	1673	1 of $69\frac{13}{18}$
Child-bed	1258	1 of $38\frac{1}{12}$	1609	1 of $41\frac{1}{5}$	1929	1 of $60\frac{10}{19}$
Diabetes					10	1 of 11679
Gout	38	1 of $1260\frac{8}{9}$	63	1 of $1051\frac{2}{3}$	398	1 of $293\frac{1}{2}$
Grief	114	1 of $420\frac{1}{4}$	90	1 of $736\frac{1}{9}$	78	1 of $1497\frac{1}{3}$
Lunatic	41	1 of $1168\frac{1}{2}$	80	1 of $828\frac{1}{5}$	339	1 of $344\frac{1}{2}$
Miſcarriage					21	1 of $5561\frac{1}{2}$
Mother, Hyſteric and Vapours	4	1 of 11978	20	1 of 3313	1	
Riſing of the Lights	529	1 of $90\frac{3}{5}$	1581	1 of $41\frac{14}{15}$	107	1 of $1091\frac{1}{2}$
Rheumatiſm					165	1 of $707\frac{3}{4}$
Sciatica	13	1 of $3685\frac{1}{6}$	2	1 of 33128	2	1 of 58395
Stoppage of the Stomach	6	1 of $7985\frac{2}{3}$	1218	1 of $54\frac{1}{3}$	1356	1 of $86\frac{1}{7}$
	7773		12215		21787	

6.4 Thomas Short's table of adult deaths listed by disease from the London bills. *Source:* Thomas Short, *New Observations, Natural, Moral, Civil, Political, and Medical on City, Town and Country Bills of Mortality* (London, 1750), p. 201. Yale University, Harvey Cushing/John Hay Whitney Medical Library.

TABLE Sixteenth, continued.

Died of outward Griefs, as Cancers, Fiſtula's, Gangrenes, King's-Evil, Leproſy, Swellings and Wens, Itch, St. *Anthony*'s Fire, Sores and Ulcers, broken and bruiſed Limbs, Impoſthume, cutting for the Stone, &c.	1312	1 of $36\frac{1}{2}$	2260	1 of $29\frac{2}{3}$	1309	1 of $89\frac{1}{5}$
Expired by unnatural Deaths, as by meer Accidents, Broken Limbs, bruiſed, burnt, or ſcalded to Death; bit by mad Creatures, drowned by Bathing, out of Boats or otherwiſe; found dead, or killed; ſlain by Falls, frightened to Death, murdered, ſhot, ſmothered, ſtabb'd, ſtarved, ſtrangled, poiſoned, over-laid, executed, exceſſive Drinking, hanged themſelves, *French* Pox, &c.	1311	1 of $36\frac{1}{2}$	2035	1 of $28\frac{1}{2}$	4101	1 of $28\frac{1}{2}$

6.5 Thomas Short's table of deaths due to casualties from the London bills. *Source:* Thomas Short, *New Observations, Natural, Moral, Civil, Political, and Medical on City, Town and Country Bills of Mortality* (London, 1750), p. 202. Yale University, Harvey Cushing/John Hay Whitney Medical Library.

A CHART of all the Fatal Diseases and Casualties in London, during 75 Years; beginning from 1701, and ending with 1776.

Collected from the London Bills of Mortality, and arranged into Five separate progressive Periods of Fifteen Years each. The Total Amount of the Five Periods, or Seventy-five Years Mortality, is added together in the Sixth Column.

Diseases and Casualties	From 1701 to 1717	From 1717 to 1732	From 1732 to 1747	From 1747 to 1762	From 1762 to 1777	Total amount of seventy-five years Mortality from 1701 to 1777
Ague	80	198	82	99	109	574
Fevers, malignant, spotted, scarlet and purple	50,955	53,330	57,995	45,621	48,594	256,085
Small Pox	22,219	34,448	29,462	29,165	36,276	151,570
Measles	1,972	2,618	2,858	3,099	3,319	13,866
Quinsy, Sore Throat	226	169	287	306	309	1,297
Pleurisy	384	602	811	407	321	3,525
Rheumatism	368	447	310	175	128	1,468
Gout	318	645	769	803	1,010	3,236
Consumption	42,541	49,680	66,009	61,749	68,949	288,928
Chin Cough, Hooping Cough, Cough	116	632	1,692	2,755	4,252	9,573
Asthma and Tissick	5,090	7,938	9,460	5,699	6,154	34,341
Apoplexy and Suddenly	2,228	3,013	3,287	3,271	3,353	15,152
Palsy	332	550	621	1,021	1,020	3,544
Lethargy	105	126	116	105	74	526
Meagrims	13	10				23
Headach	21	32	6	18		77
Lunatick	412	513	777	1,126	1,048	3,876
Spleen and Vapours	53	52	20		10	125
Rising of the Lights	1,219	1,239	197	39	10	2,074
Stoppage of the Stomach	4,139	2,557	2,286	304	179	9,465
Vomiting and Looseness	820	682	248	134	120	2,004
Cholic, Gripes, and Twisting of the Guts	13,668	11,032	3,739	1,475	796	29,710
Flux	178	200		252	341	971
Bloody Flux	133	248	167	94	93	745
Worms	697	662	161	115	56	1,691
Jaundice	1,261	1,798	2,032	1,729	2,089	8,909
Gravel, Stone and Strangury	789	868	700	421	429	3,205
Diabetes	37	48	19	16	5	125
Dropsy and Tympany	11,626	15,430	16,036	13,410	14,038	70,506
Livergrown	76	95	75	23		269
French Pox	917	1,372	1,663	997	1,016	5,965
Scurvy	63	28	14	59	42	226
Evil	1,020	919	426	197	198	2,360
Leprosy	19	53	69	39	15	195
Rash	77	128	47	59	24	341
Itch			42	31	11	84
Childbed	3,560	3,894	3,412	3,005	3,186	17,057
Abortion and Stillborn	8,746	10,231	8,793	8,820	10,241	46,831
Chrisoms and Infants	850	315	606			1,771
Miscarriage			47	56	49	152
Convulsions	91,660	114,718	111,966	85,196	89,221	492,761
Headmold-shot and water in the Head	609	2,374	2,013	1,022	337	6,355
Teeth	18,478	25,199	20,274	13,978	11,918	89,847
Thrush	839	1,191	1,512	1,391	1,101	6,034
Scald Head	9	15	29	22		75
Rickets	3,916	1,383	954	112	194	6,559
Inflammation	8	67	698	894	1,394	3,061
Imposthume	790	694	387	191	68	2,130
St. Anthony's Fire		73	36	63	69	241
Gangrene and Mortification	1,071	2,857	3,404	3,083	3,023	13,438
Canker	138	181	123	77	61	580
Cancer	1,041	1,059	774	682	719	4,275
Sores and Ulcers	695	485	402	253	236	2,071
Fistula	360	208	210	134	119	1,025
Bursten and Ruptures	310	309	304	163	140	1,226
Swelling and Wen	6		47	49	37	139
Killed by Falls, Bruises, Fractures and other Accidents	828	917	926	1,084	1,065	4,820
Self-murder	445	667	693	555	509	2,869
Murdered	132	109	147	71	77	539
Stabbed, Killed, Wounded, Shot, etc.	13	32	13		2	60
Executed			495	495		990
Drowned	900	1,193	1,451	1,718	1,781	7,043
Burnt	90	54	90	127	132	493
Scalded	15	36	45	51	40	191
Stifled, Suffocated and Smothered	16	34	62	90	68	276
Overlaid	814	1,180	1,293	414	95	3,799
Found dead	386	547	668	336	133	2,082
Grief		14	8	87	77	421
Frightened				13	2	45
Surfeits	684	131	59	31	27	932
Starved		17	96	53	57	223
Excessive Drinking	19	267	678	189	69	1,222
Bleeding	80	69	57	70	114	397
Poisoned		7	7	24	10	40
Bit by Mad Dogs and Cats		3	14	15	6	38
Bedridden		104		56	105	265
Aged	27,333	34,708	30,058	25,109	22,032	139,248

6.6 William Black's table of deaths by diseases and casualties from the London bills (1701–1776). Source: William Black, An Arithmetical and Medical Analysis of the Diseases and Mortality of the Human Species (London 1789), p. 43. Yale University, Harvey Cushing/John Hay Whitney Medical Library.

precisely these sorts of observations that led physicians and others to examine what factors might be responsible for such changes.

Almost 40 years after Short's work, William Black analyzed the London bills in his *An Arithmetical and Medical Analysis of the Diseases and Mortality of the Human Species* (1789). Begun as a lecture to the Medical Society of London, founded by the Quaker Lettsom in 1773, Black's ideas were developed into a book. It enjoyed immediate high praise because it was the only work to include a numerical account of insanity, a disease on individuals' minds because of George III's illness.[39]

Black, like Jurin and Short, considered arithmetic to be the path to certain knowledge. "When opinions are litigated in either medicine or surgery, and a thousand different leaders hoist their separate standards, assigning different causes, prognosticks, and modes of cures," Black charged in his colorful (and eminently quotable) prose, "what tribunal can possibly decide truth in this clash of contradictory assertions and conjectures; or by what clue can medical wanderers find their way through the labyrinth of prognosticks and therapeuticks, except by medical arithmetick and numbers?"[40] Comparison was central to Black's vision of medical arithmetic, just as it was to Jurin's. "Although it may not shew the best mode of cure that may hereafter be invented," Black admitted, medical arithmetic will "by comparison, determine the best that has yet been discovered, or in use."[41] Finally, arithmetic would free physicians "from the reins and fetters of ancient or of modern metaphysicks."[42]

Black summarized the London bills of mortality for 75 years (1701–1776) in one table. (See Figure 6.6.) Unlike Short, Black started with the eighteenth century because London was significantly smaller in the seventeenth century and plague dominated the bills for many years. Black divided his summary into six 15-year periods, which were clearly labeled as column heads. He chose 15-year periods on the assumption that London's population numbered roughly 700,000, and the population of Britain and Ireland roughly 15 times that, or 10 million. So mortality figures compiled for each 15-year period from the London bills represented the total mortality for Britain and Ireland in any one year.[43] Like Short, Black did not follow the alphabetical order of the London bills; instead he grouped similar diseases together. For example, Black listed febrile diseases at the beginning of the table; halfway down on the left, he put together stomach and intestinal disorders. Unlike Short, Black did not label these divisions nor place the groups in separate tables.

Trends in the incidence of each disease, deduced from his tables, were central to Black's analysis. For instance, he observed the high rate of mortality due

---

[39] See Chapter 4, "Inoculation outside London."
[40] Black, *An Arithmetical and Medical Analysis*, p. vii.
[41] Black, *An Arithmetical and Medical Analysis*, p. viii.
[42] Black, *An Arithmetical and Medical Analysis*, p. viii.
[43] Black, *An Arithmetical and Medical Analysis*, p. 38.

to consumption (one-fifth to one-sixth of all deaths in London; from 42,541 deaths for the years 1701–1717 to 68,949 for the years 1762–1777); however, he cautioned that the term consumption was too vague and that many other wasting diseases were grouped under its head.[44] Other classifications were also suspect. Black noted the decline of "surfeit" (from 684 deaths to 27) but decided that "good eating and gormandizing" could not possibly be "worn out of fashion in this metropolis." "Stoppage of the stomach," too, no longer accounted for many deaths (from 4,139 deaths to 179), and here Black poked fun at the searchers. "It would baffle the ingenuity of an antiquarian," he wrote, "to decypher the true import of this term: severe sickness, or the word Abracadabra, would be full as intelligible."[45] In sum, Black's book amounted to a running discussion of the leading causes for each illness, including environmental factors and individual behavior.

Roughly a decade after Black's *Arithmetical and Medical Analysis* appeared, William Heberden, Jr., physician and Fellow of the Royal Society, published *Observations on the Increase and Decrease of Different Diseases, and Particularly of the Plague* (1801). Heberden's observations were based on tables he constructed from the London bills of mortality and from accounts taken from London hospitals, such as the Smallpox Hospital and the Lying-In Hospital. Significantly, he began his treatise (after a few notes qualifying the reliability of the bills of mortality) with 26 pages of tables cataloging mortality by different years and by weeks within specific years. (See Figures 6.7 and 6.8.)

Heberden was quite candid about the importance of the tabular method:

The two preceding Tables exhibit a method in which such observations may safely be conducted. For, whatever errors be supposed to have crept into the registers from which they are formed, yet when taken together, and considered on an extensive scale, they must be admitted to constitute a very unexceptionable basis for medical reasoning. And the several objects being thus brought nearer to each other, and seen as it were side by side, the judgment may be formed not only much more easily, but, it is apprehended, much more certainly also, than could be done in any other manner. Another great advantage resulting from such tables is, that they do of themselves often suggest conclusions, which correct, or perhaps wholly contradict, the expectations raised upon no better foundation than vague conjecture, or popular opinion.[46]

These were precisely the same virtues Graunt had ascribed to his table of casualties in 1662.

Using his tables, Heberden observed that the number of deaths from dysentery sharply decreased over the eighteenth century, while those attributed to

[44] Black, *An Arithmetical and Medical Analysis*, p. 93.
[45] Black, *An Arithmetical and Medical Analysis*, pp. 158–159.
[46] William Heberden, Junior, *Observations on the Increase and Decrease of Different Diseases, and Particularly of the Plague* (London : T. Payne, 1801), pp. 29–30.

TABLE I.

Years - -	1701	1702	1703	1704	1705	1706	1707	1708	1709	1710	Average
CHRISTENED	15616	15687	15448	15895	16145	15369	16066	15862	15220	14928	15623
BURIED - -	20471	19481	20720	22684	22097	19847	21600	21291	21800	24620	21461
Flux Colic Gripes - - }	60.8	67	53	56	52.6	50.4	45.9	41.1	42.4	32.9	50.2
Small Pox -	53.1	15.9	43.3	66.1	49.7	36	49.9	79.2	46.6	126.7	56.6
Apoplexy Palfy Suddenly - }	8	6.9	7.6	6.4	7.1	7.8	7.2	8	7.4	6.6	7.3
Meafles - -	0.2	1.4	2.4	0.5	14.5	18	1.7	5.9	4	7.3	5.5
Childbed Mifcarriage }	10.9	11.4	10.5	11.7	13	11.9	11.9	11.5	9.8	8.8	11.1

Years - -	1711	1712	1713	1714	1715	1716	1717	1718	1719	1720	Average
CHRISTENED	14706	15660	15927	17495	17234	17421	18475	18307	18413	17479	17111
BURIED - -	19833	21198	21057	26569	22232	24436	23446	26523	28347	25454	23909
Flux Colic Gripes - - }	36.7	32.5	33.8	30.2	32.3	33.9	35.8	39.1	39.5	38.3	35.2
Small Pox -	45.7	92.5	76.8	106	48	99.4	94.4	71	114.1	56.7	80.4
Apoplexy Palfy Suddenly - }	9	7.4	9.3	7.5	8.4	7.5	10.3	8.5	8.5	9.9	8.6
Meafles - -	4.8	3.6	2.9	5.2	1.3	11	1.5	18.5	8.5	8.3	6.5
Childbed Mifcarriage }	9.8	9.8	8.4	11.6	12.5	9.4	10.3	9.9	10.3	10.2	10.2

6.7 William Heberden's table of deaths by diseases from the London bills (1701–1720). *Source:* William Heberden, *Observations on the Increase and Decrease of Different Diseases*...(London, 1801), p. 2. Yale University, Harvey Cushing/John Hay Whitney Medical Library.

apoplexy increased. To demonstrate this observation, Heberden did what had become a familiar practice – he grouped several similar diseases into a single category, including griping of the guts, bloody flux, and colic for each decade from 1700 to 1800 and created a new table that vividly captures this significant change. (See Figure 6.9.) He attributed the dramatic decline in dysentery to "the improvements which have gradually taken place, not only in London,

TABLE II.

Weekly Bills of Mortality. 1763.	Whole Number buried.	Under two years.	Above sixty years.	Apoplexy, Palsy, Suddenly.	Childbed and Miscarriage.	Consumptions.	Fever.	Colic, Flux, Gripes, Looseness.	Measles.	Small Pox.
4 Jan. - -	641	197	93	11	2	113	73	9	0	106
11 Jan. - -	565	162	84	6	3	104	55	5	0	108
18 Jan. - -	583	146	86	11	8	118	61	1	0	107
25 Jan. - -	621	149	105	5	13	103	62	3	2	113
1 Feb. - -	687	216	128	14	10	129	59	2	3	125
8 Feb. - -	612	152	120	5	8	106	76	4	1	84
15 Feb. - -	520	146	86	4	6	93	43	2	3	96
22 Feb. - -	551	158	86	6	5	108	69	3	1	79
1 Mar. - -	469	126	65	6	5	108	54	1	2	67
8 Mar. - -	513	153	86	3	7	103	64	0	0	65
15 Mar. - -	404	98	76	3	0	93	29	1	2	51
22 Mar. - -	552	157	87	3	3	114	75	2	1	73
29 Mar. - -	443	135	59	4	3	106	53	3	2	52
5 Apr. - -	448	131	79	6	6	85	62	1	2	57
12 Apr. - -	484	147	78	5	4	108	63	0	3	57
19 Apr. - -	477	141	68	6	7	83	49	0	8	61
26 Apr. - -	505	140	76	5	6	105	83	0	7	54
3 May - -	461	135	70	3	9	101	36	0	7	61
10 May - -	567	159	85	9	12	105	68	0	12	77
17 May - -	484	155	60	6	3	81	70	0	15	52
24 May - -	452	152	70	5	2	88	54	2	14	49
31 May - -	537	179	72	7	10	118	43	1	15	67
7 June - -	524	174	70	7	7	87	69	1	23	64
14 June - -	537	167	75	6	2	90	64	0	31	62
21 June - -	466	142	58	6	3	83	72	0	36	57
28 June - -	552	159	74	2	4	104	71	1	34	83

6.8 William Heberden's table of weekly mortality listed by age and disease from the London bills (1763). *Source:* William Heberden, *Observations on the Increase and Decrease of Different Diseases*...(London, 1801), p. 8. Yale University, Harvey Cushing/John Hay Whitney Medical Library.

but in all great towns, and in the manner of living throughout the kingdom; particularly with respect to cleanliness and ventilation."[47]

[47] Heberden, *Observations on the Increase and Decrease of Different Diseases,* p. 35. D.V. Glass argued that Heberden commited a "howler" because he neglected to notice that the decrease in deaths attributed to "griping in the guts" corresponded to an increase in deaths attributed to "convulsions." The late

From 1700 to 1710 the average is about 1,070 annually.

1710 to 1720 - - - - - -	770
1720 to 1730 - - - - - -	700
1730 to 1740 - - - - - -	350
1740 to 1750 - - - - - -	150
1750 to 1760 - - - - - -	110
1760 to 1770 - - - - - -	80
1770 to 1780 - - - - - -	70
1780 to 1790 - - - - - -	40
1790 to 1800 - - - - - -	20

6.9 William Heberden's table of dysentery deaths (1700–1800). *Source:* William Heberden, *Observations on the Increase and Decrease of Different Diseases . . .* (London, 1801), p. 34. Yale University, Harvey Cushing/John Hay Whitney Medical Library.

From accounts of the British Lying-In Hospital in Brownlow Street, Heberden showed that maternal mortality had decreased from 1 in 42 deaths for the decade 1749–1758, to 1 in 288 deaths for the decade 1789–1798. (See Figure 6.10.) He offered no reasons for this decline. His clearly structured table also provided figures for the number of births divided by sex, the number of twins, the number of stillborns, and the number of infant deaths. And he argued that the 1751 Act of Parliament to restrain the distillation of spirits had had a positive effect on health. As evidence, he pointed to the drop in the number of deaths attributed to dropsy and excessive drinking.[48]

Growing awareness of changes in disease incidence, an awareness informed by contemporary studies of mortality, thus emboldened medical arithmeticians to speculate about the causes of such changes and to hope for general improvement. European experience with pestilential disease, especially plague, during the eighteenth century seemed to warrant a certain degree of optimism regarding human ability to control mortality. By the end of the eighteenth century, British medical men felt confident enough to bury the plague as a disease of the past. The London bills of mortality, as an historical record of the plague, showed convincingly that the last outbreak in England had occurred in 1665.

Reflection on the reasons for this change led some to attribute plague's demise to specific human actions. William Black, for instance, asserted that "widened

nineteenth-century historian and physician Charles Creighton argued that convulsions probably signified infantile diarrhea. See D.V. Glass, *Numbering the People: The Eighteenth-Century Population Controversy and the Development of Census and Vital Statistics in Britain* (London and New York: Gordon & Cremonesi, 1973), p. 119; and Charles Creighton, *A History of Epidemics in Great Britain*, 2 vols. (Cambridge: Cambridge University Press, 1891), vol. 2, pp. 747–758.

[48] Heberden, *Observations on the Increase and Decrease of Different Diseases*, p. 45.

A. D.	No. of Women Delivered	Boys Born.	Girls Born.	Total No. of Children Born.	Women had Twins.	Children Still-born.	Children Died.	Women Died.	PROPORTION of DEATHS. Of the Women.	Of the Children.
1749	3	3		3						
1750	175	93	84	177	2	11	5	3		
1751	337	181	160	341	4	15	9	12		
1752	433	236	201	437	4	22	27	14		
1753	284	141	146	287	3	10	21	10		
1754	321	175	151	326	5	9	66	12	1 in 42	1 in 15.
1755	370	190	185	375	5	8	34	9		
1756	370	188	184	372	2	8	10	3		
1757	478	262	219	481	3	12	22	7		
1758	521	277	254	531	10	6	16	8		
1759	472	253	226	479	7	12	14	6		
1760	427	228	206	434	7	11	58	26		
1761	390	197	198	395	5	20	31	12		
1762	397	199	199	398	1	8	38	7		
1763	414	209	212	421	7	15	32	10	1 in 50	1 in 20.
1764	366	191	178	369	3	15	17	7		
1765	560	311	258	569	9	12	20	9		
1766	588	293	304	597	9	25	17	10		
1767	571	303	272	575	4	7	10	4		
1768	588	301	288	589	1	5	2	3		
1769	561	292	280	572	11	14	13	7		
1770	472	225	249	474	2	13	9	28		
1771	541	266	282	548	7	17	14	4		
1772	596	320	286	606	10	25	17	4		
1773	627	336	298	634	7	19	14	4	1 in 53	1 in 42.
1774	553	292	266	558	5	36	3	18		
1775	570	295	280	575	5	22	13	21		
1776	543	276	275	551	8	26	9	3		
1777	602	312	293	605	3	24	24	6		
1778	572	281	298	579	7	19	18	11		

6.10 William Heberden's table of maternal mortality (1749–1800). *Source:* William Heberden, *Observations on the Increase and Decrease of Different Diseases* . . . (London, 1801), pp. 40–41. Yale University, Harvey Cushing/John Hay Whitney Medical Library.

streets, ventilation, cleanliness, a more plentiful supply of water and many other causes, have all contributed to the extinction of this exotick incendiary."[49] He also applauded the development of quarantine, but criticized other state actions, namely, the policy of locking both sick and healthy within a house until all

[49] Black, *An Arithmetical and Medical Analysis*, pp. 65–66. For a similar opinion, see Heberden, *Observations on the Increase and Decrease of Different Diseases*, pp. 69–77.

A. D.	No. of Women Delivered.	Boys Born.	Girls Born.	Total No. of Children Born.	Women had Twins.	Children Still-born.	Children Died.	Women Died.	PROPORTION of DEATHS. Of the Women.	Of the Children.
1779	563	310	257	567	4	31	8	3		
1780	566	310	259	569	3	33	4	8		
1781	524	275	255	530	6	26	9	14		
1782	549	298	260	558	9	15	14	13		
1783	587	308	288	596	9	33	17	5	1 in 60	1 in 44.
1784	550	283	272	555	5	24	10	14		
1785	435	231	212	443	8	24	16	6		
1786	597	333	276	609	12	35	19	9		
1787	564	290	283	573	9	36	18	9		
1788	578	296	287	583	5	25	10	10		
1789	599	296	308	604	5	42	12	1		
1790	622	317	313	630	8	34	5	7		
1791	621	325	303	628	7	39	2	1		
1792	610	312	306	618	8	29	4	1		
1793	590	300	297	597	7	24	12	1	1 in 288	1 in 77.
1794	583	286	305	591	8	26	6	2		
1795	612	310	310	620	8	32	13	2		
1796	627	326	305	631	4	24	4	1		
1797	619	332	293	625	6	25	9	3		
1798	566	285	292	577	11	31	12	2		
1799	521	282	248	530	9	21	7	1	1 in 938	1 in 118.
1800	417	211	210	421	4	18	1	0		
Total -	26202	13642	12871	26513	311	1073	795	391		

Proportion of Boys to Girls born in the Hofpital is about 19 to 18.
　　　Children Still-born in ditto, about - - 1 to 25.
　　　Women having had Twins, about - - 1 to 84.

6.10 (*cont*)

were dead or recovered, a policy that he regarded as "extremely erroneous and impolitick" and which contributed to contagion.[50]

MORTALITY BY AGE AND PLACE

In addition to changes in the mortality of different diseases, arithmeticians were interested in mortality rates of different ages and places. "To know at what period of life each disease is most fatal to mankind, is manifestly a sort of

[50] Black, *An Arithmetical and Medical Analysis*, p. 67.

intelligence the most important, both to the patient and the physician," asserted John Haygarth in 1774.[51] Graunt and Jurin had grouped diseases into different age categories, which had depended upon common observational knowledge about the periods of life during which diseases generally affected individuals. Thus, for example, they grouped "Teeth and Convulsions" under the heading of infant and childhood diseases. This informal way of categorizing was replaced by a more exact method. The London bills of mortality listed age of death beginning in 1728, and over the course of the eighteenth century, especially after 1750, a growing number of parish clerks throughout Europe began to include age of death in their registers. This information enabled medical arith-meticians to be much more precise about the mortality of diseases at different ages and emboldened them to suggest policy recommendations based on these figures.

In 1662 John Graunt had created the first life table, but it was not until Edmond Halley's paper of 1693 that the numbers were based on accounts (taken from Breslau) in which age of death had been recorded.[52] (Halley's table is discussed in Chapter 7.) Life tables generally showed the number of individuals alive out of a given population for each year of age. As mentioned in Chapter 1, life tables were instrumental in putting annuities on a more firm evidential basis, and physicians and others studied them to glean information about mortality patterns. Life tables also clearly influenced the way individuals thought about mortality.[53] Mathematicians such as Abraham DeMoivre, Richard Price, and Antoine Déparcieux could rely on a growing number of accounts that listed age of death to calculate life expectancy figures (or probabilities of life). By the second half of the century, one could consult a life table in order to find out one's life expectancy at any age.

An example of one way to use a life table is found in the private writings of the Montpellier physician François Boissier de Sauvages.[54] Throughout his life, Sauvages kept a Livre de Maison – a journal containing notes from his readings, copies of letters, and jottings about various medical topics. Sauvages's interest in mathematics emerges clearly from these pages; they are full of measurements, numbers, and ratios. He wrote about mortality rates in French hospitals and English hospitals, the specific gravity of blood and other bodily fluids, and fig-ures concerning the incidence of smallpox and the risk of smallpox inoculation.

[51] John Haygarth, "Observations on the Bill of Mortality, in Chester, for the Year 1772," *Philosophical Transactions* 64 (1774): 71.

[52] Edmond Halley, "An Estimate of the Degrees of the Mortality of Mankind, Drawn from Curious Tables of the Births and Funerals at the City of Breslaw," *Philosophical Transactions* 17–18 (1693): 596–610.

[53] Robert Favre examined this fascinating idea in *La mort dans la littérature et la pensée françaises au siècle des lumières* (Lyon: Presses Universitaires de Lyon, 1978), chap. 1.

[54] I thank Colin Jones for bringing this document to my attention.

After some remarks on Déparcieux's work on annuities, Sauvages calculated and recorded each of his children's life expectancies in a table.[55]

mes enfants	année	mois	vie moyenne	
Nicolay	12	0	41	
Victoire	10	4	43	
François	8	8	43	9
Lucie	7	6	43	5
Mariange	0	1	0	
Sylvie	4	5	44	4
Boissier (meurt en naissance)				
...	0	7	34	
	43	7	250	1

These calculations were based solely on the age of each of his children; he did not include observations on the health of his children, whether sickly or robust, in his assessment of how long they might live.

The very great number of infant and child deaths was one of the most striking observations made time and again using a life table. Graunt thought over one-third of the children born in London died before age six. By 1750 Thomas Short was able to construct a life table for the London population based on figures taken from the bills of mortality. (See Figure 6.11.) He compared his table with Graunt's and noted that a greater number of children died under the age of six than in Graunt's time (45 of 100 versus 36 of 100), and he observed "the shocking Effects of our new and delicate Ways of nursing and rearing Children" where "some are denied all Breast, and must be brought up with the Spoon; many [others] must not draw at the Mother's Breast, but must have a strange nurse, the Cheapness of whose Wages are considered more than the Goodness of her Constitution."[56] Short thus enlisted life tables in the cause of denouncing wet-nursing in order to curb infant mortality.

In his observations on Manchester, the physician Thomas Percival provided a geographical spectrum of infant and child mortality, ranging from the most deadly, urban London, to the most healthy, the countryside:

Great towns are in a peculiar degree fatal to children. Half of all that are born in London die under three, and in Manchester under five years of age; whereas at Royton, a manufacturing township in the neighbourhood of Manchester, the number of children dying under the age

---

[55] François Boissier de Sauvages, "Livre de Maison," Archives départementales de l'Hérault, 10 F51, p. 169. Antoine Déparcieux, *Essai sur les probabilités de la durée de la vie humaine* (Paris, 1746). Boissier de Sauvages's math is incorrect in this table; the total for "vie moyenne" should be 249 years, 6 months.
[56] Short, *New Observations*, pp. 195–196.

TABLE FIFTEENTH.

For 15 Years, *viz.* from *January* 1, 1728, to *January* 1, 1743, being monthly; and begins with *January*, and ends with *December*.

Died under 2 Years old.	From 2 to 5	From 5 to 10	From 10 to 20	From 20 to 30	From 30 to 40	From 40 to 50	From 50 to 60	From 60 to 70	From 70 to 80	From 80 to 90	From 90 to 100	From 100 and upwards, Totals.
12593	2678	1306	1232	3021	3576	3730	3480	2625	1988	1203	250	37682
12550	2918	1275	1139	2852	3125	3409	3086	2508	1997	1072	226	36157
12681	3254	1267	1039	2905	3423	3450	3823	2281	1855	1002	146	37126
12731	3184	1168	1021	2728	3247	3088	2549	2107	1496	775	148	34242
12268	3194	1269	1004	2494	2991	3046	2628	2174	1427	768	147	34410
11363	3073	1239	1048	2353	2597	2803	2164	1726	1129	595	107	30197
10063	2889	1195	952	2261	2748	2622	2259	1558	1021	528	114	28210
12684	2897	1170	926	2241	2426	2755	2543	1555	1049	481	102	30829
13563	3101	1168	1081	2401	2933	2850	2558	1787	1212	617	104	33375
13832	3067	1190	1080	2344	3215	3125	2372	2030	1439	786	108	34590
12010	2867	1169	1097	2685	3378	3255	2924	2313	1511	850	122	34181
12319	3055	1297	1136	2617	3416	3609	3090	2504	1876	846	187	35952
148657	36179	14713	12755	30902	37075	37742	33476	25168	18000	9523	1761	40595

The Number of those of all Ages that died yearly for the last 15 Years, taken at a Medium.

9910	2411	980	851	2060	2471	2516	2231	1677	1200	634	117	27058

Of which died in 100 taken at a Medium.

$36\frac{6}{10}$	9	$3\frac{6}{10}$	$3\frac{2}{10}$	$7\frac{6}{10}$	$9\frac{1}{10}$	$9\frac{3}{10}$	$8\frac{2}{10}$	$6\frac{2}{10}$	$4\frac{4}{10}$	$2\frac{4}{10}$	$\frac{4}{10}$	100

The Ages of every 100 that died in *Graunt's* Time, taken at a Medium. P. 84.

Under 6	6 to 16	16 to 26	26 to 36	36 to 46	46 to 56	56 to 66	66 to 76	76 to 86	Total
36	24	15	9	6	4	3	2	1	100

6.11 Thomas Short's life table from the London bills (1728–1743). *Source:* Thomas Short, *New Observations, Natural, Moral, Civil, Political, and Medical on City, Town and Country Bills of Mortality* (London, 1750), p. 192. Yale University, Harvey Cushing/John Hay Whitney Medical Library.

of three years, is to the number of children born only as one to seven; and at Eastham, a parish in Cheshire, inhabited by farmers, the proportion is considerably less.[57]

Percival attributed the high level of child mortality in Manchester to manufacturing: "It is a common but injurious practice in manufacturing countries, to confine children, before they have attained a sufficient degree of strength, to sedentary employments, in places where they breathe a putrid air, and are debarred the free use of their limbs." Percival subtly denounced child labor, commenting that people generally "spare their horses and cattle, till they arrive at a due size and vigour," and that a similar treatment of children might be in order.[58]

One of the correspondents of the Société Royale de Médecine in Paris, Associé Regnicole Raymond, submitted a topography for Marseilles that included figures of infant and child mortality that were startlingly high, confirming the general view that cities were deadly to infants. According to his figures, 10 of 18 children born died before age six.[59]

Even though most people viewed cities as unhealthy, there were some who thought the conditions were improving. Heberden, who had attributed the decline in dysentery to improved sanitation, summarized the London bills for the entire eighteenth century and found that the number of infant deaths (under age two) had decreased steadily since 1728, when ages were first reported in the bills. Part of the decline he attributed to the 1767 Act of Parliament, which required all London parish infants to be nursed in the countryside until age six. In effect, many infant deaths that would have been recorded in London were now recorded in country parishes. Heberden hoped "that as this decrease began to take place before the date of the act in question, so its continuance since may in part be with justice attributed to the greater salubrity of the town."[60]

Medical arithmeticians also paid close attention to mortality in the prime of life. Haygarth, with the help of physicians and parish clerks in Chester, constructed a table for the year 1772 with deaths by age and disease. (See Figure 6.12.) The table revealed clearly the high number of deaths attributed to consumption. "It is a matter of astonishment," Haygarth observed, "that, between the ages of 10 and 50, more people die of consumptions, than of all other diseases." Because the years between age 10 and age 50 were the most productive in an individual's life, Haygarth asserted, "it becomes therefore an enquiry, of the most striking consequence to society, to discover the cause, in order to prevent the fatality, of a disease, which make such dreadful havock among mankind."[61]

[57] Thomas Percival, "Observations on the State of Population in Manchester, and Other Adjacent Places, Concluded," *Philosophical Transactions* 65 (1775): 324–325.
[58] Percival, "Observations... Concluded," p. 325.
[59] Raymond, "Sur la topographie médicale de Marseille & de son territoire, & sur celle des lieux voisins de cette ville," *Histoire de la Société Royale de Médecine,* 1777–1778 (Paris, 1780), pp. 66–67.
[60] Heberden, *Observations on the Increase and Decrease of Different Diseases,* p. 33.
[61] Haygarth, "Observations... for the Year 1772," pp. 72–73.

TABLE II.   DISEASES.   [To be placed facing p. 56.]

DISEASES. I. FEBRILE DISEASES.	Under 1 Year	Betw. 1 & 2	2-3	3-5	5-10	10-15	15-20	20-30	30-40	40-50	50-60	60-70	70-80	80-90	90-100	Total
Fever (G. 5, 6.) —	3		1	1	2		2	1	3	3	1	4				21
Jail Fever (5.) —						1	1									2
Mortification (7.) —									1		1					2
Pleurify (12.) —					1											1
Inflam. of the Bowels (16.)									1							1
Gravel and Stone (19.) —											1					1
Rheumatic Fever (22) —						1										1
Teething (Sauv. 198.) —	2	1														3
Gout (23) —											1					1
St. Anthony's Fire (24.) —	1															1
Small Pox (26.) —	4	2	4	4	2											16
Measles (28.) —		2														2
Miliary Fever (29.) —								1								1
Consumption (35.) —	2	3	2		2	4	6	12	10	6	9	3	3			62
Hæmorrhage (37.) —							1		1							2
II. NERVOUS DISEASES.																
Apoplexy (40.) —							1		1	1	1	3	1			8
Palfy (41.) —									1	1	4	3				9
Swoon (42.) —						1	1									2
Indigestion (43.) —									1	1	1					3
Convulfions (48, 50.)	50	16	5	3		1				1						76
Afthma (52.) —									1	3	10	10	2			26
Chincough (53.) —	12	15	3	2	1											33
Colic (55.) —												1				1
Purging and Vomiting (56.)						1										1
Infanity (63.) —						1										1
III. DISEASES of the HABIT.																
Weaknefs of Infancy (65.)	3	9	3	2												17
Decay of Age (66.) —											2	5	22	17	4	50
Dropfy (71, 75.) —										3	4	2	1			10
Dropfy of the brain (72.)			1				1									2
Rickets (79.) —	3	2	1	1												7
King's Evil (80.) —					1		1									2
Jaundice (87.) —											1					1
IV. LOCAL DISEASES.																
Cancer (114.) —									1		1	1				3
Ulcer of the bladder (134.)										1						1
Unknown difeases —	1	1			1		1		1	1						6
Cafualties —							1		1	1						3
Total —	81	51	19	14	8	6	10	23	17	21	26	32	47	20	4	379

MORBORUM GENERA.
CLASSIS I. PYREXIÆ.
G. 5. 6. Typhus, Synochus.
G. 5. Typhus carcerum.
G. 7. Sphacelus.
G. 12. Pluritis.
G. 16. Enteritis.
G. 19. Nephritis.
G. 22. Rheumatifinus.
(Sauvag. G. 198. Odontalgia dentitionis.)
G. 23. Arthritis,
G. 24. Eryfipelas,
G. 26. Variola.

G. 28. Rubeola.
G. 29. Miliaria.
G. 35. Phthifis.
G. 37. Menorrhagia lochialis.
CLASSIS II. NEUROSES.
G. 40. Apoplexia.
G. 41. Paralyfis.
G. 42. Synchope (puerperalis.)
G. 43. Dyfpepfia.
G. 48. 50. Convulfio. Epilepfia.
G. 52. Afthma.
G. 53. Pertuffis.
G. 55. Colica.

G. 56. Cholera.
G. 63. Mania.
CLASSIS III. CACHEXIÆ.
G. 65. Tabes, atrophia infantilis.
G. 66. Atrophia, fenilis.
G. 71, 75. Afcites. Anafarca.
G. 72. Hydrocephalus.
G. 79. Rachitis.
G. 80. Schrophula.
G. 87. Icterus.
CLASSIS IV. LOCALES.
G. 114. Cancer.
G. 134. Ulcus (Sauv. G. 156. Pyuria.)

6.12 John Haygarth's table of deaths by disease for Chester (1772). *Source:* John Haygarth, "Observations on the Bills of Mortality in Chester, for the Year 1772," *Philosophical Transactions* 64 (1774), unnumbered fold-out table. Burndy Library, Dibner Institute for the History of Science and Technology.

Finally, tables that included age of death allowed arithmeticians to calculate the average life span of individuals for a specific geographical area. This became one of the most common measures of salubrity developed during the long eighteenth century. "It [the average life span] is the just measure of the salubrity of countries or of habitations," wrote the Société Royale de Médecine correspondent Raymond. "Combined with the fecundity of marriages, it is the basis and perspective of endemic science."[62]

His fellow countryman, Jean-Baptiste Moheau, agreed. Moheau surveyed numerous communities throughout France and created tables displaying information about the geography of a specific locale, the occupations of its inhabitants, and the average expected duration of life ("vie commune"). These tables facilitated comparisons along a number of axes. For example, mountainous regions certainly had longer average life spans than low-lying, marshy areas, but the variations within each category remained considerable nonetheless. In the table labeled "Habitations sur le sommet des montagnes," average life span ranged from 40 years 8 months in the town of Grand-Bois located on the west coast of France, to a miserable 16 years and 5 months in Seillons, a hamlet situated on rocky terrain with stagnant water. In fact, the mortality at Seillons almost surpassed that of all the maritime and marshy locales Moheau surveyed for the table entitled "Habitations dans les contrées marécageuses, maritimes." Only La Napoule, with the incredibly low average life span of 8 years, fared worse. (See Figures 6.13 and 6.14.) From these tables, Moheau concluded that inhabitants of hilly or mountainous regions enjoyed longer lives than did those who lived in marshy areas. Nothing surprising, but the tables provided a level of proof absent from many earlier discussions of health and geography: "If this table does not produce a complete proof, it is at least an excellent model for studies that can confirm or demolish inductions."[63]

Without information about age of death, medical arithmeticians had to develop other methods of measuring salubrity. Thomas Percival, for example, in his study of Manchester published in the *Philosophical Transactions,* used the proportion of the number of deaths to total population in a given year. Manchester and Liverpool, two early manufacturing towns, had experienced tremendous population growth in the latter part of the eighteenth century, and Percival tried to measure their salubrity by calculating the ratio of deaths to total population.[64] His figures indicated that 1 out of 56 died in country parishes outside of Manchester, and that 1 of 28 died in Manchester. "And it must afford matter of astonishment even to the physician and philosopher," Percival commented,

[62] Raymond, "Sur la topographie médicale de Marseille," p. 115.
[63] Moheau, *Recherches et considérations,* p. 163.
[64] Thomas Percival, "Observations on the State of Population in Manchester, and Other Adjacent Places," *Philosophical Transactions* 64 (1774): 54–66.

198   *Recherches & Confidérations*
Suite de la T A B L E I I.

SITUATION ET NATURE DU SOL, ET INDUSTRIE
DES HABITANS.

LIEUX.	*HABITATIONS fur le fommet des montagnes.*	VIE COMMUNE.	
		Ans.	*Mois.*
CABRIERS..	Sur un roc vers le Sud-Ouest, entouré de montagnes nues à l'Est. Terroir sec, peu fertile.	31	5
GRAND-BOIS.	Découvert, fur-tout du côté de l'Ouest. .	40	8
LE CASTELLET.	Sur un roc, vers le Sud, & quelque peu à l'Ouest. Terroir fertile en vin & en huile, à deux lieues au Nord-Nord-Ouest de Toulon. . .	29	
SEILLONS..	Sur un roc nu, un peu au Sud. Terroir labourable, eaux ftagnantes dans la plaine. Hameau très-pauvre.	16	5
SIX-FOURS.	Sur une montagne ifolée & prefqu'Ifle. Terroir sec.	34	3
VENELLES..	Aſſez élevé à une demi-lieue au Nord d'Aix.	36	

6.13 Jean-Baptiste Moheau's table of life expectancies for mountainous areas
(1778). *Source:* Jean-Baptiste Moheau, *Recherches et considérations sur la population de
la France* (Paris, 1778), p. 198. Yale University, Harvey Cushing/John Hay Whitney
Medical Library.

when he reflects that the inhabitants of both live in the same climate, carry on the same
manufactures, and are chiefly supplied with provisions from the same market. But his surprize
will give place to concern and regret, when he observes the havoc produced in every large
town by luxury, irregularity, and intemperance; the numbers that fall annual victims to
the contagious distempers, which never cease to prevail; and the pernicious influence of
confinement, uncleanliness, and foul air on the duration of life.[65]

[65] Percival, "Observations... Concluded," pp. 323–324.

fur la Population. **201**

Suite de la T a b l e I I.

S i t u a t i o n   e t   n a t u r e   d u . S o l , e t   i n d u s t r i e
d e s   H a b i t a n s.

LIEUX.	*H a b i t a t i o n s* dans des contrées marécageufes, maritimes.	VIE COMMUNE.	
		Ans.	*Mois.*
BERRE. . . .	Au fond & au Nord-Eft d'un grand étang mari-time.	2 5	2
Fos.	Près de la mer, & fur une colline entourée de marais de l'Eft à l'Oueft par le Sud.	17	3
FRÉJUS. . . .	Terroir marécageux, à une demi-lieue de la mer, ayant au Nord de hautes montagnes. . .	2 2	1
LA NAPOULE.	Sur une plage maré-cageufe.	8	
RAMATUELLE.	Sur la plage. . . .	19	7

LIEUX.	*H a b i t a t i o n s* dans des contrées marécageufes, méditerranées.	VIE COMMUNE.	
		Ans.	*Mois.*
CORBIERES.	Au Nord, & tout près de la Durance, découvert vers l'Eft, & dominé à l'Oueft par une colline.	17	6
JOUQUES. . .	Au Sud de la Durance, près des çanaux d'arro-fage.	20	7
PERROLES. .	Au Sud, & tout près de la Durance.	27	4
CUERS. . . .	A l'abri des vents du Nord, terroir complanté de vignes & d'orangers. Quelques eaux croupif-fantes.	2 1	

6.14 Jean-Baptiste Moheau's table of life expectancies for marshy areas (1778). *Source:* Jean-Baptiste Moheau, *Recherches et considérations sur la population de la France* (Paris, 1778), p. 201. Yale University, Harvey Cushing/John Hay Whitney Medical Library.

Once again, Percival's figures confirmed the insalubrious nature of urban living. Short also tried to calculate the salubrity of parishes outside of London, and he, too, had to develop other methods, for example, the ratio of the number of christenings to burials. In a table covering more than 160 country parishes throughout England in two different time periods, Short presented

		PERIOD Firſt.				PERIOD Second.		
Workſop	Nottingham	1538	1737	f. d. o.	31 to 20			o
Beely Chapple	Derby Peak	138		h. m. r.	10 5			o
Catthorp	Warwickſhire	1573	1640	d. g. o.	18 11	1644	1733 23 to 20	o
Stoke Damarel	Devon	1595	1640	cl. h. d. r.	35 28	1670	1739 22 13	f.
Churſtow	Devon	1543	1643	ne. rf. d.	82 49		75 22 19	o
Foxton	Leiceſter	1560	1640	wt. w. wy. c.	10 6	1653	1736 39 29	o
Slawſton	Leiceſter		50	h. o. d.	14 8	1649	1742 64 45	o
Medbourn, c. Holt	Leiceſter	1588	1634	l. d. h. d.	48 29	1635	1738 13 10	vf.
Stoke Hammond	Buckinghamſh.		106	d. o.	65 42	1649	1737 24 19	o
Wefton, c. Sutton	Northampton		69	cl.-f. cy.	56 31	1646	1736 37 27	o
Walcote	Norfolk	1558	1644	d. o.	55 33	1645	1742 39 32	o
Thribergh	York	1599	1647	l. o. d.	29 19	1648	1733 51 40	o
Wiſper	York	1574	1629	v. hy. d.	85 56	1629	1743 19 14	o
Eccington	Derby	1559	1640	v. d. g.	40 23	1645	1735 37 27	f.
N. Luffenham	Rutland	1573	1645	f. d. o.	83 45	1646	1742 95 78	f.
Hope	Derby Peak	1600	1642	v. ls. d. h.	28 19	1700	1734 27 22	f.
Bradfield	York	1559	1649	m. r. d. o.	43 29	1650	1733 23 19	f.
Kirkanſton	York	1578	1642	o.	6 4	1658	1733 5 4	o
Bacton	Norfolk	1558	1644	o. d. le.	53 33		1732 48 39	o
Mercet	Rutland		61	o. s. d.	59 38	1651	1742 40 35	o
Raunds	Northampton		30	o. d. le.	81 54	1646	1700 13 11	b
Darly	Derby Peak	1610	1644	m. ls. d.	77 54	1644	1735 29 22	o
Bolton on Dern	York	1619	1643	o. d. g.	35 22	1643	1737 11 9	o
Bamburrow	York	1561	1642	l. d.	65 43	1643	1732 37 33	o
Newton Farrers	Devon	1600	44	h. d. le.	77 54	1645	1738 93 77	o

Difference betwixt Births and Burials in both Periods, as 11 to 7½   as 8 to 6 $\frac{4}{10}$.

6.15 Thomas Short's table of salubrity. *Source:* Thomas Short, *New Observations, Natural, Moral, Civil, Political, and Medical on City, Town and Country Bills of Mortality* (London, 1750), p. 6. Yale University, Harvey Cushing/John Hay Whitney Medical Library.

topographical information: elevation (high or low), soil condition (sandy or claylike), and so on. (See Figure 6.15.) Short explained how to read his table:

Consists of two Periods separated by a double black Line. The Columns of each Table, after the first and second, are the same in both Periods. Column first, the Names of the Country Parishes or Villages, whose Registers are extracted in the following Table. Column second, the Names of the Counties in which they lie. Column third, the Number of Years for which we have the Register during the first Period, or preceding 1644–45 – or 46, &c. including both Years specified; except in either Period there was a Chasm in the Register, or it was neglected, or ill kept. In that Case we only take the Number of Years that may be depended upon. Column fourth, the Soil or Situation of each Parish, where observe h. stands for high, l. for low, d. for dry, o. for open. g. for Gravle, or gravelly; s. for Sand, or sandy; m. for mountainous, r. for rocky, ls. for Lime-stone, s. South, n. North, e. East, w. West, wt. wet, c. Sea-coast, rs. rich Soil, le. light Earth, Land, or Soil, wy. woody, oy. ouzy, sy. springy, or full of Springs; cy. Clay, or clayie; v. various Soils, e. enclosed, my. marshy, or fenny. Column fifth, the prime Proportion of Christenings to Burials, according to the two or three first Figures or Numbers only, without regard to the lesser or Fractions. Column sixth, the number of Years in the second Period; in both Periods the first Year in each, is the Year when our Abstract begins, the other the Year it ends with. Column seventh, the Proportions between the Baptisms and Buryings in that Time. Column eighth, in the second Period, shews in what Parishes there are Dissenters, and whether a few, several, many, or none at all, by the Letters f. s. m. o.[66]

In his discussion of this table, Short correlated topographical features with the ratio of christenings to burials. Thus, "A dry, open, elevated, gravely Soil, we see obtains the next place after the dry, rocky, and mountainous; some such in this Table have 154 Christenings to 98 Burials; and the dry, high, Gret-Stone, has 100 of the former to 63 of the latter."[67] Compare this to the unhealthy "Forest Registers, where the Christenings, even in the first period, exceed not 109 to 95 Burials, which is scarce one 8th Increase."[68] And predictably, "Low Habitations, especially on stiff Clay, rotten Earth, or near a Level with the Sea, great Rivers, Marshes, Lakes, or putrid standing Waters. These are the worst of all." Burials in these places, according to Short, either are equal to or greater than the number of christenings.[69]

Another table provided a more fine-grained analysis of the burials and christenings by dividing each category by sex and by including information about the number of marriages. Using this table, Short calculated several ratios to assess the salubrity and fertility of each parish. Indications of salubrity included: 1) fewer marriages to the number baptized; 2) greater disproportion between the number of males and females baptized (the more salubrious, the more males); 3) a lower rate of infant and child mortality; 4) a larger number of emigrants; 5) a higher number of children per marriage; and 6) a larger disproportion between christenings and burials.[70]

Seasonal, as well as geographical, considerations were also addressed by medical arithmeticians. (As indicated in Chapter 5, some of the work in medical meteorology, for example John Rutty's book, examined the effects of seasons as well as weather on mortality.) John Haygarth, using Cullen's nosology, constructed a table that "shews, at one view, what diseases were most fatal in each month."[71] Examining the table, one gets little sense of a pattern, which is perhaps why Haygarth gave no further comments on this table. (See Figure 6.16.)

William Heberden's table, by contrast, is much clearer. (See Figure 6.17.) He sought to link cause of death with the chronological variables of age and weekly as well as seasonal variation. His table indicated that mortality was greatest in the months of January, February, and March, and the lowest in June, July, and August. Heberden's comment on this observation was blunt and affirmed his assertion that tables would correct common false opinions: "I believe this is

---

[66] Short, *New Observations,* pp. 4–5.   [67] Short, *New Observations,* p. 17.
[68] Short, *New Observations,* p. 17.   [69] Short, *New Observations,* p. 19.
[70] Short, *New Observations,* p. 59.
[71] John Haygarth, "Bill of Mortality for Chester for the Year 1773," *Philosophical Transactions* 65 (1775): 87.

TABLE III.   Diseases of different Months.

DISEASES I. Febrile Diseases.	Jan.	Feb.	March	April	May	June	July	Aug.	Sept.	Oct.	Nov.	Dec.	Total
Fever (CULLEN'S GENERA 5,6.)	1	4	6	4		5	1	2		3	1	6	33
Imposthume (G. 7.)												1	1
Angina pectoris (G. 7.)					1								1
Mortification (G. 7.)		1		1		1	1			1	1	2	8
Quinsey (G. 10.)				1									1
Infl. of the bowels (G. 16.)				1	1	1					1		4
Gravel and stone (G. 19.)					1								1
Teething (Sauv. 198)	1					1							2
Small-pox (G. 26.)										1			1
Thrush (G. 33.)					1								1
Consumption (G. 35.)	5	11	8	6	10	5	5	3	1	1	8	10	73
Hæmorrhage (G. 37.)		1											1
II. NERVOUS DISEASES.													
Sudden death (G. 40.)						1		1		2		3	7
Palsy (G. 41.)	1	1	2	2							2		8
Swoon (G. 42.)			1										1
Indigestion (G. 43.)			1	2				1	1				5
Convulsions (G. 48, 50.)	8	7	3	11	6	7	4	6	3	2	3	9	69
Asthma (G. 52.)	2	3	5	2					2			2	16
Chinkcough (G. 53.)	4	3		1				1		1			10
Colic (G. 55.)		1									2		3
Loosenefs (G. 57.)											1		1
Infanity (G. 63.)			1	1	1								3
III. DISEASES of the HABIT.													
Weaknefs of infancy (G. 65.)		2	1	1	2	2	1			1		3	13
Decay of age (G. 66.)	3	10	7	8	8	5	2		3	4	6	6	62
Dropsy (G. 71, 75.)	2		1	1	2	1		2	1		2	1	13
Dropsy of the brain (G. 72)			1										1
Jaundice (G. 87.)									1	1			2
IV. LOCAL DISEASES.													
Cancer (G. 114.)	1									1			2
Unknown difeafes.					1						1		2
Cafualties.		1				3						3	7
Total,	28	45	37	42	33	33	14	16	12	18	27	47	352

6.16 John Haygarth's table of monthly mortalities by disease, following Cullen's nosology, for Chester (1775). *Source:* John Haygarth, "Bills of Mortality for Chester for the Year 1773," *Philosophical Transactions* 65 (1775): 90. Burndy Library, Dibner Institute for the History of Science and Technology.

	Under 2 Years.	From 2 to 5.	From 5 to 10.	From 10 to 20.	From 20 to 30.	From 30 to 40.	From 40 to 50.	From 50 to 60.	From 60 to 70.	From 70 to 80.	From 80 to 90.	90 and upwards.	TOTALS.
Jan. -	12,593	2,678	1,306	1,232	3,021	3,576	3,730	3,480	2,625	1,988	1,203	250	37,682
Feb. -	12,550	2,918	1,275	1,139	2,852	3,125	3,409	3,086	2,708	1,997	1,072	226	36,157
March	12,681	3,254	1,267	1,039	2,905	3,423	3,450	3,823	2,281	1,855	1,002	146	37,126
Apr. -	12,731	3,184	1,168	1,021	2,728	3,247	3,088	2,549	2,107	1,496	775	148	34,242
May -	12,268	3,194	1,269	1,004	2,494	3,991	3,046	2,628	2,174	1,427	768	147	33,410
June -	11,363	3,073	1,239	1,048	2,353	2,597	2,803	2,164	1,726	1,129	595	107	30,197
July -	10,063	2,889	1,195	952	2,261	2,748	2,622	2,259	1,558	1,021	528	114	28,210
Aug. -	12,684	2,897	1,170	926	2,241	2,426	2,755	2,543	1,555	1,049	481	102	30,829
Sept. -	13,563	3,101	1,168	1,081	2,401	2,933	2,850	2,558	1,787	1,212	617	104	33,375
Oct. -	13,832	3,069	1,190	1,080	2,344	3,215	3,125	2,372	2,030	1,439	786	108	34,590
Nov. -	12,010	2,867	1,169	1,097	2,685	3,378	3,255	2,924	2,313	1,511	850	122	34,181
Dec. -	12,319	3,055	1,297	1,136	2,617	3,416	3,609	3,090	2,504	1,876	846	187	35,952
Total -	148,657	36,179	14,713	12,755	30,902	37,075	37,742	33,476	25,168	18,000	9,523	1,761	405,951

6.17 William Heberden's table of monthly mortalities listed by age from the London bills. *Source: William Heberden, Observations on the Increase and Decrease of Different Diseases . . .* (London, 1801), p. 47. Yale University, Harvey Cushing/John Hay Whitney Medical Library.

234 *Recherches & Confidérations*

TABLE II. *Queſt.* 8. *Chap.* 11.

Mois Climatériques ſuivant les âges.

MOIS.	Juſques & compris 15 ans.		De 15 à 60.		Au deſſus de 60.	
	ISLE DE RÉ, 8 Par.	FRANCE 8 Par.	ISLE DE RÉ, 8 Par.	FRANCE, 8 Par.	ISLE DE RÉ, 8 Par.	FRANCE, 8 Par.
JANVIER. .	321	287	94	·176	129	108
FEVRIER...	293	280	92	142	90	83
MARS....	278	325	103	174	92	103
AVRIL....	239	290	99	212	104	106
MAI.....	212	267	95	170	82	88
JUIN.....	221	293	90	168	76	60
JUILLET...	194	306	70	98	65	49
AOUST. . .	363	341	89	120	59	44
SEPTEMBRE.	567	441	106	134	71	78
OCTOBRE..	542	392	121	174	110	78
NOVEMBRE.	429	273	99	163	82	78
DÉCEMBRE.	307	253	97	149	118	87
TOTAL.	3966	3748	1155	1880	1078	962

6.18 Jean-Baptiste Moheau's table of monthly mortalities listed by age (1778).
Source: Jean-Baptiste Moheau, *Recherches et considérations sur la population de la France* (Paris, 1778), p. 234. Yale University, Harvey Cushing/John Hay Whitney Medical Library.

contrary to the received opinion, which may perhaps have been handed down from those ages, when the authority of Hippocrates, and Galen, superseded the evidence of the clearest facts."[72]

[72] Heberden, *Observations on the Increase and Decrease of Different Diseases,* p. 46.

Likewise, Moheau asserted that it was necessary to know which months were more deadly so that individuals could be more cautious in health matters and so that employers could assign less laborious tasks. Moheau's table showed that in France, the months of September and October were the most deadly, that of July, the least. (See Figure 6.18.) For those under the age of 15, the beginning of autumn was the most dangerous, while for adults, winter and the beginning of spring held the most perils.[73]

In their analyses of age, season, and place of death, medical arithmeticians utilized quantification and tables to investigate salubrity. What emerged from their studies was a sense that mortality was highly variable and that death depended on a great variety of factors. Still, there were identifiable and consistent patterns: The countryside was more healthy than the city; infants and children experienced high rates of mortality everywhere. These facts may have been known before, but with numbers, arithmeticians could now measure the changes in established patterns over time and perhaps influence those changes for the better.

VARIATIONS IN MORTALITY BETWEEN THE SEXES

Numerical differences between the sexes had been a long-standing concern of political and medical arithmeticians. In the seventeenth century, attention focused on births. In his analysis of the London bills of mortality, Graunt had calculated that there were 14 boys christened for every 13 girls. He observed that even though more men than women died by violence, there still would be a husband for every woman; hence, he concluded, polygamy was unnecessary, unnatural, and ungodly. When John Arbuthnot revisited the subject in the early eighteenth century, his analysis of 82 years of the London bills of mortality revealed a different ratio for male to female christenings: 13 to 12 (see Chapters 1 and 2). The constancy of this ratio, Arbuthnot argued, was a sign of divine providence, an idea taken up and popularized by Reverend William Derham in his Boyle lectures of 1711 and 1712, later published under the title *Physico-Theology*.[74]

By the mid–eighteenth century, medical arithmeticians had begun to shift their focus away from christenings and toward burials. In comparing mortality figures for men and women at different ages, they discovered that life was more deadly to men than to women. Thomas Short, for example, found that males

run greater Hazard of Abortion between their Conception and Birth, are in more Peril at their Birth, seeing there are 10 still-born and chrysom Males, to 7 Females; they run greater Danger in Childhood, seeing 62 Boys die to 53 Girls; in greater Danger in Celibacy, for 12 Boys to 11 Girls, die; in more Peril in a Marriage State, seeing above 15 married Men die for 10 married Women: All which Dangers are increased by living in Cities or great Towns.

---

[73] Moheau, *Recherches et considérations*, p. 177.   [74] William Derham, *Physico-Theology* (London, 1713).

172   *Medical Arithmetic and Environmental Medicine*

TABLE I.   DEATHS.

Ages	Males.	Females.	Ages.	Batchelors	Husbands	Widowers	Maids.	Wives.	Widows.	Total.
Under : Month, —	8	6	20-25.	2	1		6	2		11
Between 1-2 Months	3	2	25-30.	1			5	5	1	12
2-3	6	5	30-35.	2	2		2	3	1	10
3-6	5	13	35-40.		1		2	2	2	7
6-9	5	8	40-45.	1	2		2	3		8
9 Months and 1 Year	7	13	45-50.	2	4	1	1	4	1	13
1-2 Years old	22	29	50-60.		13	2	4	3	4	26
2-3	6	13	60-70.	1	7	2	3	11	8	32
3-4	2	3	70-80.	3	11	7	4	4	18	47
4-5	6	3	80-90.		2		4		14	20
5-10	5	3	90-100						4	4
10-15	4	2								
15-20	2	8								
Total of the above Ages	81	108	Total of each Condition.	12	43	12	33	37	53	190

108
81
Total 379

6.19 John Haygarth's mortality table by age, sex, and marital status (1774). *Source:* John Haygarth, "Observations on the Bills of Mortality in Chester, for the Year 1772," *Philosophical Transactions* 64 (1774): 76. Burndy Library, Dibner Institute for the History of Science and Technology.

With such an overwhelming catalog, Short could not but reach the very same conclusion that Graunt and Arbuthnot had: "Seeing the Dangers of Males, *in & extra uterum,* are so much greater than that of Females, then Polygamy is a most ridiculous, monstrous Custom."[75]

Short's denunciation of polygamy was anomalous by the mid–eighteenth century. After 1750, physicians concerned themselves less with arguments about design and the relations between the sexes and more with the greater levels of mortality experienced by men than by women. "It is a matter of curiosity, to observe how much longer women live than men," John Haygarth wrote in his observations on the bills of mortality of Chester for 1772. "This fact is well established," he continued, "by former observations on this subject, and is confirmed by the following register."[76] (Figure 6.19.)

While Haygarth accepted this difference between the sexes as "a fact," others saw it as an observation in need of explanation. John Howlett, for one, argued that men *should* live longer because their constitutions were "more firm and

[75] Short, *New Observations,* pp. 72–73.   [76] Haygarth, "Observations . . . for the Year 1772," p. 71.

robust." Yet all evidence pointed to the contrary. Howlett admitted that some men were exposed to greater dangers than women (for example soldiers, sailors, fishermen, and colliers), but the numbers were not large enough to explain the discrepancy fully.[77] In the end, Howlett resorted to moral reasons:

There is one cause still behind universally allowed to operate, and which alone, perhaps is fully adequate to the effect. Men are in general especially in large and populous towns, more intemperate than women, both in eating and drinking, and are likewise more commonly chargeable with every other irregularity and licentiousness of conduct. To these therefore may their greater mortality be most frequently imputed; and thus this singular circumstance of register evidence becomes a serious topic of moral admonition.[78]

While women generally fared better throughout life than men, childbirth provided one widely recognized risk borne solely by women. La Condamine had argued that the chances of dying from inoculation were substantially less than those of childbirth, giving the figure that 1 in 60 women died in childbirth. During the last decades of the eighteenth century, several physicians constructed accounts of the risks of childbirth using records from various hospitals and lying-in homes. Perhaps the most sobering were those presented by Jacques Tenon in his *Mémoires sur les hôpitaux de Paris*. After summarizing various accounts from British lying-in hospitals where the proportion of women dying in childbirth ranged from 1 in 51 1/9 to 1 in 131, he reported the figure from the Paris Hôtel-Dieu: 1 in 15 2/3. "Such a serious assertion needs to be supported by facts," Tenon admitted. "As proof, we offer the following table provided by a gentleman, both knowledgeable and dedicated, who volunteered to extract the figures personally from the registers of the Hôtel-Dieu."[79] (See Figure 6.20.) The table provided information not only about maternal mortality but also about stillbirths and seasonal variations. "It is a matter of serious concern that, in no region of Europe, in no town, no village, nor hospital, is the loss as high as among women in childbed at the Paris Hôtel-Dieu," Tenon concluded. "The knowledge of a skillful and vigilant midwife who looks after these women is no match for the insalubrity of this institution."[80] His proposals to improve this horrendous situation were simple: one woman per bed (typically, three women shared a bed four feet wide), separation of healthy from ill women (especially those with fevers), and prevention of "evil-smelling and contagious miasmas."[81]

Classificatory systems of mortality were critical to contemporary recognition of changing disease patterns, and they became increasingly complex in a process of continual iteration. Early tables classifying death suggested certain relationships,

[77] John Howlett, "Observations on the Increased Population, Healthiness, Etc. of Maidstone," ([Maidstone], 1782), p. 16; reprinted in Glass, *The Development of Population Statistics*.
[78] Howlett, *Observations*, p. 17.
[79] Jacques Tenon, *Memoirs on Paris Hospitals*, trans. with an Introduction, Notes, and Appendices by Dora B. Weiner (1788; Science History Publications, 1996), p. 226.
[80] Tenon, *Memoirs on Paris Hospitals*, p. 232.   [81] Tenon, *Memoirs on Paris Hospitals*, p. 232.

ANNÉE 1776.	Enfans nés.	Enfans morts nés.	Accouchées mortes.
Janvier	141.	18.	8.
Février	168.	9.	3.
Mars.............	132.	9.	2.
Avril	146.	8.	9.
Mai...............	140.	12.	2.
Juin	101.	5.	1.
Juillet.	124,	9.	8.
Août	108.	8.	7.
Septembre	96.	14.	0.
Octobre..........	125.	9.	0.
Novembre.........	123.	7.	1.
Décembre	130.	13.	10.
	1534.	121.	51.

ANNÉE 1777.	Enfans nés.	Enfans morts nés.	Accouchées mortes.
Janvier.	147.	8.	5.
Février	135.	7.	4.
Mars	150.	9.	5.
Avril............	167.	11.	2.
Mai	147.	6.	6.
Juin	129.	10.	6.
Juillet.	115.	7.	8.
Août	108.	9.	2.
Septembre	114.	10.	15.
Octobre..........	118.	18.	9.
Novembre.........	103.	10.	31.
Décembre	120.	9.	39.
	1549.	114.	132.

6.20 Jacques Tenon's table of maternal mortality in Paris (1788). *Source:* Jacques Tenon, *Mémoires sur les hôpitaux de Paris* (Paris, 1788), p. 261. Yale University, Harvey Cushing/John Hay Whitney Medical Library.

which then were investigated by more detailed accounts. Tables that initially listed only cause of death became further refined by including considerations of age, sex, geographical location, and time of year. Classifications of mortality enabled researchers to identify differences, which then required explanations. By the end of the eighteenth century, writers demonstrated in their accounts that mortality patterns had changed, and that human actions were in part responsible for these changes. Tables, thus, brought order and understanding and the suggestion of control to the experience of death and reflected a certain optimism about forestalling it. "Faithful and minute registers of mortality, and of the various diseases most fatal to mankind, at different ages," Haygarth noted, "must evidently be of the most important consequence, to the politician, the philosopher, and the physician, in their several endeavours to relieve the miseries, and promote the happiness of human nature."[82]

[82] Haygarth, "Observations . . . for the Year 1772," p. 67.

PART THREE

Political Arithmetic

7

Count, Measure, Compare:
The Depopulation Debates

In his brilliantly satirical *Lettres persanes* (1721), the French philosophe Charles Louis de Secondat, Baron de Montesquieu (1689–1755) asked somewhat seriously whether the modern world was less populated than the ancient world and answered a resounding yes. "After a calculation as exact as may be in the circumstances," he asserted without providing any evidence of such calculations, "I have found that there are upon the earth hardly one-tenth part of the people which there were in ancient times. And the astonishing thing is, that the depopulation goes on daily: if it continues, in ten centuries the earth will be a desert."[1] Montesquieu not only saw the world's population as declining, but even more fundamentally, regarded it as changing. Population had a history as well as a future.

In mercantilist writings, population had generally been treated as a static or finite entity, and questions focused on geographical comparison: Was London larger than Paris? Was Holland more densely populated than England? By contrast, Montesquieu focused attention on temporal comparison and the dynamics of population – what the French called the movement of population. His dire prediction for a dramatic decline in population was regarded by contemporaries with alarm and propelled the subject of depopulation into the realm of public controversy throughout Europe.[2]

---

[1] Montesquieu, Charles de Secondat, Baron de, *Lettres persanes,* trans. John Davidson (London: George Routledge & Sons [1721]), Letter CXII. D.V. Glass discusses the depopulation controversy in Britain in *Numbering the People: The Eighteenth-Century Population Controversy and the Development of Census and Vital Statistics in Britain* (London and New York: Gordon & Cremonesi, 1973), pp. 21–26.

[2] For a general overview of the place of population in eighteenth-century discourse, see Sylvana Tomaselli, "Moral Philosophy and Population Questions in Eighteenth Century Europe," *Population and Resources in Western Intellectual Traditions,* ed. Michael S. Teitelbaum and Jay M. Winter, supplement to *Population and Development Review,* vol. 14 (Cambridge: Cambridge University Press, 1989), pp. 7–29; Joshua Cole, *The Power of Large Numbers: Population, Politics, and Gender in Nineteenth-Century France* (Ithaca and London: Cornell University Press, 2000), chap. 1, pp. 21–54; and Hervé Hasquin, "Le débat sur la dépopulation dans l'Europe des lumières," in M. Moheau, *Recherches et considérations sur la population de la France (1778),* reedition annotated by Eric Vilquin (Paris: Institut National d'Études Démographiques, Presses Universitaires de France, 1994) pp. 397–424.

By midcentury, works such as the political economist Victor Riqueti, Marquis de Mirabeau's *L'Ami des hommes ou traité de la population* had widely popularized the idea of depopulation.[3] "In 1756, the book of *L'Ami des hommes* appeared," commented one critic in 1788, "and nearly everyone believed in the depopulation of France based on the words of the author."[4] For Mirabeau, deserted villages and emptied countryside provided visible evidence of depopulation, and all that seemingly remained subject to debate were the causes and consequences of this decline. He explored a variety of contributing factors and concluded that the blame lay in a "decline of agriculture on the one hand, and on the other hand, luxury and too much consumption by a small number of inhabitants." He dismissed clerical celibacy, emigration to the New World, and war, while maintaining that "the measure of subsistence is that of the population." In other words, agriculture was key: "People multiply like rats in a barn if they have the means to subsist."[5]

Mirabeau's emphases on the decline of agriculture and the rise of luxury were shared by many. Luxury in particular was widely condemned as corrosive to fertility. In Britain, the most popular exposition of its ill effects, Reverend John Brown's *An Estimate of the Manners and Principles of the Times* (1757), went through three editions its first year.[6] Commerce, according to Brown, "brings in Superfluity and vast Wealth; begets Avarice, gross Luxury, or effeminate Refinement among the higher Ranks, together with general Loss of Principle." Fewer wealthy marry because of an indulgence in "Vanity and Effeminacy." And among the urban "lower ranks," luxury brought impotency through "Intemperance and Disease."[7] Brown, unlike his French counterparts, provided some empirical evidence of depopulation from country parish registers that showed no increase in population from 1710 until midcentury. But in general, his target was luxury, and depopulation served mainly as evidence of its corrosive nature.

Besides luxury, British commentators pointed to the rise of manufacturing as a cause of depopulation. Robert Wallace, moderator of the General Assembly of the Church of Scotland, anonymously published *A Dissertation on the Numbers of Mankind in Ancient and Modern Times in Which the Superior Populousness*

---

[3] Victor de Riqueti, Marquis de Mirabeau, *L'Ami des hommes ou traité de la population*, 2 vols. (Darmstadt: Scientia Verlag Aalen, 1970 [Avignon, 1758–1760]), p. 11.

[4] Louis Messance, *Nouvelles recherches sur la population de la France* (1788); cited in Jacques and Michel Dupâquier, *Histoire de la démographie* (Paris: Perrin, 1985), p. 178. Many other works addressing depopulation in the 1760s and 1770s were also qualitative. In 1767, for instance, the Abbé Pierre Jaubert provided a lengthy account of the causes of depopulation (corruption of morals, war, emigration), and the means to remedy these problems. But he made only one reference to a census: one ordered by the Parlement of Bordeaux *to be* taken. [P. Jaubert], *Des causes de la dépopulation et des moyens d'y remédier* (Londres & Paris, 1767), p. 5.

[5] Mirabeau, *L'Ami des hommes*, pp. 12, 16.

[6] On the reception of Brown's *Estimate*, see James Bonar, *Theories of Population from Raleigh to Arthur Young*, p. 183; cited in Glass, *Numbering the People*, p. 40.

[7] D.V. Glass, *Numbering the People*, p. 26; citing Brown, Vol. 1, p. 153.

of Antiquity is Maintained in 1753. While he did not agree with some of Montesquieu's more grandiose claims about population during antiquity, Wallace did believe that employment in manufacturing tended to reduce population, and hence, contemporary populations might be less than in former times. The philosopher David Hume also challenged Montesquieu's views of antiquity and reasoned that war, manners, and less-developed trade and manufacturing operated as checks to the growth of the ancient population.[8] Nonetheless, Hume conceded that perhaps antiquity had been more populous because of the absence of certain deadly diseases. Ancient Greece and Rome had been plagued with disease, but on comparison, Hume decided "the disadvantage is much on the side of the moderns." The absence of smallpox alone might account for greater population in antiquity. "The tenth or the twelfth part of mankind, destroyed every generation [by smallpox], should make a vast difference, it may be thought, in the numbers of the people," Hume concluded; "and when joined to venereal distempers, a new plague diffused everywhere, this disease is perhaps equivalent, by its constant operation, to the three great scourges of mankind, war, pestilence, and famine."[9] Wallace, likewise, regarded smallpox as critical and explicitly cited James Jurin's figures on smallpox mortality as evidence of a recent natural cause of depopulation.[10]

In addition to its close association with disease, luxury, and poor agriculture, depopulation was also seen as a symptom of other more serious ills. Montesquieu argued precisely this in his *Esprit des lois* (1748), in which he studied the effect of government on population. Republics, he argued, were the most densely populated countries, whereas despotic governments brought desolation.[11] Again, he did not present any quantitative evidence for these claims, but his opinions were once more highly influential; depopulation became an accepted sign of despotism.[12] Numerous philosophes were quick to embrace this view, thereby ensuring the debate on depopulation a prominent role in discussions about the goodness of government during the 1750s and 1760s.[13]

Most prominently, Jean-Jacques Rousseau invoked Montesquieu's argument in his chapter "The Signs of a Good Government" in *The Social Contract* (1762). Rousseau stated unequivocally that the number of people was the best measure

---

[8] David Hume, "Of the Populousness of Ancient Nations," in *Essays: Moral, Political and Literary (1741–1742)*, in T.H. Green and T.H. Grouse, eds., *The Philosophical Works of David Hume*, 4 vols., Vol. 3 (London: Longmans, Green and Co., 1874), pp. 381–443.

[9] Hume, "Of the Populousness of Ancient Nations," pp. 382–383.

[10] Robert Wallace, *A Dissertation on the Numbers of Mankind, in Ancient and Modern Times in Which the Superior Populousness of Antiquity is Maintained*, 2d ed (Edinburgh, 1809) [1st ed., 1753], pp. 83–84.

[11] See Montesquieu, *Esprit des lois* (1748), Book XXIII.

[12] One historian has noted that Montesquieu's "conclusions themselves, for the most part, were contradicted by facts. . . . In spite of this affirmation it appears that in treating the question of population, he shared in many respects the prejudices of his contemporaries [that France was depopulated]." Antonin Puvilland, *Les doctrines de la population en France au XVIIIe siècle – De 1695 à 1776* (Lyon, 1912), p. 76.

[13] J.C. Perrot, "Les économistes, les philosophes, et la population," in *Histoire de la population française*, ed. Jacques Dupâquier (Paris: Presses Universitaires de France, 1988), vol. 2, p. 517.

of the quality of government, and the greater the population, the better the state:

> What is the object of any political association? It is the protection and the prosperity of its members. And what is the surest evidence that they are so protected and prosperous? The numbers of their population. Then do not look beyond this much debated evidence. All other things being equal, the government under which, without external aids like naturalization and immigration, the citizens increase and multiply most, is infallibly the best government. That under which the people diminishes and wastes away is the worst. Calculators, this is your problem: count, measure, compare.[14]

Rousseau's injunction to "count, measure, compare" marks a significant departure in the depopulation debates. Numerous causes and symptoms of depopulation had been mooted, ranging from war, disease, and emigration to changing forms of government, the increase in luxury, and the rise of manufacturing. But the very fact of depopulation had never before been questioned. Now, attention focused on counting.

In their efforts to determine the number of people, political arithmeticians developed techniques similar to those used by the medical arithmeticians: a reliance on parish registers for figures of births, deaths, and marriages; correspondence networks to collect local figures; the use of preprinted forms to encourage standardization of accounts; and the calculation of various ratios to represent aspects of different populations. A comparison of the depopulation controversies in England and France can shed new light on the different styles of political arithmetic.

COUNTING THE PEOPLE: CENSUSES AND VITAL REGISTRATION

The oldest (and perhaps the most obvious) way to ascertain the population was to count it, and in practice, that required some agency of government – national, provincial, municipal – to do the counting. The most common reason for a government to count was taxation. The very word itself, *census* in English, *cens* in French, derives from the Latin *censere* – to assess – from the Roman practice of enrolling persons and their property for taxation. Throughout the seventeenth and eighteenth centuries, British and French government censuses, although advocated, were rarely carried out successfully. One reason was popular opposition – censuses usually preceded new forms of taxation. Another obstacle was religious. Critics often mobilized biblical injunctions against enumeration. In the Old Testament, 70,000 perished because King David counted the people

---

[14] Jean-Jacques Rousseau, *The Social Contract*, trans. Maurice Cranston (New York: Penguin Books, 1982 [1762]), p. 130. I have changed one word of Cranston's translation: He translated *calculateurs* as "statisticians"; I have inserted the less anachronistic word calculators.

of Israel.[15] This fear of retribution from God or government was very real during the seventeenth and eighteenth centuries.[16]

Censuses were not the only sources of numbers. Since the sixteenth century, English and French parish clergy had been required to keep registers of vital events. These registers were not quantitative; instead, they were lists of names, along with the particular vital event (baptism, burial, or marriage). The primary purpose of vital registration was for legal questions regarding inheritance and kinship. However, over the long eighteenth century, political and medical arithmeticians began mining the registers in novel and interesting ways. In the case of population, the number of baptisms or burials for each parish could be tallied from the registers, and these figures could be used to calculate population by means of a universal multiplier (a figure that represented the proportion of births, or burials, to a total population). During the second half of the eighteenth century, political arithmeticians seized upon the multiplier method, in large part because censuses remained politically impossible. By the end of the century, however, some were arguing that this method of calculating population was, in fact, more accurate than a census could ever be.

Britain

In 1538, Thomas Cromwell, Lord Chancellor to Henry VIII, issued an injunction requiring the Anglican clergy of every parish to keep registers of all the baptisms, weddings, and funerals they oversaw. While these registers were used to establish one's age or one's parents, especially in questions of inheritance, they were ecclesiastical and not statutory records. During the reign of Queen Elizabeth, a 1597 decree directed parish clergy to send copies of the registers to the diocesan registrar every year in order to provide insurance against loss or corruption of the original registers. Taken together, these royal statutes provided the basis for vital registration in England until the nineteenth century. Numerous problems, however, cropped up with this arrangement. Some clergy complied, but not all. Most significantly, the growth of nonconformist religions meant that the births, marriages, and deaths of a significant part of the population were not recorded in the Anglican registers.

Such omissions in the registers eventually led to proposals to reform them. As we have seen, William Petty, in the late seventeenth century, outlined improvements to vital registration, as well as the establishment of a nationwide census. But little was done in these matters until the mid–eighteenth century, when Henry Pelham succeeded Robert Walpole as prime minister. Pelham (prime minister from 1746 until his death in 1754) instituted a variety of reforms,

---

[15] See 2 Samuel 24 and 1 Chronicles 21.
[16] Patricia Cline Cohen, "Death and Taxes: The Domain of Numbers in Eighteenth Century Popular Culture," in Stephen Cutcliffe, ed., *Science and Technology in the Eighteenth Century* (n.p., n.d.), pp. 51–53.

including a new calendar (the Gregorian calendar, used in most of continental Europe), a new marriage act, and an effective gin law.[17]

In 1752, John Fielding put forth *A Plan of the Universal Register Office*, and the following year a bill was proposed in Parliament for establishing a national census on the grounds that it would "be of publick Utility."[18] The bill specified procedures to be carried out by the overseers of the poor and the parish clergy, who were, respectively, to number the people and to register vital events. It provided sample forms, but individual parishes would be saddled with the costs of producing these forms. Accuracy of the clerical registers was to be ensured by comparing the Register Book with individual notices written by the parish minister for each vital event (birth, marriage, death); this was to be done by "audibly read[ing] over" the two sets of documents.[19] In addition, the bill affirmed the work of the Company of Parish Clerks in compiling the London bills of mortality, but required a new form. The Company also was enjoined to set the price of the weekly bill at not more than one penny, and the yearly bill at one shilling.[20]

Two new forms were introduced in the 1753 parliamentary bill. The census form distinguished between sexes and among three age groups (under 20, between 20 and 60, over 60). It asked for the number of poor (again distinguished by sex) receiving alms. The form required that the overseers enter the number for each category expressed in figures and in words (e.g., 84 and eighty-four), again reflecting Parliament's concern with accuracy. The vital registration form was designed to facilitate the recording of information, but abstracting or generalizing cumulative totals was difficult. It was arranged chronologically, not by vital event, and included a column for cause of death.

The parish minister was requested to prepare a yearly summary of the causes of death, and a new bill of mortality was proposed as part of the parliamentary bill. It had certain features that distinguished it from Graunt's Table of Casualties, most importantly, the inclusion of age of death as a column head. Entitled "An Abstract of the Marriages, Births, and Deaths, and also the Age, Sex, and Disease, of those who have died in the Parish of _____ in the County of _____ from the Twenty-fourth Day of June _____ to the Twenty-fourth Day of June_____ ," the new form emphasized comparison between different age groups, rather than across different years.[21] In this sample bill of mortality, the number of diseases

---

[17] W.A. Speck, *Stability and Strife: England, 1714–1760* (Cambridge, Mass.: Harvard University Press, 1977), pp. 254–257.

[18] John Fielding, *A Plan of the Universal Register Office* (London, 1752); "A Bill, with the Amendments, for Taking and Registering an Annual Account of the Total Number of People, and the Total Number of Marriages, Births, and Deaths; and Also the Total Number of Poor Receiving Alms from Every Parish, and Extraparochial Place, in Great Britain," reprinted in D.V. Glass, ed., *The Development of Population Statistics* (Farnborough, Hants, Eng.: Gregg International Publishers, 1973), p. 1.

[19] "A Bill for Taking and Registering an Annual Account of the Total Number of People," pp. 4–5.

[20] "A Bill for Taking and Registering an Annual Account of the Total Number of People," p. 12.

[21] This form is reproduced in Glass, *The Development of Population Statistics*.

and casualties listed was reduced from 81 to 40. Deaths resulting from causes other than disease were grouped together under the single head of "casualty," whereas in Graunt's table, multiple categories appeared, ranging from "found dead in the streets" to "Hanged, and made away themselves." According to the Quaker physician John Fothergill, several eminent physicians met to consider the list of diseases in the bills and "rejected all synonymous and obsolete terms, and proposed to give such an explanation of those that were retained, as might enable those whose duty it might become to make report, to do it with much more precision than it had been done hitherto."[22]

The parliamentary bill was defeated in large part because its opponents argued that a census would destroy an individual's liberty and place too much knowledge and power in the hands of government.[23] As one pamphlet writer complained, there could only be three uses for such knowledge about the British population: to decide whether to naturalize foreigners, to know how many men might be drafted for land or sea service, and to calculate how many "may be taken away for the plantations." The latter two purposes involved, to this author, the exercise of excessive government power and, thus, were contrary to the liberties of Englishmen.[24] Such sentiments were widely shared. When another bill for registering vital events was proposed five years later, it too was defeated.[25]

Despite the failure in Parliament of attempts to have the government collect vital accounts, many individuals continued to support the idea of a census and better vital registration, particularly those interested in annuities. Traditionally, annuities had provided a means of raising money for the Crown and were often used to finance war and other costly undertakings. Outside of government, interest in annuities began to grow in the seventeenth century because of their value and reliability as financial instruments for securing property across generations, an issue of increasing importance to the new commercial classes whose wealth did not lie in land. In exchange for an initial lump-sum payment, a person would receive an annual amount for the duration of his or her life. What is striking to modern eyes about pre–eighteenth-century annuities is that they were not based on the age of the annuitant. In other words, a 3-year-old and a 50-year-old could purchase the same annuity, even though the payout to

---

[22] John Fothergill, "Some Remarks on the Bills of Mortality in London; with an Account of a Late Attempt to Establish an Annual Bill for this Nation," in *Medical Observations and Inquiries,* vol. 4, p. 214; reprinted in Fothergill's *Works* (London, 1784), p. 294.

[23] For a discussion of this incident, see Peter Buck, "People Who Counted: Political Arithmetic in the Eighteenth Century," *Isis* 73 (1982): 28–45; and D.V. Glass, *Numbering the People,* pp. 11–40.

[24] [Anon.], *A Letter to a Member of Parliament, on the Registering and Numbering the People of Great Britain* (London: W. Owen, 1753), pp. 8–14; reprinted in D.V. Glass, *The Development of Population Statistics.*

[25] "A Bill for Obliging all Parishes in This Kingdom to Keep Proper Registers of Births, Deaths, and Marriages; and for Raising Therefrom a Fund towards the Support of the Hospital for the Maintenance and Education of Exposed and Deserted Young Children" (1758), reprinted in Glass, *The Development of Population Statistics.*

Age. Curt.	Per. fons.	Age. Curt.	Per. fons.	Age. Curt.	Per. fons.	Age. Curt.	Per. fons.	Age. Curt.	Per. fons.	Age. Curt.	Per. fons.	Age.	Persons.
1	1000	8	680	15	628	22	585	29	539	36	481	7	5547
2	855	9	670	16	622	23	579	30	531	37	472	14	4584
3	798	10	661	17	616	24	573	31	523	38	453	21	4270
4	760	11	653	18	610	25	567	32	515	39	454	28	3964
5	732	12	646	19	604	26	560	33	507	40	445	35	3604
6	710	13	640	20	598	27	553	34	499	41	436	42	3178
7	692	14	634	21	592	28	546	35	490	42	427	49	2709
												56	2194
												63	1694
												70	1204

Age. Curt.	Per. fons.	Age. Curt.	Per. fons.	Age. Curt.	Per. fons.	Age. Curt.	Per. fons.	Age. Curt.	Per. fons.	Age. Curt.	Per. fons.	Age.	Persons.
43	417	50	346	57	272	64	202	71	131	78	58	77	692
44	407	51	335	58	262	65	192	72	120	79	49	84	253
45	357	52	324	59	252	66	182	73	106	80	41	100	107
46	387	53	313	60	242	67	172	74	98	81	34		
47	377	54	302	61	232	68	162	75	88	82	28		
48	367	55	292	62	222	69	152	76	78	83	23		34000
49	357	56	282	63	212	70	142	77	58	84	20	Sum Total.	

7.1 Edmond Halley's life table (1693). *Source:* Edmond Halley, "An Estimate of the Degrees of Mortality of Mankind, ..." *Philosophical Transactions* 17 (1693): 600. Burndy Library, Dibner Institute for the History of Science and Technology

the 3-year-old could potentially be vastly greater than the original lump-sum amount.[26]

Beginning in the late seventeenth century, several well-known mathematicians developed life tables that could, in principle, put the calculation of annuities on an empirical basis. As shown in Chapter 1, Graunt created a life table based largely on his estimate that the rate of mortality was roughly proportional at each age. Edmond Halley (1656–1742), the royal astronomer and Fellow of the Royal Society, improved on Graunt's idea by incorporating empirical information about age of death taken from the bills of mortality of the German city Breslau. Halley's calculations and life table appeared in two essays published in the *Philosophical Transactions*.[27] (See Figure 7.1.)

Halley divided his life table into two columns: "Age Current" and "Persons." At age one, there were 1,000 persons living. By age two, 145 persons had died, leaving 855 survivors. By age seven, 308 persons had died, leaving 692 of the original 1,000, and so on. The two columns on the very right of the table listed the empirical figures from Breslau that Halley used in his calculations. Halley outlined several uses for his table, such as calculating the number of fighting men, "the differing degrees of Mortality, or rather Vitality in all Ages," and finally, the annuities and price of insurance upon lives.[28]

---

[26] Geoffrey Clark, *Betting on Lives: The Culture of Life Insurance in England, 1695–1775* (Manchester and New York: Manchester University Press, 1999); Daston, *Classical Probability in the Enlightenment* (Princeton, N.J.: Princeton University Press, 1988), pp. 121–125.

[27] "An Estimate of the Degrees of the Mortality of Mankind, Drawn from Curious Tables of the Births and Funerals at the City of Breslaw; with an Attempt to Ascertain the Price of Annuities upon Lives. By Mr. E. Halley, R.S.S.," *Philosophical Transactions* 17 (1693): 596–610; and "Some Further Considerations on the Breslaw Bills of Mortality," *Philosophical Transactions* 17–18 (1693): 654–656.

[28] Halley, "An Estimate of the Degrees of Mortality," pp. 600–604.

Halley's work was taken up by several mathematicians over the course of the eighteenth century. Abraham De Moivre, Anton Deparcieux, Thomas Simpson, Corbyn Morris, James Dodson, and Richard Price, for example, employed the new calculus of probabilities to the problem of annuities.[29] This work has been thoroughly studied in recent histories of probability. The equally important efforts to collect vital accounts – the very data on which calculations of probability were based – has not received such close examination.[30] Many mathematicians encouraged, even demanded at times, the collection of vital information in order to increase the accuracy of their calculations. Corbyn Morris, for example, published a set of proposals in 1751 to improve the London bills of mortality.[31] Two years later in a letter to the *Philosophical Transactions,* James Dodson, the Master of the Royal Mathematical School in Christ's Hospital, applauded Morris's proposals and called for some additional changes in order to give "a greater degree of certainty to the calculations of the values of annuities on lives." Specifically, Dodson highlighted the different rates of mortality between women of childbearing age and men of the same age. To this end, Dodson made two suggestions: first, that "complaints peculiarly incident to the female sex" be added to the lists of diseases; and second, that the age category 40–50 (which Morris had suggested for registering deaths) be broken into two (40–45 and 45–50), "the design of this being to fix the periods, that are fatal to the fair sex, with more certainty."[32] This is the same kind of issue medical arithmeticians addressed in their tables cataloging age and cause of death.

This concern with accuracy and precision in the collection of vital information was typical. Richard Price, the nonconformist minister and outspoken supporter of the American and French revolutions, wrote widely on annuities, the national debt, and population. Improving the collection of bills of mortality in London and in parishes and towns throughout England, he thought, "would give the precise law according to which human life wastes in its different stages, and thus supply the necessary *data* for computing accurately the values

---

[29] Abraham De Moivre, *Annuities for Life* (London, 1725); Anton Deparcieux, *Essai sur les probabilités de la durée de la vie humaine* (Paris, 1746); Thomas Simpson, *The Doctrine of Annuities and Reversion* (London, 1742); Corbyn Morris, *An Essay towards Illustrating the Science of Insurance* (London, 1747); James Dodson, "A Letter to the Right Honourable George Earl of Macclesfield, P.R.S. concerning the Value of an Annuity for Life, and the Probability of Survivorship," *Philosophical Transactions* 48 (1754): 487–499; and Richard Price, *Observations on Reversionary Payments* (London, 1769).

[30] Lorraine Daston, "The Domestication of Risk: Mathematical Probability and Insurance 1650–1830," in Lorenz Krüger, Lorraine J. Daston, and Michael Heidelberger, eds., *The Probabilitistic Revolution,* Vol. 1 (Cambridge, Mass.: MIT Press, 1987), pp. 237–260; Daston, *Classical Probability in the Enlightenment,* chap. 3; Jacques and Michel Dupâquier, *Histoire de la démographie,* chap. 6; Anders Hald, *History of Probability and Statistics and Their Applications before 1750* (New York: John Wiley & Sons, 1990), chaps. 9 and 25. For an account of De Moivre's mathematics, see Ivo Schneider, "Der Mathematiker Abraham De Moivre (1667–1754)," *Archive for History of Exact Sciences* 5 (1968–1969): 177–317.

[31] Corbyn Morris, *Observations on the Past and Present Growth and Present State of the City of London* (London, 1751).

[32] "A Letter from Mr. James Dodson to Mr. John Robertson, F.R.S. concerning an Improvement of the Bills of Mortality, 13 January 1752," *Philosophical Transactions* 47 (1753): 333, 340. Read to the RS on 16 January 1752.

of all *life-annuities* and *reversions*."[33] He himself collected data on mortality from parishes in Northampton and corresponded with many of the medical arithmeticians, including John Haygarth and Thomas Percival, who supplied Price with figures.[34] In these ways, Price was an atypical mathematician but a very typical arithmetician.

The renewed interest in the London bills of mortality led Thomas Birch, the secretary to the Royal Society, to publish in 1759 a volume that reprinted the London bills of mortality from 1657 through 1758, as well as Graunt's *Natural and Political Observations* and Petty's *Another Essay in Political Arithmetic*.[35] Birch's volume made it much easier for arithmeticians throughout England to analyze the London bills. It also marked the historical moment when medical and political arithmetic became established intellectual fields within English society. By reissuing Graunt and Petty, Birch was setting in place the standard historical narrative that has been followed in one way or another every since.

France

The French government had conducted periodic censuses for different regions of the country dating back to the middle ages. Although infrequently conducted, and usually for only one specific region at a time, there was at least one for most regions of France by the seventeenth century.[36] During Louis XIV's reign, censuses were stepped up in order to increase tax revenues. One of the king's chief advisors, the celebrated military engineer Sébastien le Prestre de Vauban, advocated an annual census, along with several new forms of taxation. Vauban's plan was part of a broad vision of reform that included the unification of weights and measures, the abolition of internal customs, and the suppression of abuses associated with tax collection – all of which would be achieved a century later during the Revolution.[37] "Without a census repeated every year, or at least every two or three years," Vauban lamented, "one cannot know precisely the

[33] Richard Price, "Observations on the Expectations of Lives, the Increase of Mankind, the Influence of Great Towns on Population, and Particularly the State of London with Respect to Healthfulness and Number of Inhabitants. In a Letter from Mr. Richard Price, F.R.S. to Benjamin Franklin, Esq; LL.D. and F.R.S.," *Philosophical Transactions* 59 (1769): 125.

[34] Peter Buck analyzes the politics of Price's work on annuities in "People Who Counted."

[35] Thomas Birch, *A Collection of the Yearly Bills of Mortality from 1657 to 1758 Inclusive* (London, 1759).

[36] For a list of these, see Guy Cabourdin and Jacques Dupâquier, "Les sources et les institutions," in *Histoire de la population française*, ed. Jacques Dupâquier (Paris: Presses Universitaires de France, 1988), vol. 2, p. 29. For an excellent discussion of these sources, see Bertrand Gille, *Les Sources statistiques de l'histoire de France – Des enquêtes du XVIIe siècle à 1870* (Paris, 1964). For general histories of censuses, demography, and the French population, see *Histoire de la population française* (Paris: Presses Universitaires de France, 1988); Jacques Dupâquier and Eric Vilquin, "Le Pouvoir royal et la statistique démographique," *Pour une histoire de la statistique* (Paris: Institut National de la Statistique et des Études Économiques, 1976), vol. 1, pp. 83–104; Jacques and Michel Dupâquier, *Histoire de la démographie*; and Jacqueline Hecht, "L'idée de dénombrement jusqu'à la révolution," *Pour une histoire de la statistique* (Paris: Institut National de la Statistique et des Études Économiques, 1976), vol. 1, pp. 21–81.

[37] P. Lazard, *Vauban 1633–1707* (Paris, 1934), pp. 544–549.

number of subjects, the true state of their wealth and poverty, what they do, how they live, their commerce and employment, if they are well or ill."[38] Although he did not use the term, Vauban was essentially describing the same approach to government that Petty advocated under the rubric of political arithmetic. Quantification would strengthen and improve royal policy.[39] But there was an important difference: Petty published many (although by no means all) of his works and addressed them to an educated public; most of Vauban's works remained unpublished and circulated only in manuscript among government officials.[40]

Throughout his career, Vauban consistently argued that a census was the only method for arriving at a precise figure for the population. In 1686, he privately printed a 12-page pamphlet entitled *Méthode générale et facile pour faire le dénombrement des peuples,* in which he outlined his ideas on conducting a census.[41] Ten years later, he provided an example of the type of census he advocated in "Description géographique de l'élection de Vézelay." This work contained a thorough description of a small election in Burgundy, that of Vézelay: its geography, crops, and products, and an enumeration of its population.[42] Vauban was careful to point out that his numbers were based on a *census,* not on an estimate. "Here is a true and sincere description of this small and poor land," Vauban wrote, "made after a very exact inquiry, founded, not on simple estimations which are nearly always faulty; but on a good, formal census, well rectified."[43]

In his "Description," Vauban included a table summarizing all his quantitative information, including figures for the number of men, women, houses, cows, and so forth for each parish in Vézelay. The table is noteworthy in one respect: It combined geographical information (the list of all the parishes within the election of Vézelay) with detailed numerical information about livestock,

---

[38] Vauban, *Note sur le recensement des peuples,* cited in Cabourdin and Dupâquier, p. 32. The historical demographer E. Vilquin first published this manuscript in 1972. Unfortunately, the original manuscript is not dated. See E. Vilquin, *Vauban et les méthodes de statistique au siècle de Louis XIV* (Paris: IDUP, 1972), cited in Cabourdin and Dupâquier, "Les sources et les institutions," p. 32; also see E. Vilquin, "Vauban, inventeur des recensements," *Annales de démographie historique,* 1975, pp. 207–257.

[39] For a discussion of Vauban's economics and his contemporaries Boisguilbert and Fenelon, see Jean-Claude Perrot, "Les économistes, les philosophes, et la population," in *Histoire de la population française,* ed. Jacques Dupâquier (Paris: Presses Universitaires de France, 1988), vol. 2, pp. 499–545. Jacques and Michel Dupâquier do not consider Vauban a political arithmetician; instead, they regard his work as contributions to descriptive statistics; see *Histoire de la démographie,* pp. 153–155.

[40] Éric Brian, *La mesure de l'état: Administrateurs et géomètres au XVIIIe siècle* (Paris: Albin Michel, 1994), pp. 159–160.

[41] The historian Edmond Esmonin rediscovered this pamphlet in the early 1950s. For his account of the discovery, see "Quelques données inédites sur Vauban et les premiers recensements de population," in E. Esmonin, *Études sur la France des XVIIe et XVIIIe siècles* (Paris: Presses Universitaires de France, 1964), pp. 260–266. (This essay was initially published in *Population,* 1954.)

[42] See Vauban, "Description géographique de l'élection de Vézelay contenant ses revenus; sa qualité; les moeurs de ses habitants; leur pauvreté et richesse; la fertilité du païs; et ce que l'on pourroit y faire pour en corriger la sterilité et procurer l'augmentation des peuples et l'accroissement des bestiaux" (1696), in Vauban, *Projet d'une Dixme Royale suivi de deux écrits financiers,* ed. E. Coornaert (Paris: F. Alcan, 1933), pp. 274–295.

[43] Vauban, "Description . . . de l'élection de Vézelay," p. 284.

houses, and vital events of the inhabitants (births, deaths, and marriages). In this regard, Vauban was much more ambitious than Graunt or Petty, who had restricted themselves to information about the human population.[44] Despite the clarity of the plan and the impressiveness of the Vézelay example, Louis XIV ignored Vauban's call for yearly censuses. Enumerations remained sporadic and uneven. In 1694, for example, the minister of finance ordered the intendants to conduct a national census prior to the establishment of a new tax, the *capitation*. But three years passed before another census was undertaken, this time as part of a set of plans entitled *Mémoires pour l'instruction du duc de Bourgogne*. This census consisted of responses to a questionnaire sent by the Duc de Beauvillier to all the intendants. According to modern demographers who have used these documents, "the majority [of *intendants*] were content with earlier figures, taken from enumerations of hearths or from the inquiry for the *capitation*."[45] Orders for a new census, thus, did not necessarily result in new enumerations. During the reign of Louis XV (1715–1774), no further general censuses were taken, although numerical information about trade and population was gathered in specific locales.[46]

While censuses were intermittent in early modern France, vital registration had a more continuous history. In 1539, at roughly the same time that Henry VIII of England announced his royal edict concerning vital registration, the royal ordinance of Villers-Coterêts was issued mandating the registration of baptisms and burials in all parishes throughout France. As in England, the clergy were responsible for maintaining the registers; however, in France, the registers were to be signed by a notary as well as by the curé. In theory, the clergy were to be enlisted by the French state, and clerical documents were to be monitored by royal officials. In practice, this was not the case. Historians and demographers who have studied these registers have never found an example of one that was, in fact, signed by a notary.[47]

---

[44] For a reproduction of this table see Vauban, *Projet d'une Dixme Royale.*
[45] Cabourdin and Dupâquier, "Les sources et les institutions," p. 35. Brian pointed out that the main object of these questionnaires was not to gather numerical information but, rather, to compile a general description of each généralité. Brian, *La mesure de l'état*, pp. 160–162.
[46] For example, while Philibert Orry, Comte de Vignory (1689–1747), was controller-general of France from 1730 to 1746, he ordered a general survey of the state of commerce and manufacturing. In a letter to the intendants dated December 1744, Orry requested information on the manufacturers and factories in each city, the number of persons employed in these industries, the number of inhabitants of each town, and the number of young men available for the military draft and capable of bearing arms, as well as an account of the resources in that area. A reply to his request can be found in the British Library. "Situation actuelle des provinces du royaume de France en l'année 1746," containing "Mémoires concernant la situation actuelle des provinces des royaume par rapport au commerce et à l'industrie des villes aux manufactures, au dénombrement des peuples et autres mémoires," British Library, Add. MS 8757. A portion of this document, "Mémoire de la généralité de Paris," is reprinted in *Mémoires des intendants sur l'état des généralités*, ed. A.M. de Boislisle (Paris, 1881), vol. 1, p. 444. For a discussion of the various inquests ordered by the French monarchy during the eighteenth century, see Brian, *La mesure de l'état*, pp. 167–168.
[47] Cabourdin and Dupâquier, "Les sources et les institutions," vol. 2, pp. 11–13. The following account of vital registration in France is largely drawn from this helpful article.

In April 1667, a new edict, formally named the ordinance of Saint Germain-en-Laye but commonly called the Code Louis, was put into effect. Among other specifications, the code called for the registration of baptisms, marriages, and burials, and the law required the curés to take the registers to a royal judge once a year, although all did not comply. Beginning in 1691 in a series of royal edicts, the Crown attempted to transfer record keeping from the Church to the royal bureaucracy. The first measure introduced the sale of offices for "clerks, keepers, and conservators of the registers of baptisms, marriages, and burials"; in 1705, the Crown sold offices for "controllers of registers and extracts of baptisms, marriages, and burials"; and in March 1709, offices for "alternative secretary clerks." Upon Louis XIV's death in May 1716, these offices came under attack from both the nobility and the clergy and were eventually suppressed in December 1716.[48] The task of vital registration returned to the clergy.[49]

In contrast to his grandfather, Louis XV introduced one noteworthy change concerning vital registration during his long reign (1715–1774). In 1736, following suggestions made by his advisor Joly de Fleury several years earlier, Louis XV issued a *Déclaration royale* that required curés to keep duplicate registers, one on official paper and one on regular paper. This specification thus allowed the curés to keep control of vital registration, but at the same time provided a means – the duplicate copy – for the state to acquire such information. The *Déclaration* formed the bureaucratic basis for the collection of vital accounts by the French state, and there were no further attempts at reform until the Revolution.[50]

Nor was there any coordinated use of the vital registers until the second half of the eighteenth century. In 1772, Abbé Joseph Marie Terray, the controller-general of France under Louis XV, requested each intendant to send a summary of the number of births, marriages, and deaths for each parish in his *generalité*, because it was "very important for the Administration to know exactly the state of the population of the realm":

It is not an enumeration by persons, dwellings [*ménages*] or households that I ask of you, that enumeration, although easy, would demand too much time and trouble to be renewed each year; what I ask is that you have sent to you each year by the clerks of the royal jurisdictions a résumé of births, marriages, deaths in all parishes. . . .[51]

---

[48] Cabourdin and Dupâquier, "Les sources et les institutions," pp. 15–16.
[49] These efforts to put vital registration in the hands of the state underscore the unclear boundary between ecclesiastical and royal functions and indicate the administrative weakness of the old regime. Royal bureaucrats were not salaried civil servants. Many offices were venal; once bought, the owners had little accountability to the king. Other officials owed their position to personal ties to the monarchy, and still others received payment from the public they served. See J.F. Bosher, "French Administration and Public Finance in Their European Setting," *The New Cambridge Modern History*, Vol. 8: "The American and French Revolutions, 1763–1793," ed. A. Goodwin (Cambridge: Cambridge University Press, 1965), pp. 565–591, esp. p. 566.
[50] Cabourdin and Dupâquier, "Les sources et les institutions," pp. 16–17.
[51] Cited and translated in Fernand Faure, "The Development and Progress of Statistics in France," in *The History of Statistics – Memoirs to Commemorate the 75th Anniversary of the American Statistical Association* (New York: The Macmillan Co., 1918), p. 263.

Significantly, Terray did *not* request a census, although he claimed (perhaps disingenuously) that a census would be easy enough. Instead, he endorsed indirect methods of calculating population.

Terray drew upon the existing bureaucracy of both clerical and state offices to collect accounts of the population. Replies to his circular are preserved in the Archives Nationales, many entered on preprinted forms entitled "Etat de la population de la Généralité _____ Année _____ ." The introduction of a printed form was itself an important innovation and insured a more consistent collection of information among the généralités.[52] The column headings were parishes, origin of the registers (*sénéchaussées,* hospitals/communities), births (boys, girls, total), marriages, deaths (men, women, total), religious professions (men, women, total), and religious deaths (monks, nuns, total). A final column was reserved for any observations thought appropriate. At the very end of this form was a table entitled "Récapitulation Particulière de l'élection de _____ ." Here, totals of the above categories were to be filled in.

Terray initially asked for numbers for the years 1770 through 1772; his inquest was continued annually by successive controller-generals until the French Revolution. The historian Éric Brian has studied the correspondence between Terray and the various intendants regarding this inquest, and he noted that Terray had to negotiate various details in order to make the accounts cohere. Did the clergy record infant deaths below a certain age? Were Protestants and Jews included? How reliable were the clerks?[53] Much as Jurin had done in his correspondence network devoted to collecting information on inoculation, Terray had to do considerable work to create comparable accounts. As discussed in the next section, the numbers collected by the controller-general's office became central to the calculations made by French political arithmeticians.

CALCULATING THE POPULATION: THE UNIVERSAL MULTIPLIER

The inability of the British and French states to establish a national census, combined with the pressing questions raised by the depopulation debates, stimulated numerous individuals both inside and outside government to try to calculate the population. During the second half of the eighteenth century, English and French political arithmeticians developed and refined a number of techniques for estimating the population. Naturally, the estimates varied, leading to several extended (and sometimes heated) exchanges about the methods of calculating population and the certainty of that knowledge. At stake were very important issues: the current and past populations, the factors causing the observed changes in population, and the measures necessary to increase population. As

---

[52] Archives Nationales, Paris F20 441. See, for example, "État de la population de la généralité de Moulins – Année 1773." Similar booklets exist for Château du Loire, Château Gantier, and de Mans.

[53] Brian, *La mesure de l'état,* pp. 172–178.

in the case of smallpox inoculation, the leading scientific societies, the Royal Society of London and the Académie Royale des Sciences in Paris, provided critical forums for discussion.

The contours of the English and French debates differed markedly, especially with respect to the social location of the arithmeticians. In France, almost all of the contributors held government positions; in Britain, the majority were Dissenters who were excluded from government because of their religion. Despite these differences, both French and English arithmeticians viewed their work as crucial to reform. Again, as in the smallpox inoculation controversy, the French arithmeticians developed more mathematically sophisticated approaches to the problem, whereas the English concentrated on refining the empirical basis for calculations. This difference can be explained in part by the resources available to each. French arithmeticians had access (sometimes limited) to the government compilations of birth and death figures from parish registers initally requested by Terray. English arithmeticians had to rely on the London bills of mortality or to collect their own data from local registers.

Britain

Political arithmeticians, beginning with William Petty, developed ingenious methods for calculating the population, all of which relied on some sort of multiplier used in conjunction with other information. Following one method, arithmeticians took the number 4 or 5 (to represent the number of persons assumed to live in each household) and multiplied it by the number of houses or hearths as given in the hearth tax records. By another method, the number of deaths recorded on the bills of mortality was multiplied by 30 to determine the population of London. Or, more commonly, the annual number of births (tallied from parish registers) was multiplied by a figure ranging from 25 to 28.[54] The multipliers for the last two methods were typically attained by taking a census of several small parishes and establishing the proportion of births or deaths to total population during an average year, that is, a year without great mortality.

The idea of a multiplier is itself noteworthy. Even though most political arithmeticians agreed that multipliers could vary considerably from community to community, they still insisted on using a single number. And while eighteenth-century writers contested the specific number, rarely did they criticize the technique of employing a universal multiplier. Debates thus focused on the choice of the multiplier (4 or 5, 27 or 28), and on the numbers drawn from tax records, parish registers, and bills of mortality.

The technique of the multiplier was used to great effect by Gregory King (1648–1712) and Charles Davenant (1656–1714), two early political

---

[54] For a brief history of the development of this method, see Cabourdin and Dupâquier, "Les sources et les institutions," p. 40. Also see Jacques and Michel Dupâquier, *Histoire de la démographie*, pp. 91–93.

arithmeticians who developed Petty's ideas.[55] King, a largely self-taught poly-math who made his living as a land and heraldry surveyor (in some ways similar to Petty), provided detailed surveys of London (1672) and Westminster (1674). In the 1680s, he worked mainly in heraldry and only took up political arithmetic in the 1690s.

In his "Natural and Political Observations and Conclusions upon the State and Condition of England," King devoted the bulk of his manuscript to numerical estimates of population, the amount of silver and gold in England, the quantity of beer consumed annually, the revenue collected from various taxes, and other quantifiable features of the realm.[56] His calculations of the population (he thought England and Wales had 5.5 million inhabitants in 1695) were based on the number of houses, a figure he took from the Hearth Office, multiplied by an average number of persons per household, which he computed from assessments of marriages, baptisms, and burials in several areas of England, although he neither revealed his calculations nor indicated his sources. One of his motivations for writing was a concern with England's ability to finance her expensive wars with Holland and France. Like Petty, King invoked the ratio of population to land area in order to compare England with its enemies. Holland, of course, came out ahead, but England fared well in comparison with France. King also examined the annual increase of population for England, while taking into account various checks to population growth, including plagues, foreign and civil wars, losses at sea, and emigration.[57]

King's manuscript was not published until 1802, although he gave a copy to Charles Davenant, who incorporated parts of it into his own *Essay upon the Probable Methods of Making a People Gainers in the Balance of Trade,* which was published in 1699. It was through Davenant's writings that eighteenth-century thinkers became familiar with King's work.[58] Davenant, a graduate of Oxford, was commissioner of the excise from 1683 through 1689, and became a member of Parliament in 1685. Although he did not create any new methods of quantifi-cation, he was an enthusiastic advocate of political arithmetic, which he defined

---

[55] See Karl Pearson, *The History of Statistics in the 17th and 18th Centuries against the Changing Background of Intellectual, Scientific and Religious Thought,* ed. E.S. Pearson (London: Charles Griffin, 1978), Chapter 4, "The Early Successors of Sir William Petty: The Political Arithmeticians," pp. 100–124.

[56] Gregory King, "Natural and Political Observations and Conclusions upon the State and Condition of England" (1690), in *Two Tracts by Gregory King,* ed. George E. Barnett, (Baltimore: Johns Hopkins University Press, 1936), p. 47.

[57] King, "Natural and Political Observations," pp. 19, 25.

[58] George Chalmers was the first to publish King's "Natural and Political Observations and Conclusions upon the State and Condition of England, 1696," as an appendix to his 1802 edition of *Estimate of the Comparative Strength of Great Britain.* A manuscript copy of King's "Natural and Political Observations and Conclusions upon the State and Condition of England, 1696" is found in the British Museum, Harl. MSS 1898.

as "the art of reasoning by figures, upon things relating to government."[59] He
followed King's approach in recommending the use of tax records in the practice
of political arithmetic:

> The Excise is a measure by which we may judge, not only what the people consume, but,
> in some sort, it lets us into a knowledge how their Numbers increase or diminish. The
> Customs are the very pulse of a Nation, from which its health, or decays, may be observ'd.
> The Hearth-money has given us a view, certain enough, of the number of families, which
> is the very Ground-work in such speculations: and these three Revenues must be the better
> guide to computers, because the accounts of them are fairly kept and stated....[60]

Davenant viewed tax records as a rich and, importantly, accurate source for vital
information about the population and its health. His attitude was very much
like Petty's in that he regarded this information as critical to state welfare; that
is, political arithmetic was a tool of royal power.[61]

There was little discussion about methods to determine England's population
before midcentury, when Parliament debated the 1753 bill proposing a national
census and a reform of vital registration. The parliamentary debates provoked a
heated exchange in the *Philosophical Transactions* between William Brakenridge
and Richard Forster (both clergymen and Fellows of the Royal Society). The
exchange is worth examining in some detail because both the methods and
sources used to calculate population were open to public scrutiny.

Brakenridge, a noted mathematician, set the tone with an article on the
number of inhabitants in London, which he had calculated from the London
bills of mortality. He began with a table listing total number of deaths for 5-year
and 10-year periods from 1704 to 1753. (See Figure 7.2.) The first column indicated the years (5-year periods above the line, 10-year periods below); the
second and third columns gave the average number of baptisms and burials
for each period within the city walls; and the fourth and fifth columns for
baptisms and burials for all parishes registered in the London bills. From this
table Brakenridge concluded that London's population had peaked between
1728 and 1743, and since then it had been on a steady decline. Adding in
estimates of the number of deaths among Dissenters, Quakers, and Jews, and
multiplying yearly total burials by 30 (the multiplier advocated by Petty, i.e.,
1 of 30 die in London per annum), Brakenridge arrived at a figure for the
total population of London: 748,350 for the period 1744–1753, and 875,760

---

[59] Charles Davenant, *Discourses on the Public Revenues and Trade* (1698), p. 127; cited in Pearson, *The History of Statistics in the 17th and 18th Centuries*, p. 118. For Pearson's evaluation of Davenant's statistics, see Pearson, pp. 113–124.
[60] Davenant, *Discourses*, p. 136; cited in Pearson, *The History of Statistics in the 17th and 18th Centuries*, p. 119.
[61] Peter Buck, "Seventeenth-Century Political Arithmetic: Civil Strife and Vital Statistics," *Isis*, 68 (1977): 67–84.

Years.	Baptifms.	Burials.	Baptifms.	Burials.
1704— 8	1870	2553	15867	22103
1709—13	1805	2551	15288	21701
1714—18	1890	2706	17586	24641
1719—23	1871	2719	18360	26978
1724—28	1829	2727	18442	27670
1729—33	1578	2532	17452	26267
1734—38	1406	2242	16762	26165
1739—43	1221	2307	15034	28219
1744—48	1062	1989	14402	23884
1749—53	1087	1790	14850	22006
1704—13	1837	2552	15577	21602
1714—23	1880	2712	18073	25809
1724—33	1703	2647	17920	27168
1734—43	1313	2320	15898	27192
1744—53	1074	1890	14626	22945

7.2 William Brakenridge's table of London burials (1704–1753). *Source:* William Brakenridge, "A Letter from the Reverend William Brakenridge, . . ." *Philosophical Transactions* 48 (1754): 789. Burndy Library, Dibner Institute for the History of Science and Technology.

for the period 1734–1743. Brakenridge then employed Petty's other method for estimating population – multiplying the number of houses by the average number of inhabitants per house (although he revised Petty's ratio of 8 to 6 inhabitants per house) – and arrived at roughly the same figures. Brakenridge deduced the number of houses from the Window Tax Office; the hearth tax had been abandonned earlier. In conclusion, Brakenridge attributed the decline in London's population to increased consumption of liquor, to "the fashionable humour of living single," and to the increase in trade in northern Britain.[62]

In a second essay in the *Philosophical Transactions,* Brakenridge extended his calculations to argue that England's population had declined, as well as London's. He used two measures: the number of houses and the amount of bread consumed. The latter measure was admittedly indirect; Brakenridge had to estimate the amount of wheat produced in England by comparing it with the amount of barley produced, which was subject to a malt tax.[63] Basing his conclusion on these two measures, he claimed that in 1710 the population of England and Wales was 5,570,000, and in 1750, 5,340,000. In a third and final essay, Brakenridge discussed more fully his interests in calculating population, and he suggested that England's wars and commerce were "rather beyond our natural strength;"

[62] William Brakenridge, "A Letter from the Reverend William Brakenridge, D.D. and F.R.S. to George Lewis Scot, Esq.; F.R.S. concerning the Number of Inhabitants within the London Bills of Mortality," *Philosophical Transactions* 48 (1754): 788–800. Glass analyzed the types of arguments and evidence Brakenridge and Forster used in his *Numbering the People,* pp. 47–51.
[63] William Brakenridge, "A Letter to George Lewis Scot, Esq; F.R.S. concerning the Number of People in England; from the Reverend William Brakenridge, D.D. Rector of St. Michael Bassishaw, and F.R.S.," *Philosophical Transactions* 49 (1756): 268–285.

they destroyed "more people than can be spared, and which, if preserved, might improve our country, and augment our power...."[64]

In 1757, Forster responded to Brakenridge's arguments by presenting evidence taken from his parish of Great Shefford in Berkshire. He compared the number of houses reported in the window tax returns with his own survey. Brakenridge had assumed that the window tax returns omitted cottages, which, he estimated, accounted for only one-quarter of the housing. Forster's survey indicated that for his parish, cottages made up fully two-thirds of the housing. Further, his survey revealed that the number of persons per house was under 5 – a significantly lower figure than Brakenridge's multiplier of 6 persons per hearth. In a subsequent essay, Forster reported that he had surveyed eight neighboring parishes in addition to Great Shefford and found a total of 588 houses, of which only 177 had paid the window tax (that is, roughly 70 percent of the houses did not pay the tax). This empirical inquiry understandably raised serious doubts about the accuracy of Brakenridge's estimates. Forster calculated a population of roughly 7,500,000 for England, 50 percent greater than Brakenridge's figure. Moreover, Forster strongly recommended to "the members of the Royal Society, who have many of them seats in Parliament, and most of them interest in those that have, to get an Act passed for perfecting registers."[65]

The discrepancy between Brakenridge's and Forster's numbers arose from the different sources they used. Brakenridge relied on numbers already compiled for other purposes, namely, the London bills of mortality and the window tax returns. Forster assembled his own figures by examining local parish registers and extrapolated his findings to the entire population of England. Brakenridge rightly objected that Forster's local measure of population growth could not accurately pertain to all parishes in England. Forster responded by describing his work as "ye method of reasoning by Induction." He continued:

> Every Body knows that Induction is an imperfect way of Argumentation; but then it is an honest one. It lays ye whole force of ye Argument before you; & therefore no body can be deceived by it. It appears to me, that ye present Philosophy (Experimental) is carried on entirely by this method; & above all, were it to be laid aside, ye Political Arithmetician wou'd be stript of ye most valuable part of his Patrimony.[66]

Induction, like numerical tables, allowed the reader to evaluate the soundness of the argument. It was, in Forster's words, "an honest" philosophical method.

---

[64] Brakenridge, "A Letter to George Lewis Scot, Esquire, concerning the Present Increase of the People in Britain and Ireland," *Philosophical Transactions* 49 (1755–1756): 886.

[65] Richard Forster, "An Extract of the Register of the Parish of Great Shefford, near Lamborne, in Berkshire, for Ten Years: With Observations on the Same: In a Letter to Tho. Birch, D.D. Secret. R.S. from the Reverend Mr. Richard Forster, Rector of Great Shefford," *Philosophical Transactions* 50 (1757): 363.

[66] Richard Forster to Rev. Birch, 2 December 1760, British Museum Add. MSS no. 4440, ff. 176–185; reprinted in Glass, *Numbering the People,* p. 79.

Forster then provided a lineage of historical precedents: "Graunt, who was, I think, ye Father of this Art, measures ye whole Nation from one Parish in Hampshire. Sr Will. Petty is full of it. King's Tables, upon which Davenant raises such a superstructure, can be built upon nothing else. Halley has measured the whole World from 5 years Bills of a Single Town in Germany."[67] Here, Forster nicely summarized the problem of what we would now call sampling procedures and honed in on the epistemologically suspect basis of induction. The political arithmeticians were all guilty on this count; nonetheless, the method remained essential. Forster cautioned, however, that this approach could be carried too far. "No Man Living has a deeper Sense of ye Merit of Mathematical Argumentation than myself," he conceded. "[T]his sort of Reasoning has been abused. Sometimes it has been applied to improper Subjects, such for instance, as Credibility, Probability, Merit, Virtue, &c."[68] Just as in the inoculation debates, where there persisted anxiety over the suitability of quantitative arguments in medicine, Forster expressed a similar concern over the very application of numbers to such subjects as credibility and virtue.

Forster's and Brakenridge's exchange in the *Philosophical Transactions* did not resolve the depopulation debate, and many of the same issues were raised again in the writings of the Dissenting minister Richard Price. Price wrote on many subjects, including politics, theology, and the national debt; he also made significant contributions to the mathematics of life insurance. In several articles to the *Philosophical Transactions* and in subsequent books, Price, relying on figures from the Window Tax Office, coupled with his own inquiries in scattered parishes, offered his own figures for England's population.[69] For the late seventeenth century, Price calculated a total population of England and Wales of roughly 6 million. By 1770, he estimated only $4\frac{1}{2}$ million – in other words, a decrease of one-quarter since the Glorious Revolution.[70] In a later work, *An Essay on the Population of England* (1780), Price studied the excise duty on liquor and found a fall in revenues, which reinforced his conclusion that the population had decreased.[71]

Many, including Arthur Young, the noted writer on agricultural matters, disputed Price's conclusions. Calling Price's assertion of depopulation an "opinion, for I can call it nothing else," Young questioned the accuracy of the numbers

---

[67] Forster to Birch, 2 December 1760, p. 79.   [68] Forster, to Birch, 2 December 1760, pp. 85–86.

[69] Richard Price, "Observations on the Expectations of Lives, the Increase of Mankind, the Influence of Great Towns on Population and Particularly the State of London with Respect to the Healthfulness and Number of Its Inhabitants," in a letter to Benjamin Franklin Esq. LL.D. and F.R.S., *Philosophical Transactions* 59 (1769): 89–125; Price, "Observations on the Proper Method of Calculating the Values of Reversions Depending on Survivorship," *Philosophical Transactions* 60 (1770): 268–276.

[70] Richard Price, *Observations on Reversionary Payments*, 1st ed. (London, 1771); 2d ed. (London, 1772); 3d ed. (London, 1773). For a discussion of Price's role in the depopulation debates, see Glass, *Numbering the People*, pp. 53–57.

[71] Richard Price, *An Essay on the Population of England*, 2d ed. (London, 1780).

taken from the Window Tax Office and the multiplier that Price had used. Young concluded that the only way "to know the real and the whole truth" was to number the people, that is, to carry out a national census.[72] To this end, he penned *Proposals to the Legislature for Numbering the People* (1771).[73] Young insisted that an accurate, precise knowledge of the population was essential to good government. This knowledge would include not only the number of people but also the different classes of persons (by vocation: those involved in agriculture, manufacturing, and commerce; by economic status: those regularly charged to the poor roles, vagrants). Coupled with information about taxes, rents, and products, knowledge about the population would allow statesmen to evaluate those conditions that promote or hinder prosperity. Inflated ideas of population or fears of depopulation might make Britain more vulnerable; "certainty in these truly important points, would be the thermometer of the state."[74] The metaphor Young invoked was telling: The thermometer had brought numerical precision to the study of meteorology; a census would bring a similar degree of precision to statecraft.

Despite Young's advocacy, Parliament once again did not enact a national census and, as in the 1750s, determinations of population remained private inquiries, rather than state-sponsored initiatives. One final example underscores the role played by individuals. William Wales, an astronomer and mathematician, who sailed on Captain Cook's second world voyage as the representative of the Board of Longitude, became interested in population issues when he was appointed Master of the Royal Mathematical School at Christ's Hospital. Wary of the pitfalls Price had encountered by basing his calculations on a limited survey, Wales devised a questionnaire about the number of houses at different periods, which he sent to correspondents throughout England. The questionnaire met with instant hostility. The public not only feared additional taxation but also objected for religious reasons. Wales shifted strategies and sent a new questionnaire (which included a table to fill in) to parish clergy in order to collect information on the annual number of baptisms and burials from their registers for three 10-year periods: 1688–1697, 1741–1750, and 1771–1780.[75] "I have met with the utmost readiness to assist me wherever I have applied," Wales noted. "And I am assured, from my own experience, that a general invitation to the clergy, and the appointment of a proper place for

[72] Arthur Young, Letter to *St. James's Chronicle*, 28 March 1772, from *Political Arithmetic* (London, 1774); reprinted in D.V. Glass, ed., *The Population Controversy* (Farnborough, Hants, Eng.: Gregg International Publishers, 1973), pp. 322, 331.

[73] [Arthur Young], *Proposals to the Legislature for Numbering the People; Containing Some Observations on the Population of Great Britain, and a Sketch of the Advantages That Would Probably Accrue from an Exact Knowledge of Its Present State. By the Author of the Tours through England* (London: W. Nicoll, 1771); reprinted in Glass, *The Development of Population Statistics*.

[74] Young, *Proposals*, p. 21.

[75] Wales's questionnaire and table are reproduced in Glass, *Numbering the People*.

the reception of their communications, would procure materials sufficient to determine this arduous problem, in political arithmetic, with great certainty."[76]

Wales forwarded to the Carlisle physician John Heysham at least 60 blank forms for information on baptisms and burials from the parishes of the County of Cumberland. Wales also requested accounts of the number of inhabitants from the same parishes in order to calculate a more accurate multiplier, explaining to Heysham:

> By taking the medium proportion between the number of births, in a great number of Cities, Towns of different sizes, and Villages, and the number of persons actually liveing in them, if I can come at extracts from near the half of the parishes in England, I think we may come nearer the absolute number of the inhabitants from thence than by any other means that has yet been proposed; unless that an actual enumeration of the whole kingdom was undertaken; which there is, at present, no hopes of. The same may be done by comparing the burials.[77]

From these returns, Wales determined that the population had *increased* over the course of the eighteenth century. Published as *An Inquiry into the Present State of Population in England and Wales* (1781), Wales's correspondence method and estimates provided a strong challenge to the earlier claims of depopulation championed by Brakenridge and Price. Wales was particularly harsh on estimates based on window tax returns and Price's calculations based on liquor duties. "[T]he pernicious practice of smuggling is carried to too great a length, not to be most severely felt in these two articles of the revenue," Wales noted, "and, therefore, . . . no dependence can be placed in calculations founded on them." Trustworthy information about the number of houses "could be expected only from an actual survey, made on the spot, by persons in no wise interested in this affair, or any others which have the least connection with it, or with any article of the revenue."[78] Wales also faulted Price for the assumption that one family resided in each house. "Your Table of the enumeration of Carlisle," Wales wrote to Heysham,

> tends to overturn (as every one else which I have seen does) Dr. Price's notion that there is no material difference between the number of houses and the number of families. In Carlisle the difference is very great indeed. But it is so in every great Town, Nottingham alone excepted, which the Dr. has produced as an example, and that town happening to prove so, has, I suppose, led him into the mistake.[79]

[76] William Wales, *An Inquiry into the Present State of Population in England and Wales* (London, 1781), p. 9; reprinted in Glass, *The Population Controversy*.
[77] William Wales to John Heysham, 10 June 1782, Heysham Collection, Carlisle City Library; published in Glass, *Numbering the People*, p. 43.
[78] Wales, *An Inquiry*, pp. 4–5.
[79] William Wales to John Heysham, 28 August 1781, Heysham Collection, Carlisle City Library; published in Glass, *Numbering the People*, p. 41.

The conclusion of Wales' inquiry – an appeal for more information – highlighted the voluntary nature of his method and was reminiscent of Jurin's advertisement concerning inoculation. "[S]uch of the clergy as this little tract many fall into the hands of," Wales wrote, "will oblige the author with the annual number of baptisms, marriages and burials, in their respective parishes."[80] His call for more information also underscored the ongoing character of his correspondence method and showed, as Wales himself remarked, "how much a single person, who is disposed to do it, may perform."[81]

Wales's book failed to secure a consensus on the issue of depopulation, and he did not publish anything further on the topic. It seemed that even with his effort to collect figures from parishes throughout England, the data remained overwhelmingly fragmentary and, hence, an inadequate base upon which to calculate total population. Frederick Morton Eden, author of *The State of the Poor* (1797), echoed this belief in a pamphlet summarizing the efforts to measure population. "He who looks for more than probabilities will be disappointed," Eden concluded. "Moral certainty cannot, in inquiries of this nature, be expected to result from investigations into the number of baptisms, burials, taxed houses, cottages, and inhabitants, in particular districts." Instead, one should look forward to the national census: "The proposed enumeration of the people will supersede the use of ingenious guesses and plausible speculations, drawn from such *data*; and (I trust) prove, beyond the possibility of doubt, that, among the distresses of the times, we have not to deplore a declining population."[82]

It was only with the French Revolution and the resulting wars that Parliament passed an act in 1800 mandating a census and vital registration in Britain; the act called such an account "expedient" – in contrast to the 1753 concern with "publick Utility." The determination of the British population became a matter of state, rather than private initiative. The impact of the depopulation controversy on the census itself was pronounced – even its title reflected its origins: "An Act for Taking an Account of the Population of Great Britain, and of the Increase or Diminution Thereof."

France

One important difference between the depopulation debates in England and France is that in the latter, there was no explicit exchange about how to calculate population. This difference had everything to do with the fact that the French arithmeticians held governmental positions and had access to similar sources of quantitative information about the population. Thus, the kinds of debates about the local, fragmentary nature of individual parish registers that marked English writings on the topic were, for the most part, absent from the French.

---

[80] Wales, *An Inquiry*, p. 79.   [81] Wales, *An Inquiry*, p. 10.
[82] Frederick Morton Eden, *An Estimate of the Number of Inhabitants in Great Britain and Ireland* (London, 1800), pp. 2–3.

In France, as in England, the earliest attempts to determine population relied on figures for the number of hearths (*feux*). One of the earliest publications listing the number of hearths was Claude Saugrain's *Dictionnaire universel de la France* (1726).[83] Saugrain's *Dictionnaire* was a three-volume work alphabetically arranged with an entry for each town in France, including the number of inhabitants. A typical entry read as follows:

Dimancheville, in Orleannois, Diocese of Orleans, Parlement of Paris, Intendance of Orleans, Election of Pithiviers, has 126 inhabitants.[84]

Saugrain gave no indication of how he arrived at the number of inhabitants; historical demographers have speculated that he multiplied the number of hearths by 4.5 to arrive at the figures he presented.[85] Earlier, Saugrain had issued *Dénombrement du royaume par Généralitez, Elections, Paroisses et Feux* (1709). This two-volume work provided the number of hearths (*feux*) for all communities, classified by elections and *généralités*. In 1720, a revised edition appeared that incorporated numbers collected in various *généralités* in the interim.[86]

In 1762, Abbé Jean-Joseph Expilly, who held a variety of governmental posts throughout his career and was a member of the Société Royale des Sciences et Belles-Lettres de Nancy, published *Dictionnaire géographique, historique et politique des Gaules et de la France,* in large part to refute the depopulationists' claims. Expilly drew on the earlier work of Saugrain and took issue with the commonly employed multiplier of 4 persons per hearth. "It is true that it is common enough that one understands by a hearth one family; but this meaning will not work in Provence, or Dauphiné, or in Brittany," he charged.[87] Instead, Expilly proposed a multiplier of 5 and argued that cities usually had closer to 6 persons per hearth, while the countryside had 4, so that 5 was an average. Using the number of hearths found in Saugrain's *Nouveau dénombrement du royaume,* Expilly calculated the population of France as 20,905,413.

Because of the inaccuracies associated with the hearth method (revealed so starkly in the English debates), the majority of works published in the second half of the eighteenth century relied upon the number of births to calculate population.[88] A good example is found in the works published under the name of Louis Messance: *Recherches sur la population des généralités d'Auvergne, de Lyon,*

[83] Jacques and Michel Dupâquier, *Histoire de la démographie,* p. 175.

[84] Claude Saugrain, *Dictionnaire universel de la France ancienne et moderne,* Vol. 1 (Paris, 1726), p. 1040.

[85] Cabourdin and Dupâquier, "Les sources et les institutions," pp. 38–39.

[86] Saugrain, *Nouveau dénombrement du royaume par généralitez, élections, paroisses et feux* (Paris, 1720).

[87] Jean J. d'Expilly, *Dictionnaire géographique, historique et politique des Gaules et de la France,* Vol. 1 (Liechtenstein: Kraus Reprint, 1978 [1762]), "Avertissement," [6 pp.], n.p.

[88] Bernard Bru, "De La Michodière à Moheau: L'évaluation de la population par les naissances," in Moheau, *Recherches et considérations sur la population de la France (1778),* reedition annotated by Eric Vilquin (Paris: Institut National d'Études Démographiques, Presses Universitaires de France, 1994), pp. 493–516; also see Bernard Bru, "Estimations Laplaciennes," in *Estimations et sondages,* ed. Jacques Mairesse (Paris: Economica, 1988), pp. 7–46.

de Rouen, et de quelques provinces et villes du royaume (1766); and *Nouvelles recherches sur la population de la France* (1788). Messance was the secretary to the intendant J.B.F. La Michodière, but scholars have plausibly argued that La Michodière was in fact the author.[89] La Michodière, one of the many enlightened bureaucrats in France during the second half of the eighteenth century, had a long and distinguished career in the French government that provided one source for his interest in population; the other was his conviction that the depopulation argument was incorrect.[90]

In order to determine the number of inhabitants, La Michodière believed that "the average number of annual births [*l'année commune des naissances*] must be a sure rule."[91] His advocacy of this technique over a census rested on pragmatic considerations. Contrary to Terray's assertion, La Michodière admitted that a census "proved difficult to carry out each century, so long as time and care required, because the fears that it could inspire in the people always prevented the inquiries ordered by the government." Births provided the best basis for calculating the population, and the information was already available from parish registers.[92] In his calculations, La Michodière relied upon the partial enumerations made by Sebastien le Prestre de Vauban at the end of the seventeenth century, and he arrived at the figure of 23,909,400 for the French population.

La Michodière's use of Vauban's enumerations, like Expilly's use of Saugrain's figures for the number of hearths, underscores the paucity of vital information available in France during the second half of the eighteenth century. A regular census remained an unattainable ideal, and pragmatic concerns led administrators to calculate the population by using multipliers. Accordingly, La Michodière and other reform-minded ministers focused on ways to increase the store of numerical information by collecting figures from the clerical registers kept throughout France – figures that would serve as a basis for calculation. And they were more successful than their counterparts in England. But how accurate or how universal the multiplier was remained subjects of heated debate.

This issue was taken up vigorously by one of La Michodière's fellow intendants, Antoine Auget, Baron de Montyon, whose *Recherches et considérations sur la population de la France* (coauthored and published under the name of his secretary Moheau) is considered a masterpiece in early demography.[93] (See Chapter 6.)

---

[89] See C.C. Gillispie, "Probability and Politics: Laplace, Condorcet, and Turgot," *Proceedings of the American Philosophical Society* 116 (1972): 11; C.C. Gillispie, *Science and Polity at the End of the Old Regime* (Princeton, N.J.: Princeton University Press, 1980), p. 47, fn. 141; and Jacques and Michel Dupâquier, *Histoire de la démographie*, pp. 177–178.

[90] For an account of La Michodière's work on population, see Bru, "Estimations Laplaciennes."

[91] Louis Messance, *Recherches sur la population des généralités d'Auvergne, de Lyon, de Rouen, et de quelques provinces et villes du royaume, avec des réflexions sur la valeur du bled tant en France qu'en Angleterre, depuis 1674 jusqu'en 1764* (Paris, 1766), p. 1.

[92] Messance, *Recherches sur la population*, pp. 2–3.

[93] For evaluations of Montyon's contributions to demography, see the excellent collection of essays appended to the new edition of his book: Moheau, *Recherches et considérations sur la population de la*

Political Arithmetic

The first part of the book is an evaluation of the various ways to calculate population. Moheau concluded that the increase or decline in the average number of annual births was the best measure of the size of population, and he invoked the familiar metaphor of a scientific instrument. "It is a thermometer that the administration cannot make too exact and one that it cannot consult too often," he explained.[94] Moheau acknowledged that the multiplier could range anywhere from 23 to 31, depending on the region in France. To demonstrate this variation, he computed figures for the universal multiplier from records of births and censuses for several towns and presented them in a series of tables. (See Figure 7.3.) One striking feature of his tables is the degree to which the calculations were carried out, that is, the precision of his figures.[95] From his investigations, Moheau concluded "that the term of proportion that seems to best suit the appreciation of the population of the realm is that of $25\frac{1}{2}$."[96]

Like the English medical arithmeticians, Moheau emphasized the reliability, certainty, and clarity of his tables. "As these tables are under the eyes of the reader," Moheau asserted, "he may adopt or contradict their consequences." Facts summarized in tables will bring about conviction, and he approvingly cited Francis Bacon on this point as the "father of the modern Philosophy."[97] Moheau also took issue with the various ingenious explanations for depopulation. Arguments about the causes and consequences of population growth or decline were vague and speculative. What was needed were calculations: "There are more men who know how to calculate than to reason. The facts strike all minds and form a body of proof, that, by its evidence, necessitates conviction."[98] This was a curious twist on the Enlightenment conception of reasoning as a form of calculation, of analysis and synthesis. In Moheau's formulation, calculation was an easier, more elementary and comprehensible task than reasoning. Figures would lead to conviction among all persons in a straightforward manner; reasoning, on the other hand, was more difficult and did not produce consensus as readily.[99]

France (1778), reedition annotated by Eric Vilquin (Paris: Institut National d'Études Démographiques, Presses Universitaires de France, 1994). Also see Joshua Cole, *The Power of Large Numbers*, pp. 31–35; Jacques and Michel Dupâquier, *Histoire de la démographie*, p. 171; Jean-Claude Perrot, "Les économistes, les philosophes, et la population," p. 530; and William Coleman, "Inventing Demography: Montyon on Hygiene and the State," in Everett Mendelsohn, ed., *Transformation and Tradition in the Sciences – Essays in Honor of I. Bernard Cohen* (Cambridge: Cambridge University Press, 1984), pp. 215–235.

[94] Moheau, *Recherches et considérations*, p. 43.

[95] This degree of precision was not unique to Moheau-Montyon. On Lavoisier's use of precise calculations, see Jan Golinski, " 'The Nicety of Experiment': Precision of Measurement and Precision of Reasoning in Late Eighteenth-Century Chemistry," in *The Values of Precision*, ed. M. Norton Wise (Princeton, N.J.: Princeton University Press, 1995), pp. 72–91.

[96] Moheau, *Recherches et considérations*, pp. 24–25. [97] Moheau, *Recherches et considérations*, pp. 8, 9.

[98] Moheau, *Recherches et considérations*, p. 8.

[99] For discussion of the relationship between calculation and intelligence in the Enlightenment, see Lorraine Daston, "Enlightenment Calculation," *Critical Inquiry* 21 (1994): 182–202.

44   *Recherches & Confidérations*

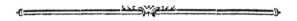

TABLE I. *Queft.* 5. *Chap.* 5.

GÉNÉRALITÉS fur lefquelles il a été opéré.	NAISSANCES pendant dix années.	NOMBRE d'habitans dénombrés	PROPORTION de l'année commune des naiffances au nombre d'habitans.	
PARIS.	684	1716	25	$\frac{1}{114}$
RIOM.	10200	25028	24	$\frac{137}{255}$
LIMOGES. . . .	3811	8862	23	$\frac{1439}{5717}$
LYON.	8262	19623	23	$\frac{3079}{4152}$
CHAMPAGNE.	220	547	24	$\frac{17}{22}$
ROUEN.	21972	60552	27	$\frac{6111}{10587}$
TOURS *. . . .	193930	458054	23	$\frac{12015}{19393}$
LA ROCHELLE.	23511	57545	24	$\frac{11186}{23521}$
TOTAL. . . .	87855	219678	24	$\frac{8358}{1805}$

* Tours n'étant compris que pour un dixieme.

7.3 Jean-Baptiste Moheau's table of multipliers (1778). *Source:* Jean-Baptiste Moheau, *Recherches et considérations sur la population de la France* (Paris, 1778), p. 44. Yale University, Harvey Cushing/John Hay Whitney Medical Library.

Several other prominent officials, including the chemist Antoine Lavoisier and the finance minister Jacques Necker, published calculations of the population based on the number of births, and like Moheau, they focused on the collection of numerical data.[100] Their figures indicated that France had not

[100] Antoine Laurent Lavoisier, *De la richesse territoriale du royaume de France* (1784); Jacques Necker, *De l'administration des finances de la France* (1784); Jean Christophe Sandrier des Pommelles, *Tableau de*

suffered depopulation over the course of the eighteenth century. In these inquiries, there was considerable cooperation between the government and the scientific community.[101] In the 1783 *Mémoires* of the Académie Royale des Sciences, for example, Du Séjour, Condorcet, and Laplace produced a report containing tables of figures for the number of towns, villages, and inhabitants.[102] Large portions of this report depended upon the efforts of the intendant La Michodière, whose papers were announced and deposited in the Académie des Sciences.[103] Entitled "Table alphabétique des villes, bourgs, villages dans différentes régions de France, Moyenne des naissances, mariages, morts sur les années 1781, 1782, 1783," La Michodière's table provided the annual number of births, deaths, and marriages of each parish of selected elections.[104] It formed the basis for the academicians' studies, and in this way the Académie supported these early demographic inquiries.

THE ROLE OF PARTIAL ENUMERATIONS

The depopulation debate encouraged the introduction, development, and evaluation of a variety of techniques to measure population. Questions about the accuracy and precision of those methods of calculation, however, led to different approaches and solutions in England and France. The work of English arithmeticians concentrated on the collection of information and was frequently

---

la population de toutes les provinces de France (1789); Louis Brion de la Tour, *Tableau de la population de la France avec les citations des auteurs* (Paris, 1789). For a discussion of these works, see Jacques and Michel Dupâquier, *Histoire de la démographie*, pp. 183–186.

[101] For accounts of the relations between the state and the scientific community, see Keith Baker, *Inventing the French Revolution* (Cambridge: Cambridge University Press, 1990); Brian, *La mesure de l'état;* and Charles C. Gillispie, *Science and Polity in France at the End of the Old Regime* (Princeton, N.J.: Princeton University Press, 1980).

[102] Similar reports were included each year in the *Mémoires de l'Académie Royale des Sciences* until 1788. See: DuSéjour, Condorcet, & Laplace, "Pour connoître la Population du Royaume, & le nombre des habitans de la Campagne, en adaptant sur chacune des Cartes de M. Cassini, l'année commune des Naissances, tant des Villes que des Bourgs & des Villages dont il est fait mention sur chaque carte," *Mémoires de l'Académie Royale des Sciences,* 1783 (Paris, 1786), pp. 703–718; ibid., 1784 (Paris, 1787), pp. 577–593; ibid., 1785 (Paris, 1788), pp. 661–689; ibid., 1786 (Paris, 1788), pp. 703–717; ibid., 1787 (Paris, 1789), pp. 601–610; ibid., 1788 (Paris, 1791), pp. 755–767. Another example of the Académie's interest in population is found in Jean Morand, "Récapitulation des baptêmes, mariages, mortuaires et enfans trouvés de la ville et faubourgs de Paris, depuis l'année 1709, jusques et compris l'année 1770," *Mémoires de l'Académie Royale des Sciences,* 1771 (Paris, 1774), pp. 830–848. In this article, Morand indicated that beginning in 1709, the city of Paris drew up abstracts of the numbers of baptisms, marriages, and deaths by month and by parish.

[103] A steady stream of correspondence from La Michodière to the Académie is preserved in the Académie's archives. For example, the Procès Verbaux of the Académie Royale des Sciences, 23 July 1785 read, "Letter of M. de la Michodière who immediately promised a register of deaths, births, and marriages for all the Realm." Procès Verbaux, Académie Royale des Sciences, T. 104 (8 jan. 1785–23 dec. 1785), entry for 23 juillet 1785. Also see entry for 31 août 1785, and T. 105 (10 jan. 1787–23 dec. 1787), entry for 5 mai 1787.

[104] De La Michodière, "Tables alphabétique des villes, bourgs, villages dans différentes régions de France, Moyenne des naissances, mariages, morts sur les années 1781, 1782, 1783," 2ème cartonnier 1785, Académie des Sciences, Paris.

geographical in orientation. Because the British state did not enumerate its population, individuals tallied their own figures, carried out their own private surveys, and published their own results in the scientific and medical press. By contrast, French arithmeticians typically worked for or with the government and advocated an enlightened approach to administration, which included having accurate numerical accounts of the population. Government officials, such as the intendant La Michodière and Controller-General Terray, concentrated their efforts on record keeping to secure accuracy, and mathematically inclined administrators, such as Messance, La Michodière, Moheau, and Montyon, made use of the figures collected by the government from parish registers. In a radical break with the tradition that held that a census was the only way to secure an accurate account of population, Moheau argued that administrators needed only approximate figures for the population and that the method of calculating population from the number of births was entirely satisfactory.

Just how satisfactory were those approximations became one of the questions the mathematician and natural philosopher Pierre Simon de Laplace considered in his investigations into the calculus of probabilities. In 1783, Laplace created a new way to look at the universal multiplier by focusing on problems of error in an article published in the *Mémoires* of the Académie Royale des Sciences,[105] one of several written by Laplace on the calculus of probabilities between 1772 and 1786.[106] In this particular paper, he presented what later became known as "Laplace's method" of calculating population.[107]

"The population of France, deduced from the annual births," Laplace asserted, is "only a probable result, and consequently susceptible to errors."[108] Using the calculus of probabilities, Laplace calculated how extensive a partial census needed to be in order to limit this error:

---

[105] Pierre Simon de Laplace, "Sur les naissances, les mariages et les morts, à Paris, depuis 1771 jusqu'en 1784; & dans toute l'étendue de la France, pendant les années 1781 & 1782," *Mémoires de l'Académie Royale des Sciences de Paris,* 1783 (Paris, 1786), pp. 693–702; *Oeuvres complètes* (14 vols, ed. l'Académie des Sciences, 1878–1912), vol. 11, pp. 35–46. For a discussion of Laplace and his work in demography, see C.C. Gillispie, *Science and Polity in France at the End of the Old Regime,* pp. 40–50. Regarding Laplace's use of probability theory in demography, see C.C. Gillispie, "Probability and Politics"; Daston, *Classical Probability in the Enlightenment,* pp. 275–278; Jacques and Michel Dupâquier, *Histoire de la démographie,* pp. 186–188.

[106] In these writings, Laplace developed what statisticians today call inverse probability – that is, reasoning from effect to cause. See Stephen M. Stigler, *The History of Statistics – The Measurement of Uncertainty before 1900* (Cambridge, Mass.: The Belknap Press of Harvard University Press, 1986), esp. Chapter 3. For a detailed discussion of Laplace's conception of probability, see Daston, *Classical Probability in the Enlightenment,* esp. pp. 267–278.

[107] See Bru, "Estimations Laplaciennes"; for a brief summary of Laplace's method, see Stephen Stigler, *The History of Statistics,* pp. 163–164, who cites the following works for technical discussions of Laplace's method: Pearson, *The History of Statistics in the 17th and 18th Centuries,* pp. 462–465; O.B. Sheynin, "P.S. Laplace's Work on Probability," *Archive for History of Exact Sciences* 16 (1976): 137–187; W.G. Cochran, "Laplace's Ratio Estimator," in *Contributions to Survey Sampling and Applied Statistics,* ed. H.A. David (New York: Wiley, 1978), pp. 3–10. Also see Laplace, *Théorie analytique des probabilités,* 1st ed. (1812), pp. 391–401.

[108] Laplace, "Sur les naissances," p. 37.

Now I find by my analysis, that to have a probability of 1000 to one, to not be mistaken by half a million in this evaluation of the population of France, it is necessary for the census which serves to limit the factor 26 [i.e., the universal multiplier] to have been 771469 inhabitants [i.e., the minimum size of the partial census].[109]

It was not until Napoleon had assumed the reigns of power that Laplace was able to put theory into practice. In his *Essai philosophique sur les probabilités,* Laplace provided an account of a partial census undertaken by the French government in 1802 upon his recommendation: "In thirty districts spread out equally over the whole of France, communities have been chosen which would be able to furnish the most exact information. Their enumerations have given 2037615 individuals as the total number of their inhabitants on the 23rd of September, 1802." He then gave figures for the same thirty districts of the annual number of births for the years 1800, 1801, and 1802, and he calculated the ratio of the population to annual births as 28 − 352845/1000000 − using the same degree of precision as Moheau. Laplace's mathematical sophistication and creativity became evident in his next question: "But what is the probability that the population thus determined will not deviate from the true population beyond a given limit?"[110] By raising this question, Laplace admitted that the results of his precise calculation were not completely accurate and, further, that he sought to define the limits of inaccuracy.

In Britain, a similar process was recommended by John Rickman, who eventually took charge of the 1801 census. He advocated enumeration in a series of proposals brought to Parliament, but conceded that it was "fraught with trouble and expence" and, in language resembling Moheau's, "attempts an accuracy not necessary, or indeed attainable, in a fluctuating subject." Moreover, since a census would not resolve the depopulation issue, he proposed that information on the number of births, burials, and marriages be collected from parish registers and that an accurate multiplier be calculated from "exact enumerations" made of three or four "distant parishes in each county . . . where almost every man is deposited in his own church yard."[111] Rickman's proposal was adopted, and in the actual census, the form for vital registration concentrated entirely on answering the question of whether Britain's population had increased or declined over the eighteenth century. The form asked for the number of burials and baptisms for each decade in the eighteenth century and, thus, endorsed the method of the universal multiplier that had been developed by the political arithmeticians.

If Rickman's census was a scientific instrument for counting the people, it was nonetheless a blunt one. For whatever it provided in terms of precise numbers

<hr>

[109] Laplace, "Sur les naissances," p. 38.
[110] Laplace, *A Philosophical Essay on Probabilities,* trans. from the sixth French edition by Frederick Wilson Truscott and Frederick Lincoln Emory (New York: Dover, 1951), p. 67.
[111] John Rickman, "Thoughts on the Utility and Facility of Ascertaining the Population," *The Commercial and Agricultural Magazine* 2 (June 1800): 391–399; reprinted in Glass, *Numbering the People,* pp. 106–113; quotations from pp. 111, 112.

of persons, it lost in detail of individual life and death. Significantly, the form for vital registration completely omitted cause and age of death, the most useful information to physicians and annuity calculators.[112] This led William Morgan, Richard Price's nephew and an important figure in the field of insurance, to charge that the 1801 census "appears to have been instituted for the mere purpose of determining a controversy."[113] Morgan, himself, did not believe that the census closed the controversy, but most other observers did. The results of the 1801 census showed the population of England and Wales to be 9.168 million people – almost double the figures calculated by Brakenridge and Price.

The degree of mathematical complexity that separated Laplace from Rickman was marked. Rickman's solution to determining an accurate multiplier was to pick three or four isolated parishes in each county, with little or no immigration and emigration, and carry out a careful count. In stark contrast, Laplace focused solely on how large a partial enumeration had to be in order to calculate the total population from the number of births within an acceptable degree of error. Rickman's solution was geographic; Laplace's probabilistic. Thus, the sophistication of the French mathematical community – already evident in their writings on inoculation – was brought to bear on the population calculations. In both countries, population became something that could be calculated, not just counted. And some even argued that calculations were, in fact, more accurate than a census.

---

[112] *An Act for Taking an Account of the Population of Great Britain, and of the Increase or Diminution Thereof* [31 December 1800], George III cap. XV; expedient, p.1.; reprinted in Glass, *The Development of Population Statistics.*

[113] In R. Price, *Observations on Reversionary Payments,* 7th ed. (London, 1812), vol. 2, pp. 211–212; cited in Glass, *Numbering the People,* p. 95.

Conclusion

In 1798, Thomas Malthus published his *Essay on the Principle of Population* in which he sought to convince the public of the threat of overpopulation after decades of debate over depopulation. Malthus's fear of overpopulation differed significantly from the long-standing anxiety over depopulation. The latter, as we have seen, was treated as a fundamental impediment to the wealth and strength of a nation, and accordingly, attention focused almost entirely on the external threats to a nation with a small or diminishing population: insufficient number of men to bear arms, too few laborers to till the fields, a decline in commerce and learning. Juxtapose this scenario with the internal threats provoked by overpopulation: hunger, death, and possible rebellion. Malthus's question was not one of good or despotic government, but of the ability to govern at all. Only an event as disruptive as the French Revolution could have produced such a radical change of perspective. The internal threats posed by the people of Paris, rather than the external threats of foreign armies, were held responsible for the excesses of the events in France. Looking around his own country, Malthus could only assume that the dislocations in population brought on by manufacturing would lead inevitably to a similar bloody outcome.

Malthus was not alone in expounding this emerging internal danger. Politicians in both Britain and France perceived the same unruly possibility, and for this reason, both governments imposed a national census in the early years of the nineteenth century. Thus, what had begun as a philosophical inquiry became central to government after 1800. A regular, comprehensive census of the people, it was assumed among politicians, increased government's control of those people. In Foucault's words, population became "an object of surveillance, analysis, intervention, modification, etc."[1]

But a census – a numbering of the people – need not be regarded solely as an instrument of centralized government discipline. Numbering the people could

---

[1] Michel Foucault, "The Politics of Health in the Eighteenth Century," in *Power/Knowledge – Selected Interviews and Other Writings, 1972–1977*, ed. Colin Gordon, trans. Colin Gordon, Leo Marshall, John Mepham, and Kate Soper (New York: Pantheon Books, 1980), p. 171.

Conclusion

also serve as a mechanism for democratic participation. The best eighteenth-century example of this is found in the Constitution of the United States, where a census formed the basis for proportional representation and a republican form of government. In this case, a census of the population placed power in the hands of the very people who were being enumerated.

This same sort of ambiguity marked the use of quantification in medicine. In a reversal of the widespread disinterest among eighteenth-century French physicians in numerical accounts, statistics became one of the hallmarks of a distinctive approach to medicine taught in the Paris hospitals beginning in the wake of the Revolution.[2] Not only were therapies and patient outcomes evaluated numerically, but in the emerging field of public health, physicians became the leading quantifiers in nineteenth-century France.[3] Foucault and others have identified and emphasized the dehumanizing features of clinical statistics (where the patient becomes just another case of a certain disease or condition). But other less pessimistic accounts of medical statistics have underscored its positive effects, most prominently the development of the random clinical trial as the best method to evaluate the efficacy of medical treatments. In these narratives, numbers become the measure of improvement in patient care.[4]

Whether in government or in hospitals, statistics of the nineteenth and twentieth centuries differ markedly from eighteenth-century political and medical arithmetic. The ability of the state and other bureaucratic institutions to provide continuity, centralization, and authenticity in record keeping increased significantly after 1800. In sharp contrast, the activities of eighteenth-century arithmeticians were voluntary, sporadic, and highly contingent on particular controversies.

In the English inoculation debates, John Arbuthnot and James Jurin created the revolutionary technique of calculating the risks of dying from inoculated and natural smallpox. The Royal Society furnished the resources for Jurin's work and an audience for the types of arguments he developed. Arbuthnot and Jurin demonstrated how the numbers of dead could be used to evaluate a medical procedure, and clearly, many were persuaded by this novel approach. Later in the century, during the controversy over inoculating the urban poor, physicians once again turned to the number of deaths attributed to smallpox (culled from the London bills of mortality) to evaluate whether inoculation had increased smallpox mortality. They constructed myriad tables, but in spite of

[2] Erwin Ackerknecht, *Medicine at the Paris Hospital, 1794–1848* (Baltimore: Johns Hopkins Press, 1967).
[3] Ann LaBerge, *Mission and Method: The Early Nineteenth-Century French Public Health Movement* (Cambridge: Cambridge University Press, 1992), chap. 2, pp. 49–81; William Coleman, *Death is a Social Disease: Public Health and Political Economy in Early Industrial France* (Madison: University of Wisconsin Press, 1982), esp. chap. 5, pp. 124–148.
[4] Ackerknecht, *Medicine at the Paris Hospital, 1794–1848*; Michel Foucault, *The Birth of the Clinic: An Archaeology of Medical Perception*, trans. A.M. Sheridan Smith (1963; New York: Vintage Books, 1975); J. Rosser Matthews, *Quantification and the Quest for Medical Certainty* (Princeton, N.J.: Princeton University Press, 1995).

their ingenuity, numerical accounts failed to secure consensus, and the whole method of using tables for demonstration came under criticism.

In France, philosophes, not physicians, promoted the practice of inoculation. The Paris Académie Royale des Sciences, like the Royal Society, provided an important venue for the development of quantitative approaches. The academician Daniel Bernoulli extended Jurin's work through the calculus of probabilities and mathematically sophisticated tables showing the risks of dying from natural smallpox at different ages and the gains to the population if inoculation were universally practiced. Jean d'Alembert, while supportive of inoculation, responded that Bernoulli's mathematical approach was not at all persuasive because probabilistic calculations about populations could not adequately represent future risks to individuals, especially mothers. The complexity of these arguments, based on the calculus of probabilities, blocked nonmathematicians from participating in the debate. Because of the high degree of specialization, most French physicians remained aloof and indifferent to quantitative arguments.

Another remarkable difference is the nearly complete absence of numerical tables in the French inoculation debates. The absence reflected the dearth of vital accounts. Consequently, Bernoulli, d'Alembert, and others called for the collection of more numbers. But even when numerical information about inoculation was available, for example in La Condamine's history of inoculation, it was embedded in the text, rather than placed in a separate table.[5] The French preferred a pleasant literary style to a shopkeeper's unadorned account.

In the case of medical meteorology, numerical tables proved useful as instruments to collect, rather than to display, observations. Tables encouraged consistency and regularity in recording information, and they facilitated comparison between sets of observations. But their design varied considerably. In some, daily weather observations remained paramount, and notes on acute diseases (those believed to be most affected by weather) were relegated to the bottom of the form. In others, the course of an individual's disease took precedence, and weather observations, at first listed alongside daily notes of symptoms, were subsequently placed in a separate table. In the most ambitious set of tables, the French physician Jean Razoux coupled daily weather observations with the numbers of patients categorized by disease and sex being treated at the Hôtel-Dieu in Nîmes. He left the bulk of conclusions to be drawn by the reader, a common conceit among advocates of numerical tables, who argued that such results were self-evident.

In environmental medicine more generally, tabulating deaths by carefully chosen categories enabled arithmeticians to observe the rise and fall of specific diseases, the effects of climate and geography on mortality, the high number

[5] Charles Marie de La Condamine, "Suite de l'histoire de l'inoculation de la petite vérole depuis 1758 jusqu'en 1765," *Mémoires de l'Académie Royale des Sciences*, 1765 (Paris, 1768), pp. 513–514.

of infant and child deaths, and the changes in maternal mortality. Tables were heralded as important new instruments to aid not only physicians but politicians as well. But some tables, for example those of Thomas Short, were too exhaustive and too exhausting for the reader. As William Black put it, "the reader must have no small portion of phlegm and resolution to follow them throughout with attention."[6]

In the depopulation controversy, almost all the participants acknowledged the pertinence and utility of quantification. But if quantification was not questioned, the actual figures presented certainly were. Critics challenged population estimates taken from religious and secular sources, as well as the methods of calculation constructed to make the estimates. These criticisms increased the pressure on government officials to collect and evaluate numerical information, hence paving the way for a national census.

In comparing quantification in England and France, a very striking contrast emerges, namely, the prominent role played by physicians in England and their virtual absence in France. In England, the writings of doctors, from Petty to Percival, Arbuthnot to Short, and Jurin to Black, predominate in medical and political arithmetic. Given their professional orientation and the availability of the London bills of mortality, the English focused on variable rates of mortality. In France, almost no doctors employed quantitative arguments or contributed to political and medical arithmetic. Instead, government administrators – from Vauban, to the Controller-Generals Orry and Terray, to the secretaries Messance and Moheau, to the intendants Montyon and La Michodière – were the chief quantifiers in eighteenth-century France. Rather than drawing on or generating bills of mortality, they concentrated their efforts on enumerations of the population, an administrative bias reflected in French political arithmeticians' concerns for fiscal matters. Mortality rates by disease were only of passing interest.

Two sorts of explanation can account for these cultural differences. The first concerns institutional structures. French physicians remained far more accountable to local faculties of medicine than did English doctors, and French medical faculties held vested interest in maintaining local control of medical practice and education in order to preserve their powerful positions. The organization of eighteenth-century French medicine thus contributed to its conservative and traditional character and impeded the introduction of new practices, such as inoculation, or new forms of argument, such as those based on numerical tables. It is no surprise that the innovative Société Royale de Médecine, founded in 1776, challenged the authority of established French medical corporations by fostering new modes of inquiry, including the collection and use of numerical information.

[6] William Black, *An Arithmetical and Medical Analysis of the Diseases and Mortality of the Human Species* (London, 1789), p. 37.

In England, by the end of the seventeenth century, the Royal College of Physicians had degenerated to such a low point that it simply did not exert control over the profession.[7] Medical practice was neither regulated nor supervised to the extent that French practice was, and physicians advanced their careers in more entrepreneurial ways. So, for example, a considerable number were members of the Royal Society, while in France, few practicing physicians were elected to the exclusive Académie Royale des Sciences.[8] The relatively open nature of the London Royal Society exposed physicians to quantitative and mathematical approaches to knowledge. In consequence, English physicians frequently embraced more wide-ranging interests and activities than did their French counterparts.

The second sort of explanation concerns the types of sources containing numerical information about different populations. The London bills of mortality, initially collected to monitor the occurrence of plague, became the major source for the writings of English political and medical arithmeticians. The bills were unique; they were the only continuous, contemporary, numerical documents concerning population. Unlike parish registers, they did not list individuals' names; rather, they provided counts of baptisms and burials. The resulting quality of anonymity, of individuals being represented by numbers as part of a group, was strikingly new and unusual.

English political and medical arithmeticians did not rely solely on the London bills of mortality, however. They also solicited and collected their own information. Correspondence networks were yet another key component to quantification. Gathering individual accounts, classifying them, and rendering them into numbers became the critical activities of English arithmeticians. In contrast, French arithmeticians generally relied on numbers already collected by the state. They did not generate new data so much as manipulate the old.

Most political and medical arithmeticians trumpeted the profound advantages of tables and calculations. Short, for example, declared that tables were vital to any understanding of the history of epidemics. Tables forged *the* link between annual accounts of baptisms and burials, disease and meteorological observations, and observations on medical practice. They made it obvious to anyone reading them which situations were the most fertile ("productive of People"). They also provided a ready means to assess the impact of "new Improvements, Trades, Manufactories &c. to Health."[9] The French secretary Moheau thought tables of mortality, if made public, would be more effective in changing people's

---

[7] See Harold Cook, *The Decline of the Old Medical Regime in Stuart London* (Ithaca, N.Y.: Cornell University Press, 1986).

[8] Alternative societies, most prominently the Société Royale de Médecine, were established in France to redress the perceived need for an official scientific society of medicine. See Roger Hahn, *The Anatomy of a Scientific Institution – The Paris Academy of Sciences, 1666–1803* (Berkeley: University of California Press, 1971), pp. 101–104.

[9] Short, *New Observations, Natural, Moral, Civil, Political, and Medical, on City, Town, and Country Bills of Mortality* (London, 1750), p. 83.

XXV. *Tables of the comparative Mortality of the* Meafles, *from* 1768 *to* 1774, *collected from the Regifter of the Collegiate* Church *in* Manchefter, *by Dr.* Percival.

T A B L E I.

Ages.	Males.	Females.	Seafons.		Total of Deaths, by all Difeafes, during fix years.
From birth to 3 months.	I	I	Jan.		
			Feb.	17	
From 3 to 6 months.	3	0	March		
			April		
1 year.	6	4	May		
2	17	14	June	51	
3	17	8	July		
			Aug.	16	
4	4	3	Sept.		
5	2	7	Oct.		
10	0	2	Nov.		
20	0	1	Dec.	7	
30	0	1			
Total	50	41		*91	3807

C.1 Thomas Percival's table of measles deaths listed by age, sex, and month (1768–1774). *Source:* Thomas Percival, "Essay on the Small-Pox and Measles," in *Medical Observations and Inquiries*, Vol. 5 (1776), p. 282. Yale University, Harvey Cushing/John Hay Whitney Medical Library.

behavior than any type of police action. "If the causes of death were published annually," Moheau explained, "this table put under the eyes of people would give a more persuasive lesson than all dissertations. The number of people drowned, or those suffocated by charcoal fumes, would inspire views of prudence and caution that the most rigid police cannot supply."[10]

By the late eighteenth century, political and medical arithmeticians had come to believe in the immediate transparency of tables. "This table requires no comments," Thomas Percival asserted after presenting one showing measles mortality

[10] Moheau, *Recherches et considérations sur la population de la France,* reedition annotated by Eric Vilquin (Paris: Institut National d'Études Démographiques, Presses Universitaires de France, 1994), pp. 242–243.

at different ages.[11] (See Figure C.1.) And indeed, this particular table was a model of conciseness and clarity that could stand without explanation. Moreover, the power, persuasiveness, and effectiveness of tables (especially as tools of investigation) had become commonplace. "Many other very important corollaries may be deduced from this and the preceding tables," Percival concluded, "but I wish rather to excite, than to anticipate the inquiries of the intelligent reader."[12] Tables, thus, were informative, instructive, and very interesting, all at the same time.

Tables, however, were only part of the greater transformation wrought by the quantification of things human. The act of counting human beings, born, diseased, or dead, perforce introduced an assumption of radical equality: Each individual of a quantified group (whether rich or poor, young or old, male or female) was considered equivalent to every other member of that group when counted. Quantification focused attention on groups, categories of people, rather than on individuals. Assigning numbers to people created anonymity as well as identity; it depersonalized, and dehumanized, and at the same time it leveled an unequal and hierarchical society. Whether one takes a pessimistic or optimistic view of numbers, the Janus-faced nature of quantification has been with us since the end of the eighteenth century.

---

[11] Percival, "Essay on the Smallpox and Measles," *Medical Observations and Inquiries*, Vol. 5 (1776), p. 283.
[12] Percival, "Essay on the Smallpox and Measles," p. 289.

BIBLIOGRAPHY

MANUSCRIPT SOURCES

Archives de l'Académie des Sciences, Paris
 MS 2eme cartonnier 1785
 MS Procès Verbaux
Archives départementale de l'Hérault, Montpellier
 D 144
 D 189
 10 F51
Archives Nationales, Paris
 F20 104
 F20 441
Bodleian, Oxford
 Rawlinson D.871
British Library, London
 Sloane MSS 4034, 4047, 406B
 Add. MSS 4440, 8757
Royal Society of London
 Classified Papers XXIII (1–2)
 Council Minutes
 Early Letters
 Letter Book
 Journal Books, XII
 Register Book Copy
 Meteorological Archives
Wellcome Institute for the History of Medicine, London
 Wellcome MS 6146

PRINTED PRIMARY SOURCES

Anonymous. *An Account of the Rise, Progress and State of the Hospital, for Relieving Poor People Afflicted with the Small Pox, and for Inoculation.* n.p., n.d. [1754].
 A Computation of the Increase of London, and Parts Adjacent; with Some Causes Thereof, and Remarks Thereon. London, 1719.

Considerations on the Propriety of a Plan for Inoculating the Poor of London at Their Own Habitations: With a View Particularly to the Arguments Urged in Defense of It, by the Author of a Late Anonymous Letter to Dr. J.C. Lettsom. London, 1779.

L'inoculation nécessaire. n.p., 1759.

A Letter to a Member of Parliament on the Registering and Numbering the People of Great Britain. London, 1753. Reprinted in D.V. Glass, ed., *The Development of Population Statistics.* Farnborough, Hants, Eng.: Gregg International Publishers, 1973.

A Letter to J.C. Lettsom, MD, FRS, SAS & c. Occasioned by Baron Dimsdale's Remarks on Dr. Lettsom's Letter to Sir Robert Barker, and G. Stacpoole, esq. upon General Inoculation. By an Uninterested Spectator of the Controversy between Baron Dimsdale and Dr. Watkinson. London, 1779.

The Medical Register for the Year 1779. London, 1779.

The New Practice of Inoculating the Small-Pox Consider'd. And an Humble Application to the Approaching Parliament for the Regulation of That Dangerous Experiment. London, 1722.

Plan of a Dispensary for Inoculating the Poor. n.p., n.d.

A Representation from the Governors of the Hospital for the Small-Pox and for Inoculation. n.p., n.d. [1756].

A Serious Address to the Public concerning the Most Probable Means of Avoiding the Dangers of Inoculation. London, 1758.

Uncertainty of the Present Population of This Kingdom; Deduced from a Candid Review of the Accounts Lately Given of It by Dr. Price, on the One Hand, Mr. Eden, Mr. Wales, and Mr. Howlett on the Other. London, 1781.

Aikin, John. "The Bill of Mortality of the Town of Warrington, for the Year 1773." *Philosophical Transactions* 64 (1774): 438–444.

Arbuthnot, John. "An Argument for Divine Providence Taken from the Regularity Observ'd in the Birth of Both Sexes." *Philosophical Transactions* 27 (1710–1712): 186–190.

An Essay concerning the Effects of Air on Human Bodies. London, 1733.

An Essay on the Usefulness of Mathematical Learning in a Letter from a Gentleman in the City to his Friend in Oxford. 2d ed. [1st ed., 1701] Oxford, 1721.

Of the Laws of Chance. London, 1692.

[Arbuthnot, John]. *Mr. Maitland's Account of Inoculating the Smallpox Vindicated, from Dr. Wagstaffe's Misrepresentations of That Practice, with Some Remarks on Mr. Massey's Sermon.* London, 1722.

[Astruc, Jean.] *Doutes sur l'inoculation de la petite vérole, proposés à la Faculté de Médecine de Paris.* n.p., 1756.

Aubrey, John. *Brief Lives.* Ed. Richard Barber. London: The Boydell Press, 1982.

[Auffray, Jean.] *Le luxe consideré relativement à la population et à l'économie.* Lyon, 1762.

Baker, George. *An Inquiry into the Merits of a Method of Inoculating the Small-Pox, Which Is Now Practised in Several Counties of England.* London, 1766.

Barrow. "An Account of the Births and Burials with the Number of Inhabitants at Stoke-Damerell in the County of Devon." *Philosophical Transactions* 39 (1735–1736): 171–172.

Bayle, Pierre. "Deux essais d'arithmetique politique touchant les villes et hospitaux de Londres et de Paris." *Nouvelles de la république des lettres,* October 1685, pp. 1144–1151.

Bell, John. *London's Remembrancer, or a True Account of Christnings and Mortality in All the Years of the Pestilence within the Cognizance of the Bills of Mortality Being XVIII Years Taken Out of the Register of the Company of Parish Clerks of London, &c.* London, 1665.

[Berkeley, George.] *The Analyst: Or, a Discourse Addressed to an Infidel Mathematician.* London, 1734.

Bernoulli, Daniel. "Essai d'une nouvelle analyse de la mortalité causée par la petite vérole et des avantages de l'inoculation pour la prévenir." *Mémoires de l'Académie Royale des Sciences,* 1760 (Paris, 1765), Part 2, pp. 1–79.

Birch, Thomas. *A Collection of the Yearly Bills of Mortality from 1657 to 1758 Inclusive.* London, 1759.

The History of the Royal Society of London. Vols. 1–4. Facsimile of London Edition of 1756–1757. Introduction by A. Rupert Hall and Marie Boas Hall. New York: Johnson Reprint Corporation, 1968.

Black, William. *An Arithmetical and Medical Analysis of the Diseases and Mortality of the Human Species.* London, 1789. Reprinted with an introduction by D.V. Glass. Farnborough, Hants, Eng.: Gregg International Publishers Limited, 1973.

Observations Medical and Political: On the Small-pox and Inoculation; and on the Decrease of Mankind at Every Age with a Comparative View of the Diseases Most Fatal to London during Ninety Years. London, 1781.

Observations Medical and Political, on the Smallpox and Inoculation; and on the Mortality of Mankind at Every Age in City and Country ... To Which Is Added a Postscript. 2d ed. London, 1781.

Bodin, Jean. *Six Books of the Commonwealth.* Trans. and Abridged by M.J. Tooley. 1576; Oxford: Basil Blackwell [1955].

Boswell, James. *Life of Samuel Johnson LLD.* 1791; New York: Modern Library, 1931.

Boylston, Zabdiel. *An Historical Account of the Small-Pox Inoculated in New England, upon All Sorts of Persons, Whites, Blacks, and of All Ages and Constitutions.* London, 1726.

Brady, Samuel. *Some Remarks upon Dr. Wagstaffe's Letter, and Mr. Massey's Sermon against Inoculating the Smallpox ... In Three Letters to a Friend.* London, 1722.

Brakenridge, William. "A Letter from the Reverend William Brakenridge, D.D. and F.R.S. to George Lewis Scot, Esq; F.R.S. concerning the Number of Inhabitants within the London Bills of Mortality." *Philosophical Transactions* 48 (1754): 788–800.

"A Letter to George Lewis Scot, Esq; F.R.S. concerning the Number of People in England; from the Reverend William Brakenridge, D.D. Rector of St. Michael Bassishaw, and F.R.S." *Philosophical Transactions* 49 (1755–1756): 268–285.

"A Letter to George Lewis Scot, Esquire, concerning the Present Increase of the People in Britain and Ireland." *Philosophical Transactions* 49 (1755–1756): 877–890.

Brieude. "Topographie médicale de la haute Auvergne." *Histoire de la Société Royale de Médecine,* 1782–1783 (Paris, 1787), pp. 257–340.

Brown, John. *An Estimate of the Manners and Principles of the Times.* 2d ed. London, 1757.

Browning, John. "The Number of People in the City of Bristol, Calculated from the Burials for Ten Years Successive, and Also from the Number of Houses." *Philosophical Transactions* 48 (1753): 217–220.

Burges, James. *An Account of the Preparation and Management Necessary to Inoculation.* London, 1754.

Butini, Jean-Antoine. *Traité de la petite vérole, communiquée par l'inoculation.* Paris, 1752.

Byrom, John. *The Private Journal and Literary Remains of John Byrom.* Ed. Richard Parkinson. Manchester: Chetham Society, 1854.

Chais, Charles. *Essai apologétique sur la méthode de communiquer la petite vérole par inoculation; où l'on tâche de faire voir que la conscience ne auroit en être blessée, ni la religion offensée.* A la Haye, 1754.

Chalmers, George. *An Estimate of the Comparative Strength of Great Britain during the Present and Four Preceding Reigns.* 2d ed. London, 1791.

Clifton, Francis. *The State of Physick, Ancient and Modern, Briefly Consider'd: with a Plan for the Improvement of It.* London, 1732.

———. *Tabular Observations Recommended as the Plainest and Surest Way of Practising and Improving Physick in a Letter to a Friend.* London, 1731.

Clinch, William. *An Historical Essay on the Rise and Progress of the Small-Pox. To Which Is Added, a Short Appendix, to Prove, That Inoculation Is No Security from the Natural Small-Pox.* London, 1725.

Colman, Benjamin. *Some Observations on the New Method of Receiving the Small-Pox by Ingrafting or Inoculating.* Boston, 1721.

Considerations on a Bill for Obliging all Parishes of This Kingdom to Keep Proper Registers of Births, Deaths, and Marriages. London, 1759.

Cotte, Louis. *Traité de météorologie.* Paris, 1774.

Cotte, R.P. "Mémoire sur la topographie médicale de Montmarenci & ses environs." *Histoire de la Société Royale de Médecine,* 1779 (Paris, 1782), pp. 61–83.

Cousin. "Sur la vertu anti-septique du quinquina." In *Receuil d'observations de médecine des hôpitaux militaires.* Ed. François-Marie-Claude Richard de Hautesierck. 2 vols. Paris, 1782, vol. 2., p. 531.

d'Alembert, Jean. *Oeuvres philosophiques, historiques et littéraires de d'Alembert.* Ed. J.F. Bastien. 18 vols. Paris, 1805.

———. *Opuscules mathématiques.* 8 vols. Paris, 1761–1780.

Davenant, Charles. *Discourses on the Public Revenues and Trade.* London, 1698.

DeBaux, Pierre. *Parallèle de la petite vérole naturelle, avec l'artificielle, ou inoculée, avec un traité intermédiare de la petite vérole fausse, volante, ou adultérine.* Avignon, 1761.

DeHaen, Anton. *Réfutation de l'inoculation servant de réponse à deux pieces qui ont paru cette année 1759. Dont la première est une dissertation lue dans la Société de l'Académie Royale des Sciences de Paris par M. de la Condamine, et la seconde, une lettre de Mr. Tyssot.* Vienne, 1759.

Delacoste, J. *Lettre sur l'inoculation de la petite vérole comme elle se pratique en Turquie et en Angleterre.* Paris, 1723.

DeMoivre, Abraham. *Annuities for Life.* London, 1725.

Déparcieux, Antoine. *Essai sur les probabilités de la durée de la vie humaine.* Paris, 1746.

Derham, William. *Physico-Theology or, a Demonstration of the Being and Attributes of God from His Works of Creation.* Reprint of 4th ed. 1716; New York: Arno Press, 1977.

d'Expilly, Jean J. *Dictionnaire géographique, historique et politique des gaules et de la France.* 1762; Liechtenstein: Kraus Reprint, 1978.

Dimsdale, Thomas. *Observations on the Introduction to the Plan of the Dispensary for General Inoculation. With Remarks on a Pamphlet Entitled "An Examination of a Charge Brought against Inoculation by DeHaen, Rast, Dimsdale, and Other Writers. By John Watkinson, MD."* London, 1778.

Thoughts on General and Partial Inoculations. London, 1776.

Dodd, William. *The Practice of Inoculation Recommended, in a Sermon Preached at St. James's, Westminster, April the 9th, 1767, on the Anniversary Meeting of the Governors of the Small-pox Hospital.* London, n.d. [1767].

Dodson, James. "A Letter from Mr. James Dodson to Mr. John Robertson, F.R.S. concerning an Improvement of the Bills of Mortality." *Philosophical Transactions* 47 (1753): 333–340.

"A Letter to the Reverend William Brakenridge, D.D. Rector of St. Mich. Bassishaw, and F.R.S. with a Table of the Value of Annuities on Lives." *Philosophical Transactions* 49 (1755–1756): 891–892.

"A Letter to the Right Honourable George Earl of Macclesfield, P.R.S. concerning the Value of an Annuity for Life, and the Probability of Survivorship." *Philosophical Transactions* 48 (1754): 487–499.

Duhamel du Monceau, H.L. "Observations botanico-météorologiques, faites au château de Denainvilliers proche Pluviers en Gâtinois pendant l'année 1754." *Mémoires de l'Académie Royale des Sciences,* 1754 (Paris, 1759), pp. 383–412.

Eden, Frederick Morton. *An Estimate of the Number of Inhabitants in Great Britain and Ireland.* London, 1800.

Faiguet de Villeneuve, Joachim. *Discours d'un bon citoyen, sur les moyens de multiplier les forces de l'Etat, & d'augmenter la population.* Brussels, 1760.

Fielding, John. *A Plan of the Universal Register Office.* London, 1752.

Forster, Richard. "An Extract of the Register of the Parish of Great Shefford, near Lamborne, in Berkshire, for Ten Years: With Observations on the Same: In a Letter to Tho. Birch, D.D. Secret. R.S. from the Reverend Mr. Richard Forster, Rector of Great Shefford." *Philosophical Transactions* 50 (1757): 356–363.

"A Letter to the Rev. Thomas Birch, D.D. Secr. R.S. concerning the Number of People of England; by the Rev. Richard Forster, Rector of Great Shefford in Berkshire." *Philosophical Transactions* 50 (1757): 457–465.

Fothergill, John. "Some Remarks on the Bills of Mortality in London with an Account of a Late Attempt to Establish an Annual Bill for This Nation." *The Works of John Fothergill.* Ed. John Coakley Lettsom. 3 vols. London, 1784.

Frewen, Thomas. *The Practice and Theory of Inoculation with an Account of Its Success. In a Letter to a Friend.* London, 1749.

Galiani, l'Abbé Ferdinand. *Correspondance.* 2 vols. Paris, 1889.

Gardeil. "Mémoire sur une épidémie qui a régné à Toulouse pendant l'automne de l'année 1772." *Histoire de la Société Royale de Médecine,* 1776 (Paris, 1779), pp. 14–22.

Graunt, John. *Natural and Political Observations Made upon the Bills of Mortality.* London, 1662.

Natural and Political Observations Made upon the Bills of Mortality. 3rd Edition, Much Enlarged. London, 1665.

Natural and Political Observations Made upon the Bills of Mortality. The Fourth Impression. Oxford, 1665.

Natural and Political Observations Made upon the Bills of Mortality. The Fifth Edition, Much Enlarged. London, 1676. Reprinted in *The Economic Writings of Sir William Petty.* Ed. Charles Henry Hull. Cambridge: Cambridge University Press, 1899.

Halley, Edmond. "An Estimate of the Degrees of the Mortality of Mankind, Drawn from Curious Tables of the Births and Funerals at the City of Breslaw." *Philosophical Transactions* 17–18 (1693): 596–610.

"Some Further Considerations on the Breslaw Bills of Mortality." *Philosophical Transactions* 17–18 (1693): 654–656.

Hatton, Edward. *An Intire System of Arithmetic: Or Arithmetic in All Its Parts.* London, 1721.

A New View of London; or, an Ample Account of That City. London, 1708.

Haygarth, John. "Bills of Mortality for Chester for the Year 1773." *Philosophical Transactions* 65 (1775): 85–90.

An Inquiry How to Prevent the Small-pox and Proceedings of a Society. Chester, 1785.

"Observations on the Bill of Mortality, in Chester, for the Year 1772." *Philosophical Transactions* 64 (1774): 67–78.

"Observations on the Population and Diseases of Chester, in the Year 1774." *Philosophical Transactions* 68 (1778): 131–154.

A Sketch of a Plan to Exterminate the Casual Small-pox from Great Britain; and to Introduce General Inoculation. Vol. 1 (Vol. 2 was never published). London, 1793.

Heberden, Thomas. "Of the Increase and Mortality of the Inhabitants of the Island of Madeira." *Philosophical Transactions* 57 (1767): 461–463.

Heberden, William. *Observations on the Increase and Decrease of Different Diseases, and Particularly of the Plague.* London, 1801.

[Hecquet, Philippe.] *Observations sur la saignée du pied, et sur la purgation au commencement de la petite vérole, des fièvres malignes & des grandes maladies. Preuves de décadence dans la pratique de médecine, confirmées par de justes raisons de doute contre l'inoculation.* Paris, 1724.

Heysham, John. *Observations on the Bills of Mortality in Carlisle, for the Year 1787.* Carlisle, 1788. Reprinted in *The Development of Population Statistics.* Ed. D.V. Glass. Farnborough, Hants, Eng.: Gregg International Publishers, 1973.

Hillary, William. "An Account of the Principal Variations of the Weather and the Concomitant Epidemical Diseases from 1726 to 1734 at Ripon," bound with his *Essay on the Smallpox.* London, 1740.

Hooke, Robert. *The Diary of Robert Hooke, M.A., M.D., F.R.S., 1672–1680.* Ed. Henry W. Robinson and Walter Adams. London: Taylor & Francis, 1935.

Hosty, A. *Extrait du rapport de M. Hosty, Docteur-Régent de la Faculté de Médecine de Paris, pendant son séjour à Londres, au sujet de l'inoculation. Extrait du Mercure de France, du mois d'Août.* Paris, 1755.

Houlton, Robert. *The Practice of Inoculation Justified. A Sermon Preached at Ingatestone, Essex, October 22, 1766, in Defence of Inoculation.* Chelmsford, 1767.

Howgrave, Francis. *Reasons against the Inoculation of the Small-Pox. In a Letter to Dr. Jurin.* London, 1724.

[Howlett, John.] *Observations on the Increased Population, Healthiness, etc. of Maidstone.* [Maidstone], 1782. Reprinted in *The Development of Population Statistics.* Ed. D.V. Glass. Farnborough, Hants, Eng.: Gregg International Publishers, 1973.

Hume, David. *Essays: Moral, Political, and Literary.* Edinburgh, 1742. In *The Philosophical Works of David Hume.* Ed. T.H. Green and T.H. Grouse. 4 vols. London: Longmans, Green and Co., 1875.

Huxham, John. *Observations on the Air and Epidemic Diseases from the Year MDCCXXVII to MDCCXXXVII Inclusive; Together with a Short Dissertation on Devonshire Colic. Translated from the Latin Original by His Son, John Corham Huxham.* 1739; London: J. Hinton, 1759.

Jaubert, P. *Des causes de la dépopulation et des moyens d'y remédier.* London and Paris, 1767.

Jurin, James. *An Account of the Success of Inoculating the Small Pox in Great Britain with a Comparison between the Miscarriages in That Practice, and the Mortality of the Natural Small Pox.* 2d ed. London, 1724.

An Account of the Success of Inoculating the Small Pox in Great Britain, for the Year 1724. London, 1725.

An Account of the Success of Inoculating the Small-Pox in Great Britain, for the Year 1725. London, 1726.

An Account of the Success of Inoculating the Small-Pox in Great Britain, for the Year 1726. London, 1727.

[Philalethes Cantabrigiensis.] *Geometry No Friend to Infidelity; or, a Defence of Sir Isaac Newton and the British Mathematicians.* London, 1734.

"A Letter to the Learned Caleb Cotesworth, MD, FRS, of the College of Physicians, and Physician to St. Thomas's Hospital, Containing a Comparison between the Mortality of the Natural Small Pox, and That Given by Inoculation." *Philosophical Transactions* 32 (1722–1723): 213–224.

A Letter to the Learned Caleb Cotesworth, MD, FRS, of the College of Physicians, and Physician to St. Thomas's Hospital. Containing a Comparison between the Mortality of the Natural Small Pox, and That Given by Inoculation. Which Is Subjoined an Account of the Success of Inoculation in New-England; As Likewise an Extract from Several Letters concerning a Like Method of Communicating the Small-Pox, That Has Been Used Time out of Mind in South Wales. London, 1723.

King, Gregory. *Two Tracts: Natural and Political Observations upon the State and Condition of England; and of the Naval Trade of England Anno 1688.* Ed. with an introduction by George E. Barnett. Baltimore: Johns Hopkins Press, 1936.

La Condamine, Charles-Marie de. *Histoire de l'inoculation de la petite vérole.* 2 vols. Amsterdam, 1773.

Lettres . . . à M. de Dr. Maty sur l'état présent de l'inoculation en France. Paris, 1764.

"Mémoire sur l'inoculation de la petite vérole." *Mémoires de l'Académie Royale des Sciences,* 1754 (Paris, 1759), pp. 615–670.

"Second mémoire sur l'inoculation de la petite vérole, contenant la suite de l'histoire de cette méthode & de ses progrès, de 1754 à 1758." *Mémoires de l'Académie Royale des Sciences,* 1758 (Paris, 1763), pp. 439–482.

"Suite de l'histoire de l'inoculation de la petite vérole depuis 1758 jusqu'en 1765." *Mémoires de l'Académie Royale des Sciences,* 1765 (Paris, 1768), pp. 505–532.

Laplace, Pierre-Simon. *A Philosophical Essay on Probabilities.* Trans. from the 6th French ed. by Frederick Wilson Truscott and Frederick Lincoln Emory, with an introductory note by E.T. Bell. New York: Dover Publications, Inc, 1951.

"Sur les naissances, les mariages et les morts à Paris, depuis 1771 jusqu'en 1784; et dans toute l'étendue de la France pendant les années 1781 et 1782." *Mémoires de l'Académie Royale des Sciences,* 1783 (Paris, 1786), pp. 693–702.

Théorie analytique des probabilités. Paris, 1812.

Lavoisier, Antoine Laurent. *De la richesse territoriale de la royaume de France.* Texts and Documents presented by Jean-Claude Perrot. Paris: Editions de C.T.H.S., 1988 [1784].

[LeHoc.] *L'Inoculation de la petite vérole renvoyée à Londres.* A la Haye, 1764.

MacKenzie, James. *The History of Health and the Art of Preserving It. The Third Edition: To Which Is Added, a Short and Clear Account of the Commencement, Progress, Utility, and Proper Management of Inoculating the Small-Pox, As a Valuable Branch of the Prophylaxis.* Edinburgh, 1760.

Macquart, Louis-Charles-Henri. *Extrait d'une question sur l'inoculation de la petite vérole.* Inserted in *Journal de Médecine* du mois de Février 1755. n.p., n.d.

Madier. "Mémoire sur la topographie médicale de Bourg-Saint-Andéol." *Histoire de la Société Royale de Médecine,* 1780–1781 (Paris, 1785), pp. 95–152.

Maitland, Charles. *Mr. Maitland's Account of Inoculating the Small Pox.* London, 1722.

Mr. Maitland's Account of Inoculating the Small Pox. 2d ed. London, 1723.

Malouin, Paul-Jacques. "Histoire des maladies épidémiques de 1754. Observées à Paris en même temps que les différentes températures de l'air." *Mémoires de l'Académie Royale des Sciences,* 1754 (Paris, 1759), p. 499.

Marx, Karl. *A Contribution to the Critique of Political Economy.* Trans. from 2d German ed. by N.I. Stone. New York: International Library Publishing Co., 1904 [1859].

Massey, Edmund. *A Letter to Mr. Maitland, in Vindication of the Sermon against Inoculation.* London, 1722.

A Sermon against the Dangerous and Sinful Practice of Inoculation. Preach'd at St. Andrew's Holborn. On Sunday, July the 8th, 1722. London, 1722.

Massey, Isaac. *Remarks on Dr. Jurin's Last Yearly Account of the Success of Inoculation.* London, 1727.

A Short and Plain Account of Inoculation with Some Remarks on the Main Arguments Made Use of to Recommend That Practice, by Mr. Maitland and Others. 2d ed. London, 1723.

[Mather, Cotton.] *An Account of the Method and Success of Inoculating the Small-Pox in Boston in New England.* London, 1722.

Mauduyt, P. J. C. "Mémoire sur le traitement électrique, administré à quatre-vingt-deux malades." *Histoire de la Société Royale de Médecine,* 1777–1778 (Paris, 1780), pp. 199–431.

Messance, Louis. *Recherches sur la population des généralités d'Auvergne, de Lyon, de Rouen, et de quelques provinces et villes du royaume, avec des réflexions sur la valeur du beld tant en France qu'en Angleterre, depuis 1674 jusqu'en 1764.* Paris, 1766.

Mirabeau, Victor de Riqueti, Marquis de. *L'Ami des hommes ou traité de la population.* 2 vols. Reimpression of the Avignon edition, 1758–1760. Darmstadt: Scientia Verlag Aalen, 1970.

Moheau, Jean-Baptiste. *Recherches et considérations sur la population de la France.* Reedition annotated by Éric Vilquin. 1778; Paris: Institut National d'Études Démographiques, Presses Universitaires de France, 1994.

Monro, Alexander. *An Account of Inoculation of Small Pox in Scotland.* Edinburgh, 1765.

Montesquieu, Charles Louis de Secondat. *De l'esprit des lois.* Paris, 1748.

Persian Letters. Trans. John Davidson. 1721; London: George Routledge & Sons.

Montucla, Jean Etienne. *Recueil de pièces concernant l'inoculation de la petite vérole, et propres à en prouver la sécurité et l'utilité.* Paris, 1756.

Morand, Jean. "Récapitulation des baptêmes, mariages, mortuaires & enfans trouvés de la ville & faubourgs de Paris, depuis l'année 1709 jusques et compris l'année 1770." *Mémoires de l'Académie Royale des Sciences de Paris,* 1771 (Paris, 1774), pp. 830–848.

Morris, Corbyn. *An Essay towards Illustrating the Science of Insurance.* London, 1747.

Observations on the Past Growth and Present State of the City of London. London, 1751.

Mourgue, Jacques-Augustin. *Essai de statistique.* Paris, an IX.

"Plan d'observations sur la cause des variations de l'atmosphere." *Mémoires de la Société Royale des Sciences de Montpellier,* 1772.

Neal, David. *A Narrative of the Method and Success of Inoculating the Small Pox in New England. By Mr. Benjamin Colman . . . To Which Is Now Prefixed, an Historical Introduction.* London, 1722.

Necker, Jacques. *De l'administration des finances de la France.* 1784.

Nettleton, Thomas. *An Account of the Success of Inoculating the Small-Pox; in a Letter to Dr. William Whitaker.* London, 1722.

"A Letter from Dr. Nettleton." *Philosophical Transactions* 32 (1722–1723): 51.

"Part of a Letter from Dr. Nettleton." *Philosophical Transactions* 32 (1722–1723): 209–212.

Noguez, Pierre. *Relation du succès de l'inoculation de la petite vérole dans la Grande Bretagne Par Mr. Jurin. Traduit de l'Anglois. Cet ouvrage est augmenté d'un discours préliminaire sur la pétite vérole, & d'une dissertation sur la Transpiration.* Paris, 1725.

Percival, Thomas. "Essay on the Small-Pox and Measles." *Medical Observations and Inquiries* 5 (1789): 283–289.

Further Observations on the State of Population in Manchester, and Other Adjacent Places. Manchester, 1774.

"Observations on the State of Population in Manchester, and Other Adjacent Places." *Philosophical Transactions* 64 (1774): 54–66.

"Observations on the State of Population in Manchester, and Other Adjacent Places, Concluded." *Philosophical Transactions* 65 (1775): 322–335.

Petty, William. *Another Essay in Political Arithmetick, concerning the Growth of the City of London* (1682). In *The Economic Writings of Sir William Petty.* Ed. Charles H. Hull. 2 vols. Cambridge: Cambridge University Press, vol. 2, pp. 451–478.

The Economic Writings of Sir William Petty. Ed. Charles Henry Hull. 2 vols. Cambridge: Cambridge University Press, 1899.

Five Essays in Political Arithmetick [1687]. In *The Economic Writings of Sir William Petty.* Ed. Charles H. Hull. 2 vols. Cambridge: Cambridge University Press, 1899, vol. 2, pp. 521–544.

Further Observations upon the Dublin Bills [1686]. In *The Economic Writings of Sir William Petty.* 2 vols. Ed. Charles H. Hull. Cambridge: Cambridge University Press, 1899, vol. 2, pp. 493–498.

Observations upon the Dublin Bills of Mortality [1683]. In *The Economic Writings of Sir William Petty.* 2 vols. Ed. Charles H. Hull. Cambridge: Cambridge University Press, 1899, vol. 2, pp. 479–491.

The Petty Papers: Some Unpublished Writings of Sir William Petty. Ed. Marquis of Lansdowne. 2 vols. London: Constable & Co., 1927.

The Petty-Southwell Correspondence, 1676–1687. Ed. Marquis of Lansdowne. London: Constable & Co., 1928.

Political Arithmetick [1690]. In *The Economic Writings of Sir William Petty.* 2 vols. Ed. Charles H. Hull. Cambridge: Cambridge University Press, 1899, vol. 1, pp. 233–313.

Two Essays in Political Arithmetick [1687]. *The Economic Writings of Sir William Petty.* 2 vols. Ed. Charles H. Hull. Cambridge: Cambridge University Press, 1899, vol. 2, pp. 501–513.

Pickering, Roger. "A Scheme of a Diary of the Weather, Together with Draughts and Descriptions of Machines Subservient Thereunto." *Philosophical Transactions* 43, no. 473 (1744): 1–18.

Pommelles, Jean Christophe Sandrier des. *Tableau de la population de toutes les provinces de France.* n.p., 1789.

Price, Richard. *An Essay on the Population of England.* 2d ed. London, 1780.

"Further Proofs of the Insalubrity of Marshy Situations." *Philosophical Transactions* 64 (1774): 96–98.

Observations on Reversionary Payments. 2 vols. 7th ed. London, 1812. [First ed., 1769].

"Observations on the Difference between the Duration of Human Life in Towns and in Country Parishes and Villages." *Philosophical Transactions* 65 (1775): 424–445.

"Observations on the Expectations of Lives, the Increase of Mankind, the Influence of Great Towns on Population, and Particularly the State of London with Respect to Healthfulness and Number of Inhabitants." *Philosophical Transactions* 59 (1769): 89–125.

"Observations on the Proper Method of Calculating the Values of Reversions Depending on Survivorship." *Philosophical Transactions* 60 (1770): 268–276.

Pulteney, Richard. "An Account of Baptisms, Marriages, and Burials during Forty Years, in the Parish of Blandford Forum, Dorset." *Philosophical Transactions* 68 (1778): 615–621.

Pylarini, Jacob. *Nova et tuta variolas excitandi per transplantationem methodus; nuper inventa et in usum tracta: que rite peracta immunia in posterum praeservantur ab hujusmodi contagio corpora.* Venice, 1715. Reprinted in *Philosophical Transactions* 29 (1716): 393–399.

Quesnay, François. "Précis de l'organisation, ou mémoire sur les états provinciaux, avec des Questions intéressantes sur la population, l'agriculture et le commerce." In Victor de Riqueti, Marquis de Mirabeau. *L'ami des hommes ou traité de la population.* Vol. 2, Part 4. Reimpression of the Avignon edition, 1758–1760. Darmstadt: Scientia Verlag Aalen, 1970.

Tableau Économique. Ed. with new material, translations, and notes by Marguerite Kuczynski and Ronald L. Meek. 1758. London: Macmillan, 1972.

Raymond. "Sur la topographie médicale de Marseille & de son territoire, & sur celle des lieux voisins de cette ville." *Histoire de la Société Royale de Médecine, 1777–1778* (Paris, 1780), pp. 66–140.

Razoux, Jean. *Tables nosologiques et météorologiques très-étendues dressés à l'Hôtel-Dieu de Nismes depuis le premier juin 1757 jusques au premier janvier 1762.* Basle, 1767.

Renaudin. "Mémoire sur le sol, les habitans et les maladies de la Province d'Alsace." In *Recueil d'observations de médecine des hôpitaux militaires.* Ed. François-Marie-Claude Richard de Hautesierck. 2 vols. Paris, 1782, vol. 2, pp. 6–48.

Richard de Hautesierck, François-Marie-Claude, ed. *Recueil d'observations de médecine des hôpitaux militaires.* 2 vols. Paris, 1766 and 1782.

Rickman, John. "Thoughts on the Utility and Facility of Ascertaining the Population." *The Commercial and Agricultural Magazine* 2 (1800): 391–399. Reprinted in *Numbering the People: The Eighteenth-Century Population Controversy and the Development of Census and Vital Statistics in Britain.* Ed. D.V. Glass. Farnborough, Hants, Eng.: Saxon House, 1973, pp. 106–113.

Rousseau, Jean-Jacques. *The Social Contract.* Trans. Maurice Cranston. 1762. New York: Penguin Books, 1982.

Rutty, John. *A Chronological History of the Weather and Seasons, and of the Prevailing Diseases in Dublin. With Their Various Periods, Successions, and Revolutions, during the Space of Forty Years. With a Comparative View of the Difference of the Irish Climate and Diseases, and Those of England and Other Countries.* London, 1770.

Saugrain, Claude. *Dictionnaire universel de la France ancienne et moderne.* Paris, 1726.

Nouveau dénombrement du royaume par generalitez, élections, paroisses et feux. Paris, 1720.

Scheuchzer, John Gasper. *An Account of the Success of Inoculating the Small-Pox in Great Britain, for the Years 1727 and 1728.* London, 1729.

Schultz, David. *An Account of Inoculation.* Trans. from the Swedish. London, 1758.

Séjour, Achille-Pierre Dionis du, Marie-Jean-Antoine-Nicolas Caritat de Condorcet, and Pierre-Simon de Laplace. "Pour connoître la Population du Royaume, et le nombre des habitans de la campagne, en adaptant sur chacune des Cartes de M. Cassini, l'année commune des Naissances, tant des Villes que des Bourgs et des Villages." *Mémoires de l'Académie Royale des Sciences,* 1783 (Paris, 1786), pp. 703–718.

Short, Thomas. *A Comparative History of the Increase and Decrease of Mankind and Several Countries Abroad According to the Different Soils, Business of Life, Use of the Non-Naturals, &c.* London, 1767.

New Observations, Natural, Moral, Civil, Political, and Medical, on City, Town, and Country Bills of Mortality. London, 1750.

[Short, Thomas.] *A General Chronological History of the Air, Weather, Seasons, Meteors &c. in Sundry Places and Different Times.* London, 1749.

Simpson, Thomas. *The Doctrine of Annuities and Reversions.* London, 1742.

Smith, Adam. *An Inquiry into the Nature and Causes of the Wealth of Nations.* Ed. Edwin Cannan. 1776; New York: The Modern Library, 1937.

Sprat, Thomas. *History of the Royal Society.* Ed. with an introduction and notes by Jackson I. Cope and Harold Whitmore Jones. 1667; St. Louis: Washington University Studies, 1959.

Stow, William. *Remarks on London: Being an Exact Survey of the Cities of London and Westminster.* London, 1722.

Süssmilch, Johann Peter. *Die Göttliche Ordnung.* Berlin, 1741.

Sutton, Daniel. *The Inoculator, or Suttonian System of Inoculation.* 1796.

Tenon, Jacques. *Memoirs on Paris Hospitals.* Trans. with an Introduction and Notes and Appendices by Dora B. Weiner. Science History Publications, 1996 [1788].

Timoni, Emanuele. "An Account or History, of the Procuring the Small Pox by Incision, or Inoculation; As It Has for Some Time Been Practised at Constantinople." *Philosophical Transactions* 29 (1714): 72–82.

Tissot, Samuel Auguste André David. *L'Inoculation justifiée ou dissertation pratique et apologétique sur cette méthode.* Lausanne, 1754.

Tour, Louis Brion de la. *Tableau de la population de la France avec les citations des auteurs.* Paris, 1789.

Tronchin, Théodore. "L'Inoculation." *Encyclopédie ou Dictionnaire Raisonné des Sciences, des Arts et des Métiers.* 1st ed. Vol. 8. Neufchastel, 1765.

Vauban, Sebastien le Prestre de. *Projet d'une Dixme Royale suivre de deux écrits financiers.* Ed. E. Coornaert. 1707; Paris: F. Alcan, 1933.

Voltaire, François Marie Arouet. *Letters concerning the English Nation.* Ed. with notes and introduction by Nicholas Cronk. 1733; Oxford: Oxford University Press, 1994.

Lettres philosophiques. Paris, 1734.

Wagstaffe, William. *A Letter to Dr. Freind Shewing the Danger and Uncertainty of Inoculating the Small Pox*. London, 1722.

Lettre au Docteur Freind: Montrant le danger et l'incertitude d'inserer la petite vérole. Anonymous trans. London, 1722.

Wales, William. *An Inquiry into the Present State of Population in England and Wales*. London, 1781. Reprinted in *The Population Controversy*. Ed. D.V. Glass. Farnborough, Hants, Eng.: Gregg International Publishers, 1973.

Wallace, Robert. *A Dissertation on the Numbers of Mankind in Ancient and Modern Times: In Which the Superior Populousness of Antiquity Is Maintained*. Edinburgh, 1753.

Watkinson, John. *An Examination of a Charge Brought against Inoculation, by DeHaen, Dimsdale, and Other Writers*. London, 1778.

Watson, William. *An Account of a Series of Experiments, Instituted with a View of Ascertaining the Most Successful Method of Inoculating the Small-Pox*. London, 1768.

Williams, Perrott. *Some Remarks upon Dr. Wagstaff's [sic] Letter against Inoculating the Small-Pox. In a Letter to Himself, Defending That Practice*. London, 1725.

Wintringham, Clifton. *Commentarium Nosologicum Morbos Epidemicos et Aeris Variationes in Urbe Eboracensi Locisque Vicinis*. London, 1733.

Wood, Anthony. *Athenae Oxonienses: An Exact History of All the Writers and Bishops Who Have Had Their Education in the Most Antient and Famous University of Oxford*. London: Knaplock, Midwinter, and Tonson, [1721].

Woodville, William. *The History of the Inoculation of the Small-Pox in Great Britain*. Vol. 1 [Vol. 2 never published]. London, 1796.

Young, Arthur. *Political Arithmetic*. London, 1774.

[Young, Arthur.] *Proposals to the Legislature for Numbering the People; Containing Some Observations on the Population of Great Britain, and a Sketch of the Advantages That Would Probably Accrue from an Exact Knowledge of Its Present State. By the Author of the Tours through England*. London: W. Nicoll, 1771. Reprinted in *The Development of Population Statistics*. Ed. D.V. Glass. Farnborough, Hants, Eng.: Gregg International Publishers, 1973.

SECONDARY SOURCES

Abraham, James Johnston. *Lettsom – His Life, Times, Friends and Descendants*. London: William Heinemann, 1933.

Ackerknecht, Erwin. *Medicine at the Paris Hospital, 1794–1848*. Baltimore: Johns Hopkins Press, 1967.

Alder, Ken. *Engineering the Revolution: Arms and Enlightenment in France, 1763–1815*. Princeton, N.J.: Princeton University Press, 1997.

Ariès, Philippe. *Western Attitudes toward Death from the Middle Ages to the Present*. Trans. Patricia M. Ranum. Baltimore: Johns Hopkins University Press, 1974.

Baigrie, Brian S., ed. *Picturing Knowledge: Historical and Philosophical Problems concerning the Use of Art in Science*. Toronto: University of Toronto Press, 1996.

Baker, Keith. *Condorcet: From Natural Philosophy to Social Mathematics*. Chicago and London: University of Chicago Press, 1975.

Inventing the French Revolution. Cambridge: Cambridge University Press, 1990.

Beattie, Lester M. *John Arbuthnot – Mathematician and Satirist*. Cambridge, Mass.: Harvard University Press, 1935.

Behar, L. "Des tables de mortalité aux XVIIe et XVIIIe siècles. Histoire – signification." *Annales de Démographie Historique* (1976): 173–200.

Bevan, William L. *Sir William Petty: A Study in English Economic Literature.* Baltimore: American Economic Association, 1894.

Boislisle, A.M. de, ed. *Mémoires des Intendants sur l'état des généralités.* Paris: Imprimerie Nationale, 1881.

Bonar, James. *Theories of Population from Raleigh to Arthur Young.* 1929; New York: Augustus M. Kelley, Reprints of Economic Classics, 1966.

Borsay, Anne. "An Example of Political Arithmetic: The Evaluation of Spa Therapy at the Georgian Bath Infirmary, 1742–1830." *Medical History* 45 (2000): 149–172.

Bosher, J.F. "French Administration and Public Finance in Their European Setting." In *The New Cambridge Modern History.* Ed. A. Goodwin. Vol. 8: *The American and French Revolutions, 1763–1793.* Cambridge: Cambridge University Press, 1965, pp. 565–591.

Bourguet, Marie-Noëlle. *Déchiffrer la France: La statistique départementale à l'époque napoléonienne.* Paris: Editions des Archives Contemporaines, 1988.

Bowker, Geoffrey C., and Susan Leigh Star. *Sorting Things Out: Classification and Its Consequences.* Cambridge and London: The MIT Press, 1999.

Bradley, L. *Smallpox Inoculation: An Eighteenth Century Mathematical Controversy.* Nottingham: University of Nottingham, 1971.

Brewer, John. *The Sinews of Power.* New York: Knopf, 1989.

Brian, Éric. *La mesure de l'état: Administrateurs et géomètres au XVIIIe siècle.* Paris: Albin Michel, 1994.

"Moyens de connaître les plumes. Étude lexicométrique." In Jean-Baptiste Moheau. *Recherches et considérations sur la population de la France.* Reedition annotated by Eric Vilquin. Paris: Institut National d'Études Démographiques, Presses Universitaires de France, 1994, pp. 383–396.

Brockliss, Laurence, and Colin Jones. *The Medical World of Early Modern France.* Oxford: Clarendon Press, 1997.

Bru, Bernard. "De La Michodière à Moheau: L'évaluation de la population par les naissances." In Jean-Baptiste Moheau. *Recherches et considérations sur la population de la France,* Reedition annotated by Eric Vilquin. Paris: Institut National d'Études Démographiques, Presses Universitaires de France, 1994, pp. 493–516.

"Estimations Laplaciennes." *Estimations et sondages.* Ed. Jacques Mairesse. Paris: Economica, 1988, pp. 7–46.

Brunton, Deborah. "'Pox Britannica': Smallpox Inoculation in Britain, 1721–1830." Ph.D. thesis, University of Pennsylvania, 1990.

Buck, Peter. "People Who Counted: Political Arithmetic in the Eighteenth Century." *Isis* 73 (1982): 28–45.

"Seventeenth-Century Political Arithmetic: Civil Strife and Vital Statistics." *Isis* 68 (1977): 67–84.

Buer, M.C. *Health, Wealth and Population in the Early Days of the Industrial Revolution.* 1926; New York: Howard Fertig, 1968.

Burn, John Southerden. *Registrum Ecclesiae Parochialis: The History of Parish Registers in England.* 2d ed. 1862; republished by East Ardsley, Eng.: EP Publishing Limited, 1976.

Bynum, W.F. "Nosology." *Companion Encyclopedia of the History of Medicine.* Ed. W.F. Bynum and Roy Porter. 2 vols. London and New York: Routledge, 1993, vol. 1, pp. 335–356.

Cabourdin, Guy, and Jacques Dupâquier. "Les sources et les institutions." In *Histoire de la population française*. Ed. Jacques Dupâquier. Vol. 2: *De la Renaissance à 1789*. Paris: Presses Universitaires de France, 1988, pp. 9–50.

Capp, Bernard. *Astrology and the Popular Press – English Almanacs, 1500–1800*. London: Faber & Faber, 1979.

Cassedy, James H. *American Medicine and Statistical Thinking, 1800–1860*. Cambridge, Mass.: Harvard University Press, 1984.

——— *Demography in Early America: Beginnings of the Statistical Mind, 1600–1800*. Cambridge, Mass.: Harvard University Press, 1969.

——— "Medicine and the Rise of Statistics." In *Medicine in Seventeenth Century England*. Ed. Allen G. Debus. Berkeley: University of California Press, 1974, pp. 283–312.

Charlot, E., and Jacques Dupâquier. "Mouvement annuel de la population de la ville de Paris de 1670 à 1821." *Annales de démographie historique* (1967): 511–519.

Christie, James. *Some Account of Parish Clerks, More Especially of the Ancient Fraternity (Bretherne and Sisterne), of S. Nicholas, Now Known as the Worshipful Company of Parish Clerks*. London, 1893.

Clark, Geoffrey. *Betting on Lives: The Culture of Life Insurance in England, 1695–1775*. Manchester and New York: Manchester University Press, 1999.

Clark, William. "On the Table Manners of Academic Examination." In *Wissenschaft als kulturelle Praxis, 1750–1900*. Ed. Hans Erich Bödecker, Peter Hanns Reill, and Jürgen Schlumbohm. Göttingen: Vandenhoeck & Ruprecht, 1999, pp. 33–67.

Cochran, W.G. "Laplace's Ratio Estimator." In *Contributions to Survey Sampling and Applied Statistics*. Ed. H.A. David. New York: Wiley, 1978, pp. 3–10.

Cohen, Patricia Cline. *A Calculating People – The Spread of Numeracy in Early America*. Chicago: University of Chicago Press, 1982.

——— "Death and Taxes: The Domain of Numbers in Eighteenth Century Popular Culture." In *Science and Technology in the Eighteenth Century*. Ed. Stephen Cutcliffe. n.p., n.d., pp. 51–69.

——— "Statistics and the State: Changing Social Thought and the Emergence of a Quantitative Mentality in America, 1790–1820." *William and Mary Quarterly* 38 (1981): 35–55.

Cole, Joshua. *The Power of Large Numbers: Population, Politics, and Gender in Nineteenth-Century France*. Ithaca and London: Cornell University Press, 2000.

Coleman, William. *Death is a Social Disease: Public Health and Political Economy in Early Industrial France*. Madison: University of Wisconsin Press, 1982.

——— "Inventing Demography: Montyon on Hygiene and the State." In *Transformations and Tradition in the Sciences: Essays in Honor of I. Bernard Cohen*. Ed. Everett Mendelsohn. Cambridge: Cambridge University Press, 1984, pp. 215–235.

Comiti, Vincent-Pierre. "Éléments historique de l'utilisation de la méthode statistique en médecine." *Histoire des sciences médicales* 13 (1979): 121–130.

Cook, Harold. *The Decline of the Old Medical Regime in Stuart London*. Ithaca, N.Y.: Cornell University Press, 1986.

Courlieu. A. *L'Ancienne Faculté de Médecine de Paris*. Paris, 1877.

Creighton, Charles. *A History of Epidemics in Great Britain*. 2 vols. Cambridge: Cambridge University Press, 1891.

Cullen, M.J. *The Statistical Movement in Early Victorian Britain*. New York: The Harvester Press, 1975.

Darmon, Pierre. *La longue traque de la vérole: Les pionniers de la médecine préventive.* Collection *Pour l'Histoire.* Paris: Perrin, 1986.

La variole, les nobles et les princes: La petite vérole mortelle de Louis XV. Brussels: Éditions Complexe, 1989.

Darnton, Robert. *The Literary Underground of the Old Regime.* Cambridge, Mass.: Harvard University Press, 1982.

Daston, Lorraine. "Baconian Facts, Academic Civility and the Prehistory of Objectivity." *Annals of Science* 8 (1991): 337–364.

Classical Probability in the Enlightenment. Princeton, N.J.: Princeton University Press, 1988.

"The Domestication of Risk: Mathematical Probability and Insurance, 1650–1830." In *The Probabilistic Revolution.* Ed. Lorenz Krüger, Lorraine J. Daston, and Michael Heidelberger. 2 vols. Cambridge, Mass.: MIT Press, 1987, vol. 1, pp. 237–260.

"Enlightenment Calculation." *Critical Inquiry* 21 (1994): 182–202.

"The Ideal and Reality of the Republic of Letters in the Enlightenment." *Science in Context* 2 (1991): 367–386.

"Rational Individuals versus Laws of Society: From Probability to Statistics." In *The Probabilistic Revolution.* Ed. Lorenz Krüger, Lorraine J. Daston, and Michael Heidelberger. 2 vols. Cambridge, Mass.: MIT Press, 1987, vol. 1, pp. 295–304.

De Beer, G.R. *Sir Hans Sloane and the British Museum.* Oxford: Oxford University Press, 1953.

DeLacy, Margaret. "Nosology, Mortality, and Disease Theory in the Eighteenth Century." *Journal of the History of Medicine* 54 (1999): 261–284.

Delaunay, Paul. *Le monde médical parisien au dix-huitième siècle.* Paris: J. Rousset, 1906.

Desrosières, Alain. *La politique des grand nombres: Histoire de la raison statistique.* Paris: Éditions la Découverte, 1993.

Dobson, Mary J. *Contours of Death and Disease in Early Modern England.* Cambridge: Cambridge University Press, 1997.

Donnelly, Michael. "On Foucault's Uses of the Notion 'Biopower.'" In *Michel Foucault, Philosopher.* Trans. Timothy J. Armstrong. New York: Routledge, 1992.

Douglas, Mary. *How Institutions Think.* Syracuse, N.Y.: Syracuse University Press, 1986.

Ducreux, M.E. "Les Premiers Essais d'évaluation de la Population Mondiale et l'idée de Dépopulation au XVIIe siècle." *Annales de Démographie Historique* (1977): 421–429.

Dulieu, Louis. *La Médecine à Montpellier.* 2 vols. Paris: Les Presses Universelles, 1972.

Dupâquier, Jacques, ed. *Histoire de la population française.* Vols. 1 and 2. Paris: Presses Universitaires de France, 1988.

Pour la démographie historique. Paris: Presses Universitaires de France, 1984.

Dupâquier, Jacques, and Michel Dupâquier. *Histoire de la démographie.* Paris: Perrin, 1985.

Dupâquier, Jacques, and Eric Vilquin. "Le Pouvoir royal et la statistique démographique." In *Pour une histoire de la statistique.* 2 Vols. Paris: Institut National de la Statistique et des Études Économiques, 1976, vol. 1, pp. 83–104.

Eisenstein, Elizabeth L. *The Printing Press as an Agent of Change: Communications and Cultural Transformations in Early-Modern Europe.* Cambridge: Cambridge University Press, 1979.

Endres, A.M. "The Functions of Numerical Data in the Writings of Graunt, Petty, and Davenant." *History of Political Economy* 17 (1985): 245–264.

Esmonin, Edmond. *Études sur la France des XVIIe et XVIIIe siècles*. Paris: Presses Universitaires de France, 1964.

"Montyon, véritable auteur des *Recherches et considérations sur la population*, de Moheau." *Population* 13 (1958): 269–282.

Estes, J. Worth. "Quantitative Observations of Fever and its Treatment before the Advent of Short Clinical Thermometers." *Medical History* 35 (1991): 189–216.

Faure, Fernand. "The Development and Progress of Statistics in France." In *The History of Statistics: Memoirs to Commemorate the 75th Anniversary of the American Statistical Association.* New York: The Macmillan Co., 1918, pp. 219–329.

Favre, Robert. *La mort dans la littérature et la pensée française au siècle des lumières*. Lyon: Presses Universitaires de Lyon, 1978.

Feldman, Theodore S. "Late Enlightenment Meteorology." In *The Quantifying Spirit in the 18th Century*. Ed. Tore Frängsmyr, J.L. Heilbron, and Robin E. Rider. Berkeley: University of California Press, 1990, pp. 143–178.

Fitzmaurice, Edmond. *The Life of Sir William Petty, 1623–1687*. London: John Murray, 1895.

Forbes, Thomas R. "By What Disease or Casualty: The Changing Face of Death in London." In *Health, Medicine and Mortality in the Sixteenth Century*. Ed. Charles Webster. Cambridge: Cambridge University Press, 1979, pp. 117–139.

Foucault, Michel. *The Birth of the Clinic*. Trans. A.M. Sheridan Smith. 1963; New York: Vintage Books, 1975.

Discipline and Punish: The Birth of the Prison. Trans. Alan Sheridan. 1975; New York: Vintage Books, 1979.

The History of Sexuality. Vol. 1: *An Introduction*. Trans. Robert Hurley. 1976; New York: Vintage Books, 1980.

The Order of Things. [An anonymous translation of *Les mots et les choses*.] 1966; New York: Vintage Books, 1970.

"The Politics of Health in the Eighteenth Century." In *Power/Knowledge: Selected Interviews and Other Writings 1972–1977*. Ed. Colin Gordon. Trans. Colin Gordon, Leo Marshall, John Mepham, and Kate Soper. New York: Pantheon Books, 1980, pp. 166–182.

Frängsmyr, Tore, J.L. Heilbron, and Robin E. Rider, eds. *The Quantifying Spirit in the 18th Century*. Berkeley: University of California Press, 1990.

Frank, Robert G., Jr. *Harvey and the Oxford Physiologists*. Berkeley: University of California Press, 1980.

Frisinger, H. Howard. *The History of Meteorology to 1800*. New York: Science History Publications, 1977.

Gay, Peter. *The Enlightenment*. 2 vols. New York: Norton, 1966, 1969.

Gille, Bertrand. *Les sources statistiques de l'histoire de France; Des enquêtes du XVIIe siècle à 1870*. Geneva: Droz, 1964.

Gillispie, Charles C. "Probability and Politics: Laplace, Condorcet, and Turgot." *Proceedings of the American Philosophical Society* 116 (1972): 1–20.

Science and Polity in France at the End of the Old Regime. Princeton, N.J.: Princeton University Press, 1980.

Gittings, Clare. *Death, Burial and the Individual in Early Modern England*. London and Sydney: Croom Helm, 1984.

Glacken, Clarence J. *Traces on the Rhodian Shore: Nature and Culture in Western Thought from Ancient Times to the End of the Eighteenth Century*. Berkeley and Los Angeles: University of California Press, 1967.

Glass, D.V. *The Development of Population Statistics*. Farnborough, Hants, Eng.: Gregg International Publishers, 1973.

"John Graunt and his 'Natural and Political Observations.'" *Notes and Records of the Royal Society* 19 (1964): 63–100.

Numbering the People: The Eighteenth-Century Population Controversy and the Development of Census and Vital Statistics in Britain. London and New York: Gordon & Cremonesi, 1973.

The Population Controversy. Farnborough, Hants, Eng.: Gregg International Publishers, 1973.

Glass, D.V., and D.E.C. Eversley, eds. *Population in History – Essays in Historical Demography*. London: Edward Arnold, 1965.

Goldgar, Anne. *Impolite Learning: Conduct and Community in the Republic of Letters, 1680–1750*. New Haven and London: Yale University Press, 1995.

Goldstein, Jan. "Foucault among the Sociologists: The 'Disciplines' and the History of the Professions." *History and Theory* 23 (1984): 170–192.

Golinski, Jan. "Barometers of Change: Meteorological Instruments as Machines of the Enlightenment." In *The Sciences in Enlightened Europe*. Ed. William Clark, Jan Golinski, and Simon Schaffer. Chicago and London: University of Chicago Press, 1999, pp. 69–93.

Making Natural Knowledge: Constructivism and the History of Science. Cambridge: Cambridge University Press, 1998.

"'The Nicety of Experiment': Precision of Measurement and Precision of Reasoning in Late Eighteenth-Century Chemistry." In *The Values of Precision*. Ed. M. Norton Wise. Princeton, N.J.: Princeton University Press, 1995, pp. 72–91.

Goodman, Dena. *The Republic of Letters: A Cultural History of the French Enlightenment*. Ithaca and London: Cornell University Press, 1994.

Goubert, Jean-Pierre. *Malades et médecins en Bretagne, 1770–1790*. Rennes: Institut Armoricain de Recherches Historiques, 1974.

Greenwood, Major. *Medical Statistics from Graunt to Farr*. Cambridge: Cambridge University Press, 1948.

Grundy, Isobel. "Medical Advance and Female Fame: Inoculation and its After-Effects." *Lumen* 13 (1994): 13–42.

Hacking, Ian. "Biopower and the Avalanche of Printed Numbers." *Humanities in Society* 5 (1982): 279–295.

The Emergence of Probability. Cambridge: Cambridge University Press, 1975.

"Karl Pearson's History of Statistics." *British Journal for the Philosophy of Science* 32 (1981): 177–183.

"Prussian Numbers, 1860–1882." In *The Probabilistic Revolution*. Ed. Lorenz Krüger, Lorraine J. Daston, and Michael Heidelberger. 2 vols. Cambridge, Mass.: MIT Press, 1987, vol. 1, pp. 377–394.

The Taming of Chance. Cambridge: Cambridge University Press, 1990.

Hahn, Roger. *The Anatomy of a Scientific Institution: The Paris Academy of Sciences, 1660–1800*. Berkeley: University of California Press, 1971.

Hald, Anders. *A History of Probability and Statistics and Their Applications before 1750*. New York: John Wiley & Sons, 1990.

236   *Bibliography*

Hankins, Thomas L. *Jean d'Alembert – Science and the Enlightenment.* Oxford: Clarendon Press, 1970.

Hannaway, Caroline. "Environment and Miasmata." In *Companion Encyclopedia of the History of Medicine.* Ed. W.F. Bynum and Roy Porter. Vol. 1. London and New York: Routledge, 1993, pp. 296–300.

"Medicine, Public Welfare and the State in Eighteenth-Century France: The Société Royale de Médecine of Paris (1776–1793)." Ph.D. thesis, Johns Hopkins University, 1974.

"The Société Royale de Médecine and Epidemics in the Ancien Régime." *Bulletin of the History of Medicine* 46 (1972): 257–273.

Hasquin, Hervé. "Le débat sur la dépopulation dans l'Europe des lumières." In Jean-Baptiste Moheau, *Recherches et considérations sur la population de la France.* Reedition annotated by Eric Vilquin. Paris: Institut National d'Études Démographiques, Presses Universitaires de France, 1994, pp. 397–424.

Hecht, Jacqueline. "L'idée du dénombrement jusqu'à la révolution." In *Pour une Histoire de la Statistique.* 2 Vols. Paris: Institut National de la Statistique et des Études Économiques, 1976, vol. 1, pp. 21–81.

Heilbron, J.L. "A Mathematical Mutiny, with Morals." In *World Changes: Thomas Kuhn and the Nature of Science.* Ed. Paul Horwich. Cambridge, Mass.: Harvard University Press, 1993, pp. 81–129.

Physics at the Royal Society during Newton's Presidency. Los Angeles: William Andrews Clark Memorial Library, 1983.

Henry, L. *Manuel de démographie historique.* Geneva and Paris: Droz, 1967.

Hill, Christopher. *The World Turned Upside Down.* New York: Penguin Books, 1975.

Hollingsworth, T.H. *Historical Demography.* Cambridge: Cambridge University Press, 1976.

Hopkins, Donald R. *Princes and Peasants: Smallpox in History.* Chicago: University of Chicago Press, 1983.

Hoppen, K. Theodore. *The Common Scientist in the Seventeenth Century – A Study of the Dublin Philosophical Society, 1683–1708.* Charlottesville: University Press of Virginia, 1970.

Hoppit, Julian. "Political Arithmetic in Eighteenth-Century England." *Economic History Review* 49 (1996): 516–540.

Jacob, Margaret C. *Scientific Culture and the Making of the Industrial West.* New York and Oxford: Oxford University Press, 1997.

Jardine, Lisa. *Francis Bacon: Discovery and the Art of Discourse.* Cambridge: Cambridge University Press, 1974.

Johannisson, Karin. "Society in Numbers: The Debate over Quantification in Eighteenth Century Political Economy." In *The Quantifying Spirit in the Eighteenth Century.* Ed. Tore Frängsmyr, J.L. Heilbron, and Robin E. Rider. Berkeley: University of California Press, 1990, pp. 343–362.

Johns, Adrian. *The Nature of the Book: Print and Knowledge in the Making.* Chicago: University of Chicago Press, 1998.

Jones, Colin. "La Vie et les revendications des étudiants en médecine à Montpellier au XVIIIe siècle." *Actes du 110e Congrès National des Sociétés Savantes.* Montpellier, 1985, pp. 117–128.

Jones, Colin, and Michael Sonenscher. "The Social Functions of the Hospital in Eighteenth-Century France: The Case of the Hôtel-Dieu of Nîmes." In Colin Jones. *The Charitable*

Imperative: Hospitals and Nursing in Ancien Regime and Revolutionary France. London and New York: Routledge, 1989, pp. 48–86.

Jordanova, Ludmilla. "Earth Science and Environmental Medicine: The Synthesis of the Late Enlightenment." In *Images of the Earth: Essays in the History of the Environmental Sciences.* Ed. L.J. Jordanova and Roy Porter. British Society for the History of Science, 1979, pp. 119–146.

Kargon, Robert. "John Graunt, Francis Bacon, and the Royal Society: The Reception of Statistics." *Journal of the History of Medicine* 18 (1963): 337–348.

Science in Victorian Manchester: Expertise and Enterprise. Baltimore: Johns Hopkins University Press, 1977.

Keynes, Geoffrey Langdon. *A Bibliography of Sir William Petty F.R.S. and of the Observations on the Bills of Mortality by John Graunt F.R.S..* Oxford: Clarendon Press, 1971.

King, Lester. *Medical Thinking – A Historical Preface.* Princeton, N.J.: Princeton University Press, 1982.

Kreager, Philip. "New Light on Graunt." *Population Studies* 43 (1988): 129–140.

"Quand une population est-elle une nation? Quand une nation est-elle un état? La démographie et l'émergence d'un dilemme moderne, 1770–1870." *Population* 6 (1992): 1639–1656.

Krüger, Lorenz, Lorraine J. Daston, and Michael Heidelberger, eds. *The Probabilistic Revolution.* 2 vols. Cambridge, Mass.: MIT Press, 1987.

Kuczynski, R.R. "British Demographers' Opinions on Fertility, 1660–1760." In *Political Arithmetic – A Symposium of Population Studies.* Ed. Lancelot Hogben. London: George Allen and Unwin, 1938, pp. 283–327.

Kuhn, Thomas S. *The Essential Tension.* Chicago: University of Chicago Press, 1977.

Kula, Witold. *Measures and Men.* Trans. Richard Szreter. Princeton, N.J.: Princeton University Press, 1986.

Kwass, Michael. *Privilege and the Politics of Taxation in Eighteenth-Century France: Liberté, Égalité, Fiscalité.* Cambridge: Cambridge University Press, 2000.

LaBerge, Ann. *Mission and Method: The Early Nineteenth-Century French Public Health Movement.* Cambridge: Cambridge University Press, 1992.

Latour, Bruno. *Science in Action.* Cambridge, Mass.: Harvard University Press, 1987.

"Visualization and Cognition: Thinking with Eyes and Hands." *Knowledge and Society: Studies in the Sociology of Culture Past and Present* 6 (1986): 1–40.

Lawrence, Susan C. *Charitable Knowledge: Hospital Pupils and Practitioners in Eighteenth-Century London.* Cambridge: Cambridge University Press, 1996.

Lazard, Pierre. *Vauban, 1633–1707.* Paris: F. Alcan, 1934.

Lazarsfeld, P.F. "Notes on the History of Quantification in Sociology: Trends, Sources and Problems." *Isis* 52 (1961): 277–333.

Lecuir, J. "Deux siècles après: Montyon, véritable auteur des *Recherches et considérations sur la population de la France,* de Moheau." *Annales de démographie historique* (1979): 195–249.

Lécuyer, Bernard-Pierre. "The Statistician's Role in Society: The Institutional Establishment of Statistics in France." *Minerva* 25 (1987): 35–55.

Le Roy Ladurie, E., and J.P. Desaive, "Étude par ordinateur des données météorologiques constituées par les correspondants de la Société Royale de Médecine (1776–1792)." In Jean-Paul Desaive, Jean-Pierre Goubert, Emmanuel le Roy Ladurie, Jean Meyer, Otto Muller, and Jean-Pierre Peter. *Médecins, climat et épidémies à la fin du XVIIIe siècle.* Paris: Mouton, 1972, pp. 23–134.

Letwin, William. *The Origins of Scientific Economics – English Economic Thought, 1660–1776.* London: Methuen, 1963.

Levasseur, Emile. *La Population Française.* 3 vols. Paris: Arthur Rousseau, 1889.

Lobo, Francis M. "John Haygarth, Smallpox and Religious Dissent in Eighteenth-Century England." In *The Medical Enlightenment of the Eighteenth Century.* Ed. Andrew Cunningham and Roger French. Cambridge: Cambridge University Press, 1990, pp. 217–253.

Luria, A.R. "Towards the Problem of the Historical Nature of Psychological Processes." *International Journal of Psychology* 6 (1971): 259–272.

Manley, Gordon. "The Weather and Diseases: Some 18th-Century Contributions to Observational Meteorology." *Notes and Records of the Royal Society of London* 9 (1952): 300–307.

Matthews, J. Rosser. *Quantification and the Quest for Medical Certainty.* Princeton, N.J.: Princeton University Press, 1995.

Maulitz, Russell C. *Morbid Appearances: The Anatomy of Pathology in the Early Nineteenth Century.* Cambridge: Cambridge University Press, 1987.

May, Maisie. "Inoculating the Urban Poor in the Late Eighteenth Century." *British Journal for the History of Science* 30 (1997): 291–305.

McCloy, Shelby T. *The Humanitarian Movement in Eighteenth-Century France.* Lexington: University of Kentucky Press, 1957.

McManners, John. *Death and the Enlightenment.* Oxford: Clarendon Press, 1981.

Mercer, Alex. *Disease, Mortality and Population in Transition: Epidemiological-Demographic Change in England since the Eighteenth Century as Part of a Global Phenomenon.* Leicester, London, and New York: Leicester University Press, 1990.

Meyer, Jean. "Une enquête de l'Académie de médecine sur les épidémies (1774–1794)." *Annales – Economies, Sociétés, Civilisations* 21 (1966): 729–749.

Miller, Genevieve. *The Adoption of Inoculation for Smallpox in England and France.* Philadephia: University of Pennsylvania Press, 1957.

  "Putting Lady Mary in Her Place: A Discussion of Historical Causation." *Bulletin of the History of Medicine* 55 (1981): 2–16.

Mitchell, Harvey. "Rationality and Control in French Eighteenth-Century Medical Views of the Peasantry." *Comparative Studies in Society and History* 21 (1979): 82–112.

Moravia, Sergio. "The Enlightenment and the Sciences of Man." *History of Science* 18 (1980): 247–268.

Murphy, Terence D. "Medical Knowledge and Statistical Methods in Early Nineteenth Century France." *Medical History* 25 (1981): 301–319.

Musson, A.E., and Eric Robinson. *Science and Technology in the Industrial Revolution.* Manchester: University of Manchester Press, 1968.

Mykkänen, Juri. "'To Methodize and Regulate Them': William Petty's Governmental Science of Statistics." *History of the Human Sciences* 7 (1994): 65–88.

Needham, Joseph. "Human Laws and Laws of Nature in China and the West." *Journal of the History of Ideas* 12 (1951): 3–30.

Oakley, Francis. "Christian Theology and the Newtonian Science: The Rise of the Concept of the Laws of Nature." *Church History* 30 (1961): 433–457.

Ogle, William. "An Inquiry into the Trustworthiness of the Old Bills of Mortality." *Journal of the Royal Statistical Society* 55 (1892): 437–460.

Pasquier, Maurice. *Sir William Petty – Ses Idées Économiques.* 1903; New York: Burt Franklin, 1971.

Pearson, Karl. *The History of Statistics in the 17th and 18th Centuries against the Changing Background of Intellectual, Scientific and Religious Thought.* Ed. E.S. Pearson. London: Charles Griffin, 1978.

Perrot, Jean-Claude. "Les économistes, les philosophes, et la population." In *Histoire de la Population Française.* Ed. Jacques Dupâquier. Vol. 2: *De la Renaissance à 1789.* Paris: Presses Universitaires de France, 1988, pp. 499–551.

"The Golden Age of Regional Statistics (Year IV – 1804)." In Jean-Claude Perrot and Stephen Woolf. *State and Statistics in France, 1789–1815.* London: Harwood Academic Publishers, 1984, pp. 1–80.

Peter, Jean-Pierre. "Aux sources de la médicalisation, le regard et le mot; le travail des topographies médicales." In *Populations et cultures: Études réunies en l'honneur de François Lebrun.* Rennes: Université de Rennes 2 Haute-Bretagne and the Institut culturel de Bretagne, 1989.

"Disease and the Sick at the End of the Eighteenth Century." In *Biology of Man in History.* Ed. Robert Forster and Orest Ranum. Trans. Elborg Forster and Patricia Ranum. Baltimore: Johns Hopkins University Press, 1975, pp. 81–124. [Originally published in *Annales- Économies, Sociétés, Civilisations* (1967): 711–751.]

Poovey, Mary. *A History of the Modern Fact: Problems of Knowledge in the Sciences of Wealth and Society.* Chicago: University of Chicago Press, 1998.

Porter, Dorothy, and Roy Porter. *Patients and Practitioners: Doctors and Doctoring in Eighteenth-Century England.* Stanford, Calif.: Stanford University Press, 1989.

Porter, Roy. *The Creation of the Modern World: The Untold Story of the British Enlightenment.* New York and London: W.W. Norton & Co., 2000.

English Society in the Eighteenth Century. Rev. ed. London: Penguin Books, 1990.

Porter, Theodore M. *The Rise of Statistical Thinking, 1820–1900.* Princeton, N.J.: Princeton University Press, 1986.

Trust in Numbers: The Pursuit of Objectivity in Science and Public Life. Princeton, N.J.: Princeton University Press, 1995.

Puvilland, Antonin. *Les Doctrines de la population en France au XVIIIe siècle – De 1695 à 1776.* Lyon: Imprimerie de "Revue judiciaire," 1912.

Ramsey, Matthew. *Professional and Popular Medicine in France, 1770–1830.* Cambridge: Cambridge University Press, 1988.

Raymond, Jean-François de. *Querelle de l'inoculation ou préhistoire de la vaccination.* Paris, 1982.

Raynaud, Maurice. *Les Médecins au temps de Molière.* 2d ed. Paris: Didier, 1863.

Razzell, Peter. *The Conquest of Smallpox: The Impact of Inoculation on Smallpox Mortality in Eighteenth Century Britain.* Sussex: Caliban Books, 1977.

Edward Jenner's Cowpox Vaccine: The History of a Medical Myth. Sussex: Caliban Books, 1977.

Essays in English Population History. London: Caliban Books, 1994.

"Population Change in Eighteenth-Century England: A Re-Appraisal." In *Population in Industrialization.* Ed. Michael Drake. London: Methuen, 1969.

Revel, Jacques. "Knowledge of the Territory." *Science in Context* 4 (1991): 133–161.

Riley, James. *The Eighteenth-Century Campaign to Avoid Disease.* New York: Macmillan, 1987.

Population Thought in the Age of the Demographic Revolution. Durham, N.C.: Carolina Academic Press, 1985.

Roche, Daniel. *Le Siècle des lumières en province: Académies et académiciens provinciaux, 1680–1789.* Paris: Mouton, 1978.

Roncaglia, Alessandro. *Petty – The Origins of Political Economy.* Trans. Isabella Cherubini. 1977; Armonk, N.Y.: M.E. Sharpe, 1985.

Rosen, George. *From Medical Police to Social Medicine: Essays on the History of Health Care.* New York: Science History Publications, 1974.

"Problems in the Application of Statistical Analysis to Questions of Health: 1700–1880." *Bulletin of the History of Medicine* 29 (1955): 27–45.

Rossi, Paolo. *Francis Bacon: From Magic to Science.* Trans. Sacha Rabinovitch. Chicago: University of Chicago Press, 1968.

Rowbotham, Arnold H. "The 'Philosophes' and the Propaganda for Inoculation of Smallpox in Eighteenth-Century France." *University of California Publications in Modern Philology* 18 (1935): 265–290.

Rudwick, Martin. "The Emergence of a Visual Language of Geology, 1760–1840." *History of Science* 14 (1976): 149–195.

Rusnock, Andrea. "Hippocrates, Bacon and Medical Meteorology at the Royal Society, 1700 to 1750." In *Reinventing Hippocrates.* Ed. David Cantor. Burlington, Vt.: Ashgate, 2001, pp. 144–161.

"The Weight of Evidence and the Burden of Authority: Case Histories, Medical Statistics and Smallpox Inoculation." In *Medicine in the Enlightenment.* Ed. Roy Porter. Wellcome Clio Medica Series. Amsterdam and Atlanta: Rodopi Press, 1995, pp. 289–315.

Rusnock, Andrea, ed. *The Correspondence of James Jurin (1684–1750), Physician and Secretary to the Royal Society.* Amsterdam and Atlanta: Rodopi Press, 1996.

Sabatier, J.C. *Recherches historiques sur la Faculté de médecine de Paris.* Paris: Deville Cavellin, 1835.

Schaffer, Simon. "A Social History of Plausibility: Country, City and Calculation in Augustan Britain." In *Rethinking Social History: English Society, 1570–1920, and Its Interpretation.* Ed. Adrian Wilson. Manchester and New York: Manchester University Press, 1993, pp. 128–157.

Schneider, Ivo. "Der Mathematiker Abraham de Moivre (1667–1754)." *Archive for History of Exact Sciences* 5 (1968–1969): 177–317.

Schumpeter, Joseph A. *History of Economic Analysis.* Ed. Elizabeth Boody Schumpeter. New York: Oxford University Press, 1954.

Shapin, Steven. *A Social History of Truth: Civility and Science in Seventeenth Century England.* Chicago: University of Chicago Press, 1994.

Shapin, Steven, and Simon Schaffer. *Leviathan and the Air-Pump: Hobbes, Boyle, and the Experimental Life.* Princeton, N.J.: Princeton University Press, 1985.

Shapiro, Barbara J. *A Culture of Fact: England 1550–1720.* Ithaca and London: Cornell University Press, 2000.

Probability and Certainty in Seventeenth-Century England. Princeton, N.J.: Princeton University Press, 1983.

Sheynin, O.B. "On the History of Medical Statistics." *Archive for History of Exact Sciences* 26 (1982): 241–286.

"P.S. Laplace's Work on Probability." *Archive for History of Exact Sciences* 16 (1976): 137–187.

Simmel, Georg. *The Philosophy of Money.* Trans. Tom Bootmore and David Frisby. 1907; London: Routledge & Kegan Paul, 1978.

Slaughter, Mary. *Universal Languages and Scientific Taxonomy in the Seventeenth Century.* Cambridge: Cambridge University Press, 1982.

Speck, W.A. *Stability and Strife: England, 1714–1760.* Cambridge, Mass.: Harvard University Press, 1977.

Spengler, Joseph J. *French Predecessors of Malthus.* Durham, N.C.: Duke University Press, 1942.

Stangeland, Charles Emil. *Pre-Malthusian Doctrines of Population: A Study in the History of Economic Theory.* New York: Columbia University Press, 1904.

Staum, Martin S. *Cabanis: Enlightenment and Medical Philosophy in the French Revolution.* Princeton, N.J.: Princeton University Press, 1980.

Stevenson, Lloyd G. "'New Diseases' in the Seventeenth Century." *Bulletin of the History of Medicine* 39 (1965): 1–21.

Stewart, Larry. *The Rise of Public Science: Rhetoric, Technology, and Natural Philosophy in Newtonian Britain, 1660–1750.* Cambridge: Cambridge University Press, 1992.

Stigler, Stephen M. *The History of Statistics – The Measurement of Uncertainty before 1900.* Cambridge, Mass.: Harvard University Press, 1986.

"The Measurement of Uncertainty in Nineteenth-Century Social Science." In *The Probabilistic Revolution.* Ed. Lorenz Krüger, Lorraine J. Daston, and Michael Heidelberger. 2 vols. Cambridge, Mass.: MIT Press, 1987, vol. 1, pp. 287–292.

Strauss, E. *Sir William Petty – Portrait of a Genius.* London: The Bodley Head, 1954.

Sutherland, J. "John Graunt: A Tercentenary Tribute." *Journal of the Royal Statistical Society,* Series A, 126 (1963): 536–556.

Thomas, Keith. "Numeracy in Early Modern England." *Transactions of the Royal Historical Society,* 5th ser., 37 (1977): 103–132.

Tomaselli, Sylvana. "Moral Philosophy and Population Questions in Eighteenth Century Europe." In *Population and Resources in Western Intellectual Traditions.* Ed. Michael S. Teitelbaum and Jay M. Winter. Supplement to vol. 14: *Population and Development Review.* Cambridge: Cambridge University Press, 1989, pp. 7–29.

Tröhler, Ulrich. "Quantification in British Medicine and Surgery, 1750–1830, with Special Reference to its Introduction into Therapeutics." Ph.D. thesis, University of London, 1978.

Tufte, Edward. *The Visual Display of Quantitative Information.* Cheshire, Conn.: Graphics Press, 1983.

Tuttle, Leslie. "'Sacred and Politic Unions': Natalism, Families, and the State in Old Regime France, 1666–1789." Ph.D. thesis, Princeton University, 2000.

Underwood, E. Ashworth. *Boerhaave's Men.* Edinburgh: Edinburgh University Press, 1977.

Vilquin, E. *Vauban et les méthodes de statistique au siècle de Louis XIV.* Paris: IDUP, 1972.

"Vauban, inventeur des recensements." *Annales de démographie historique* (1975): 207–257.

Walford, Cornelius. "Early Bills of Mortality." *Transactions of the Royal Historical Society* 7 (1878): 212–248.

Wear, Andrew. "Making Sense of Health and the Environment in Early Modern England." In *Medicine in Society: Historical Essays.* Ed. Andrew Wear. Cambridge: Cambridge University Press, 1992, pp. 119–147.

Webster, Charles. *The Great Instauration.* London: Gerald Duckworth, 1975.

Webster, Charles, ed. *Health, Medicine, and Mortality in the Sixteenth Century.* Cambridge: Cambridge University Press, 1979.

Westergaard, H., ed. *Contributions to the History of Statistics.* London: P.S. King and Son, 1932.

Williams, Elizabeth. *The Physical and the Moral: Anthropology, Physiology, and Philosophical Medicine in France, 1750–1850.* Cambridge: Cambridge University Press, 1994.

Wise, M. Norton, ed. *The Values of Precision.* Princeton, N.J.: Princeton University Press, 1995.

Woolf, Stuart J. "Towards the History of the Origins of Statistics: France, 1789–1815." In Jean-Claude Perrot and Stuart J. Woolf. *State and Society in France, 1789–1815.* New York: Harwood Academic Publishers, 1984.

Wrigley, E.A., and R.S. Schofield. *The Population History of England, 1541–1871.* Cambridge, Mass.: Harvard University Press, 1981.

Zilsel, Edgar. "The Genesis of the Concept of Physical Law." *Philosophical Review* 51 (1942): 242–279.

INDEX

Other titles in the series (*continued from the front of the book*)

Bilharzia: A History of Imperial Tropical Medicine, JOHN FARLEY
Preserve Your Love for Science: Life of William A. Hammond, American Neurologist, BONNIE E. BLUSTEN
Patients, Power, and the Poor in Eighteenth-Century Bristol, MARY E. FISSELL
AIDS and Contemporary Society, EDITED BY VIRGINIA BERRIDGE AND PHILIP STRONG
Science and Empire: East Coast Fever in Rhodesia and the Transvaal, PAUL F. CRANEFIELD
The Colonial Disease: A Social History of Sleeping Sickness in Northern Zaire, 1900–1940, MARYINEZ LYONS
Mission and Method: The Early Nineteenth-Century French Public Health Movement, ANN F. LABERGE
Meanings of Sex Differences in the Middle Ages: Medicine, Science, and Culture, JOAN CADDEN
Public Health in British India: Anglo-Indian Preventive Medicine, 1859–1914, MARK HARRISON
Medicine before the Plague: Practitioners and Their Patients in the Crown of Aragon, 1285–1345, MICHAEL R. MCVAUGH
The Physical and the Moral: Anthropology, Physiology, and Philosophical Medicine in France, 1750–1850, ELIZABETH A. WILLIAMS
A Social History of Wet Nursing in America: From Breast to Bottle, JANET GOLDEN
Pupils and Practitioners in Eighteenth-Century London, SUSAN C. LAWRENCE
Charity and Power in Early Modern Italy: Benefactors and Their Motives in Turin, 1541–1789, SANDRA CAVALLO
International Health Organisations and Movements, 1918–1939, PAUL WEINDLING
The Progress of Experiment: Science and Therapeutic Reform in the US, 1900–1990, HARRY M. MARKS
Sir Arthur Newsholme and State Medicine 1885–1935, JOHN M. EYLER
The Transformation of German Academic Medicine, 1750–1820, THOMAS H. BROMAN
Public Health in the Age of Chadwick, Britain, 1800–1854, CHRISTOPHER HAMLIN
Making Sense of Illness: Studies in Twentieth Century Medical Thought, ROBERT A. ARONOWITZ
Last Resort: Psychosurgery and the Limits of Medicine, JACK D. PRESSMAN
The Midwives of Seventeenth-Century London, DOREEN EVENDEN
Spreading Germs: Disease Theories and Medical Practice in Britain, 1865–1900, MICHAEL WORBOYS